Contributions to Statistics

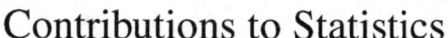

For further volumes:
http://www.springer.com/series/2912

Gilbert MacKenzie • Defen Peng

Editors

Statistical Modelling in Biostatistics and Bioinformatics

Selected Papers

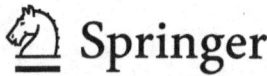 Springer

Editors
Gilbert MacKenzie
Defen Peng
Centre of Biostatistics
University of Limerick
Limerick
Ireland

ISBN 978-3-319-35764-5   ISBN 978-3-319-04579-5 (eBook)
DOI 10.1007/978-3-319-04579-5
Springer Cham Heidelberg New York Dordrecht London

Printed on acid-free paper

Springer is part of Springer Science+Business Media (www.springer.com)

Preface

This volume contains an appreciation of John Nelder, FRS, inventor of Generalized Linear Models (GLMs) and hierarchical generalized linear models HGLMs, and 14 papers on statistical modelling. The range of topics covered is diverse, but falls squarely into the following classification: (a) survival and event history modelling, (b) longitudinal and time series modelling, (c) statistical model development and (d) applied statistical modelling. The themes are representative of modern statistical model development and several celebrate John Nelder's various contributions to the subject.

The volume owes its genesis, in part, to the 3rd International Workshop on Correlated Data Modelling held at the University of Limerick in Ireland (www3.ul.ie/wcdm07) and in equal measure to Science Foundation Ireland's Biostatistics and Bioinformatics research programme, BIO-SI (www3.ul.ie/bio-si) based in the Centre of Biostatistics, University of Limerick, Ireland. The combination of these contributions has led to an interesting compilation of papers on statistical model development. In particular we would like to thank Professor Roger Payne for contributing a paper on the new class of Hierarchical Generalised Non-Linear Models. There is also emphasis on important emerging areas such as Bioinformatics and Statistical Genetics.

We are particularly grateful to members of the BIO-SI project without whose various contributions this volume could not have been compiled. Professor Defen Peng of Zhongnan University of Economics and Law, PRC and BIO-SI Research Fellow, was invited to serve as a guest editor, and she has contributed an interesting paper on the classical problem of reference subclass choice in categorical regression models.

We are also pleased that this volume has been produced by Springer—a recognized academic publishing house. This should have the effect of raising awareness and encouraging participation in the WCDM workshops and in the BIO-SI project. Accordingly, we have been fortunate to have attracted Springer's interest and we gratefully acknowledge Veronika Rosteck, Associate Editor, Statistics, Springer Heidelberg, Germany, for her encouragement and assistance with this project.

Many people worked hard to complete the volume. Foremost amongst these we must thank the team in the Centre of Biostatistics (Dr. Emma Holian, Dr. David Ramsey and the students) who organised the WCDM workshop. Of course, this would not have been possible without the sterling efforts of Alessandra Durio and the late Ennio Isaia (see Postscript) in Torino. Professors John Hinde (NUIG, Ireland) and Jianxin Pan (Manchester, UK) also gave valuable advice and support.

We have of course to thank all of the sponsors of the workshop for their support, especially the Irish Statistical Association (www.istat.ie) and Science Foundation Ireland (www.sfi.ie), which kindly supported the workshop with grants. The editors also acknowledge the financial support of SFI's BIO-SI research programme (www3.ul.ie/bio-si.) and the Research Office in the University of Limerick.

Limerick, Ireland   Gilbert MacKenzie
Limerick, Ireland   Defen Peng
Autumn 2013

Acknowledgements: An Appreciation—John Nelder, FRS

We pause to remember John Ashworth Nelder, FRS (Figs. 1 and 2), "John" to those of us who knew him and admired his contribution to Statistical Modelling and more widely to Statistical Science. John died on Saturday, August 7, 2010, aged 85 years. He had retired from Rothamsted, Ronald Fisher's stomping ground, aged 60, having already had an outstanding career which included, *inter alia*, the development of the family of Generalized Linear Models (GLMs) with his collaborator Robert MacLagan Wedderburn, a (Scottish) colleague at the Experimental Research Station.

Inimitably, John's research output in "statistical mathematics" continued undiminished from Imperial College, London, where he held a visiting Professorship. With Professor Youngjo Lee (Seoul National University, South Korea) John built on his earlier work on Generalised Linear Models and together they developed the theory of Hierarchical Generalised Linear Models (HGLMs).

Their first paper was read to the Royal Statistical Society in 1996. No longer were the random effects in mixed models confined to the Gaussian stable, but were generalised to the Exponential Family: Exponential Family response (Y) and Exponential Family error (u). Mixed models would never be the same again. Inference was generalised to a hierarchical likelihood containing random effects unlike standard likelihood methods advocated by Fisher. One consequence was that a new method of estimating the dispersion parameters was required and this problem was neatly solved by an appeal to the Cox–Reid adjustment method of creating an adjusted profile likelihood. Later this technique would come to be viewed as a nuisance parameter elimination technique of great utility.

In many ways the 1996 paper was a *tour de force*, but curiously it was not well received. Doubts were cast on the technique's ability to cope with matched pairs (binary data) in small samples and the Bayesian fraternity did not fully grasp the hierarchical arguments which allowed Lee and Nelder to treat random parameters as fixed effects. Moreover, H-likelihood inference did not require the use of a prior. And, in any case, the problem could always be cast in a Bayesian mould. It was to be fully 5 years before the 2001 Biometrika paper, which first introduced the notion of double hierarchical generalised linear models, DHGLMs, began to redress the balance of opinion. It took another 5 years to the seminal 2006

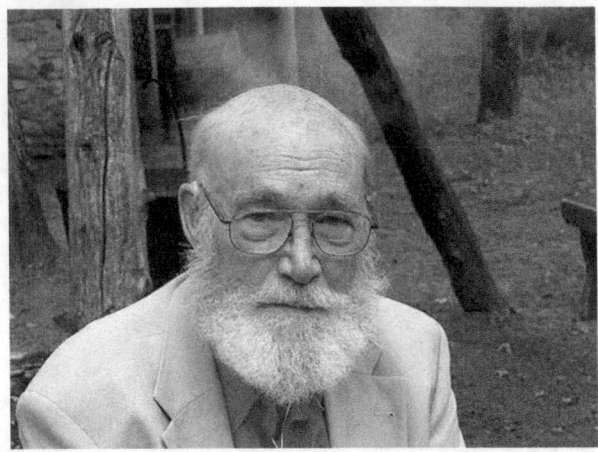

Fig. 1 John Ashworth Nelder, FRS, July 2006

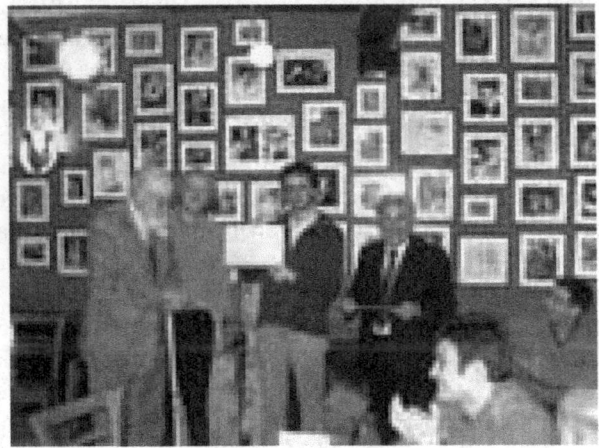

Fig. 2 John Nelder presenting prizes at WCDM, Torino, 2004

paper, entitled Double Hierarchical Generalised Linear Models, again read to the Royal Statistical Society to demonstrate the power of the method. DHGLMs have a HGLM for the location parameters and another linked HGLM for the dispersion parameters, the latter being a natural extension of Nelder and Lee's ideas on *structural dispersion*. This paper dealt with many criticisms of the H-likelihood method and *so-called* counter examples. These transpired to be largely bogus due to various misunderstandings of the 1996 paper.

It is worth remarking that there are very close links with the development of *covariance modelling* techniques. It is natural from an optimality perspective to wish to model the mean and covariance structure with the same rigor. Unsurprisingly, it turns out that many covariance models are related to DHGLMs, although typically, in the longitudinal data setting, the modelling is undertaken in the observation, rather than in the latent, space.

Once again, the 2006 paper was not without its critics. However, that the H-likelihood idea worked well, in more general classes of models than claimed by Lee and Nelder in their 2006 paper, was known to statisticians working on survival analysis, where many models lie beyond the censored Exponential Family and involve frailty. Some of these findings appear in the now classic 2006 book by Lee, Nelder and Pawitan and are due in large measure to the sterling work of Professor Il Do Ha.

Younger statisticians may take heart from this story. Little of lasting value in statistical model development is built overnight and it has taken Lee and Nelder more than a decade to place the H-likelihood idea on a recognised footing. John Nelder, never completely satisfied, was often heard to remark that the work was far from complete and there was still much to be done. Such tenacity was part of John Nelder's nature, from which we can all draw inspiration.

Limerick, Ireland   Gilbert MacKenzie
Limerick, Ireland   Defen Peng
Herts, UK   Roger Payne

Contents

Contributors

Rita Allais Department of Social-Economic, Mathematical & Statistical Sciences, University of Turin, Turin, Italy

Norma Bargary Department of Mathematics & Statistics, University of Limerick, Limerick, Ireland

Marco Bosco Department of Management, University of Turin, Turin, Italy

Caroline Brophy Department of Mathematics & Statistics, National University of Ireland Maynooth, Maynooth, Co Kildare, Ireland
UCD School of Mathematical Sciences, Environmental & Ecological Modelling Group, University College Dublin, Dublin, Ireland

Susana Conde Department of Mathematics, Imperial College, London, UK

J. Connolly UCD School of Mathematical Sciences, Environmental & Ecological Modelling Group, University College Dublin, Belfield, Dublin, Ireland

Alessandra Durio Department of Economics & Statistics "S. Cognetti de Martiis", University of Turin, Turin, Italy

A. Augusto F. Garcia Department of Genetics, Luiz de Queiroz College of Agriculture, University of São Paulo, São Paulo, Brazil

D. Gibson Department of Plant Biology, Center for Ecology, Southern Illinois University, Carbondale, IL, USA

Il Do Ha Faculty of Information Science, Daegu Haany University, Gyeongsan, South Korea

John Haywood School of Mathematics, Statistics and Operations Research, Victoria University of Wellington, Wellington, New Zealand

John P. Hinde School of Mathematics, Statistics and Applied Mathematics, National University of Ireland, Galway, Ireland

Philip Hougaard Biostatistics, Lundbeck, Valby, Denmark

Ennio Isaia Department of Statistics & Applied Mathematics, University of Turin, Turin, Italy

Joseph Lynch The Centre for Biostatistics, University of Limerick, Limerick, Ireland

Gilbert MacKenzie The Centre for Biostatistics, University of Limerick, Limerick, Ireland

Marie-José Martinez Team MISTIS, INRIA Rhône-Alpes & Laboratoire Jean Kuntzmann, Montbonnot, Saint-Ismier Cedex, France

Roger W. Payne Department of Computational and Systems Biology, Rothamsted Research, Harpenden, Herts, UK
VSN International, Hemel Hempstead, Herts, UK

Defen Peng The Centre for Biostatistics, University of Limerick, Limerick, Ireland

David Ramsey Department of Computer Science and Management, Wrocaw University of Technology, Wrocaw, Poland

John Randal School of Economics and Finance, Victoria University of Wellington, Wellington, New Zealand

P.W. Wayne Harvard Medical School, Osher Center for Integrative Medicine, Boston, MA, USA

Jing Xu Department of Mathematics, Statistics & Economics, Birkbeck College, London, UK

Introduction

Gilbert MacKenzie and Defen Peng

1 Preamble

The aim of this book is to provide the reader with an interesting selection of papers on modern statistical model development in bio-statistics and bio-informatics. The book also attempts to celebrate, in passing, the work of John Nelder who made an enormous contribution to statistical model development. The papers presented herein have been compiled from several sources. The majority contribution by numbers stems from Science Foundation Ireland's BIO-SI project (www3.ul.ie/bio-si) centred in the Universities of Limerick and Galway in Ireland. However, the volume has also been exceptionally fortunate to attract papers from several distinguished international statisticians who had participated in a Workshop on Correlated Data Modelling held in the University of Limerick (www3.ul..ie/wcdm07). The various papers offered represent a refreshing blend of experience and youth as the next generation of researchers begin to contribute.

Accordingly, it is with great pleasure that the Editors introduce the material.

2 Contributions

The contributed papers have been arranged naturally into four groups, namely:

- Survival and event history analysis.
- Longitudinal analysis and time series.
- Statistical model development.
- Applied statistical modelling.

G. MacKenzie (✉)
The Centre for Biostatistics, University of Limerick, Limerick, Ireland
e-mail: gilbert.mackenzie@ul.ie

G. MacKenzie and D. Peng (eds.), *Statistical Modelling in Biostatistics and Bioinformatics*, Contributions to Statistics, DOI 10.1007/978-3-319-04579-5_1, © Springer International Publishing Switzerland 2014

2.1 Survival and Event History Analysis

The survival section presents an interesting mixture of papers on this evergreen topic. The first paper from Professor Philip Hougaard provides a thorough review of recent developments in multivariate survival analysis covering the gamut of modelling settings including parametric and semi-parametric models and right and interval censoring schemes. The paper is non-technical and succeeds in emphasising the key ideas while providing insight into known pitfalls. Altogether an excellent introduction to the area and a most apt leading paper.

The next paper by MacKenzie and Ha deals inter alia with non-proportional hazards (non-PH) parametric survival models introducing two new log-normal frailty models via the Generalised Time-Dependent Logistic model (GTDL) (MacKenzie 1996). The authors employ the H-likelihood method of estimation which has the advantage of conveniently avoiding intractable integrations. The paper picks up an important theme based on the notion of a *canonical scale*. Lee et al. (2006) argue that H-likelihood estimation requires the random effects and fixed effects to be placed on the same scale (canonical), but MacKenzie and Ha show that this requirement is strictly unnecessary as inference is similar in both GTDL frailty models, even when the random effects are on a different scale. This paper illustrates that the H-likelihood method works well beyond the envelope claimed by Lee et al. (2006).

The third paper in this section explores the idea of *structural dispersion*. Lynch and MacKenzie develop the idea of Gamma frailty models starting from Weibull and GTDL basic hazards when analysing survival from a large number of incident cases of breast cancer in 13 local health authorities in the West Midlands of the UK. The resulting models are both non-PH and have structural dispersion models of the subject-specific form $\sigma_i^2 = \exp(\omega_i) = \exp(x_i'\beta)$ for the frailty variances, σ^2. These models show superior fit compared to routine frailty models $\sigma_i^2 = \sigma^2$ for $i = 1, \ldots, n$ patients and compared to the basic survival models. The fact that the variance of the random effects may be subject-specific, yet controlled by baseline fixed effects, seems a plausible alternative to conventional schemes.

The last paper deals with a type of discrete survival analysis. Martinez and Hinde argue that discrete survival times can be viewed as ordered multicategorical data. They use a continuation-ratio model which is particularly appropriate when the ordered categories represent a progression through different stages, such as survival through various times. This particular model has the advantage of being a simple decomposition of a multinomial distribution into a succession of hierarchical binomial models. In a clustered data context, they incorporate random effects into the linear predictor of the model to account for uncontrolled experimental variation. Assuming a normal distribution for the random effects, an EM algorithm with adaptive Gaussian quadrature is used to estimate the model parameters. This approach is applied to the analysis of grouped toxicological data obtained from a biological control assay. This paper illustrates the variety of methods available in the field of survival analysis.

2.2   Longitudinal and Time Series

The opening paper presents a thoughtful analysis of visitor arrivals in New Zealand. Haywood and Randal demonstrate the poor performance, with seasonal data, of existing methods for endogenously dating multiple structural breaks. Motivated by iterative nonparametric techniques, they present a new approach for estimating parametric structural break models that performs well. They suggest that iterative estimation methods are a simple but important feature of this approach when modelling seasonal data. The methodology is illustrated by simulation and is then used to analyse a monthly short-term visitor arrival time series to New Zealand, in order to assess the effect of the 9/11 terrorist attacks. While some historical events had a marked structural effect on trends in those arrivals, they show that 9/11 did not.

Continuing the time series theme Allais and Bosco present an application of Generalized Linear Models to the prevention of risks of insolvency of an automotive financial service. In order to forecast the performance of instalment payments of the customers, they resort to a logit multivariate regression model. Before fitting the model, they resort to sample logits, Generalized Additive Models and univariate logistic regression in order to identify the subset of best predictors and verify the assumption of the statistical model. For the estimated model, they use Wald statistics to assess the significance of the coefficients, the Likelihood Ratio to test the goodness of fit of the model, and the Odds Ratio to interpret the estimated coefficients. In order to verify the goodness of fit of the model, they employ classification tables and the Receiver Operating Characteristic curve. Finally, they validate the fitted model by means of a predictive-test on a training set.

Xu and MacKenzie return to the joint mean-covariance modelling theme in a longitudinal setting where the mean is subject to some constraints. A data-driven method for modelling the intra-subject covariance matrix is developed in the context of constrained marginal models arising in longitudinal data. A constrained iteratively re-weighted least squares estimation algorithm is applied. Some key asymptotic properties of the constrained ML estimates are given. They analyze a real data set in order to compare data-driven covariance modelling methods with classical menu-selection-based modelling techniques under a constrained mean model, extending the usual regression model for estimating generalized autoregressive parameters. Finally, they demonstrate, via a simulation study, that a correct choice of covariance matrix is required in order to minimise not only the bias, but also the variance, when estimating the constrained mean component.

2.3   Statistical Model Development

In this section the emphasis is firmly on the development of new classes of model and or statistical methods.

Professor Payne introduced Hierarchical generalized non-linear models. Hierarchical generalized linear models allow non-Normal data to be modelled in situations when there are several sources of error variation. He extends the familiar generalized linear models to include additional random terms in the linear predictor. However, he does not constrain these terms to follow a Normal distribution nor to have an identity link, as is the case in the more usual generalized linear mixed model. He thus provides a much richer set of models that may seem more intuitively appealing. Another extension to generalized linear models allows nonlinear parameters to be included in the linear predictor. The fitting algorithm for these generalized nonlinear models operates by performing a nested optimization, in which a generalized linear model is fitted for each evaluation in an optimization over the nonlinear parameters. The optimization search thus operates only over the (usually relatively few) nonlinear parameters, and this should be much more efficient than a global optimization over the whole parameter space. This paper reviews the generalized nonlinear model algorithm, and explains how similar principles can be used to include nonlinear fixed parameters in the mean model of a hierarchical generalized linear model, thus defining a *hierarchical generalized nonlinear model.*

Durio and Isaia argue that it is well known that in all situations involving the study of large data sets where a substantial number of outliers or clustered data are present, regression models based on M-estimators are likely to be unstable. Resorting to the inherent properties of robustness of the estimates based on the Integrated Square Error criterion, a technique of regression analysis which consists in comparing the results arising from L_2 estimates with the ones obtained by applying some common M-estimators. The discrepancy between the estimated regression models is measured by means of a new concept of similarity between functions and a system of statistical hypothesis. A Monte Carlo Significance test is introduced to verify the similarity of the estimates. Whenever the hypothesis of similarity between models is rejected, a careful investigation of the data structure is required in order to check for the presence of clusters, which can lead us to consider a mixture of regression models. Concerning this, they show how the L_2 criterion can be applied in fitting a finite mixture of regression models. The theory is outlined and the whole procedure is applied to a case study concerning the evaluation of the risk of fire and the risk of electric shocks arising in electronic transformers.

Bargary et al. develop the idea of model-based clustering using orthogonal regressions. They note that finite mixture models have been used extensively in clustering applications, where each component of the mixture distribution is assumed to represent an individual cluster. The simplest example describes each cluster in terms of a multivariate Gaussian density with various covariance structures. However, using finite mixture models as a clustering tool is highly flexible and allows for the specification of a wide range of statistical models to describe the data within each cluster. These include modelling each cluster using linear regression models, mixed effects models, generalized linear models, etc. This paper investigates the use of mixtures of orthogonal regression models to cluster biological data arising from a study of the sugarcane plant.

Peng and MacKenzie consider the evergreen problem of choosing the reference subclass in categorical regression models. They show how to choose the reference subclass optimally and note that this choice requires the use of secondary criteria. They derive the optimal design allocation of observations to subclasses and provide a statistic, based on the generalized variance and its distribution for measuring the discrepancy between the optimal allocation and any observed allocation occurring in an observational studies in the context of the general linear model. They then extend their methods to generalized linear models. The focus is on techniques which maximize the precision of the resulting estimators. They explore the general form of the optimal design matrix for general linear models with categorical regressors, and propose an algorithm to find the optimal design matrix for generalized linear models when the design matrix is of high dimension. They note that the proposed statistic, a measure of discrepancy, can be used to show if secondary criteria for the choice of reference subclasses are needed in parametric categorical regression models. They illustrate their methods by means of simulation studies and the analysis of a set of lung cancer survival data.

2.4   Applied Statistical Analysis

The papers in this section derive their main thrust from applications but nevertheless contain a substantial element of model development and/or review.

David Ramsey reviews tests for detecting selective sweeps. The emigration of humankind from Africa and the adoption of agriculture have meant that the selective pressures on humankind have changed in recent evolutionary times. A selective sweep occurs when a positive mutation spreads through a population. For example, a mutation that enables adults to digest lactase has spread through the Northern European population, although it is very rare in the African population. Since neutral alleles that are strongly linked to such a positive mutation also tend to spread through the population, these sweeps leave a signature, a valley of low genetic variation. He reviews the development of statistical tests for the detection of selective sweeps using genomic data, particularly in the light of recent advances in genome mapping and considers directions for future research.

Brophy et al. discuss issues that arise in the analysis of reproductive allocation (RA) in plants when predicting from complex models. Communicating models of RA requires predictions on the original scale of the data and this can present challenges if transformations were used during the modelling. It is also necessary to estimate without bias the mean level of RA as this may reflect a plant's ability to contribute in the next generation. Several issues can arise in modelling RA including the occurrence of zero values and the clustering of plants in stands which can lead to the need for more complex models. They present a two-component finite mixture model framework for the analysis of RA data with the first component being a censored regression model on the logarithmic scale and the second component being a logistic regression model. Both components contained random error terms to allow for potential correlation between grouped plants. They implement the models using data from an experiment carried out to assess environmental factors on reproductive allocation and detail the issues that arose in predicting from the model. They also present a bootstrap analysis to generate standard errors for predictions from the model and to test for comparisons among predictions.

Conde and MacKenzie review methods for searching high-dimensional contingency tables and present some recent developments. The review deals with the main ideas and is relatively non-technical providing a natural book-end to the volume. They present a review focussed on model selection in log-linear models and contingency tables. The concepts of sparsity and high-dimensionality have become more important nowadays, for example, in the context of high-throughput genetic data. In particular, they describe recently developed automatic search algorithms for finding optimal hierarchical log-linear models (HLLMs) in sparse multi-dimensional contingency tables in R and some LASSO-type penalized likelihood model selection approaches. The methods rely, in part, on a new result which identifies and thus permits the rapid elimination of non-existent maximum likelihood estimators in high-dimensional tables. They are illustrated using a set of high-dimensional comorbidity data.

Overall, the papers contained in this volume represent a level of variety and strength in statistical model development which would have no doubt pleased John Nelder.

References

Lee, Y., Nelder, J. A., & Pawitan, Y. (2006). *Generalised linear models with random effects: Unified analysis via h-likelihood*. London: Chapman and Hall.
MacKenzie, G. (1996). Regression models for survival data: The generalised time dependent logistic family. *Journal of the Royal Statistical Society, 45*, 21–34.

Part I
Survival Modelling

Multivariate Interval-Censored Survival Data: Parametric, Semi-parametric and Non-parametric Models

Philip Hougaard

Abstract Interval censoring means that an event time is only known to lie in an interval (L,R], with L the last examination time before the event, and R the first after. In the univariate case, parametric models are easily fitted, whereas for non-parametric models, the mass is placed on some intervals, derived from the L and R points. Asymptotic results are simple for the former and complicated for the latter. This paper is a review describing the extension to multivariate data, like eruption times for teeth examined at visits to the dentist. Parametric models extend easily to multivariate data. However, non-parametric models are intrinsically more complicated. It is difficult to derive the intervals with positive mass, and estimated interval probabilities may not be unique. A semi-parametric model makes a compromise, with a parametric model, like a frailty model, for the dependence and a non-parametric model for the marginal distribution. These three models are compared and discussed. Furthermore, extension to regression models is considered. The semi-parametric approach may be sensible in many cases, as it is more flexible than the parametric models, and it avoids some technical difficulties with the non-parametric approach.

Keywords Bivariate survival • Frailty models • Interval censoring • Model choice

1 Introduction

Interval-censored survival data refer to survival data, where the times of events are not known precisely; they are only known to lie in given intervals. The event could, for example, be HIV infection, or outbreak of a disease. Interval censoring typically

P. Hougaard (✉)
Biostatistics, Lundbeck, DK-2500 Valby, Denmark
e-mail: PHOU@lundbeck.com

G. MacKenzie and D. Peng (eds.), *Statistical Modelling in Biostatistics and Bioinformatics*, Contributions to Statistics, DOI 10.1007/978-3-319-04579-5_2,
© Springer International Publishing Switzerland 2014

arises because the status of an individual is not known at all times, due to it being necessary to make a specific measurement in order to find out whether the event has happened. Such a measurement could be bioanalytical analysis of a blood sample or an X-ray. It turns out that instead of knowing all examinations at all times, it is sufficient to know that the event time is in an interval of the form $(L_i, R_i]$, where the left endpoint is the time last seen without the disease, and the right endpoint is the first time seen with the disease. Subjects with the disease at the first examination has $L_i = 0$, and subjects that are never observed to have the disease have $R_i = \infty$, that is, are right-censored. For many diseases (for example, diabetes type II), the natural time scale is age. Interval censoring is in contrast to the standard survival data setup, where all event times are either known precisely, or they happen after the end of observation (that is, right-censored data).

This paper will give a brief overview of the univariate case (Sect. 2), but the real purpose is to consider models for multivariate data. An introduction to modelling multivariate data is in Sect. 3, without reference to how data are collected. The interval censoring way of observing data is then described in Sect. 4. This paper describes and compares three different ways of modelling multivariate interval-censored data. The fully parametric models are described in Sect. 5, the non-parametric models in Sect. 6, and the semi-parametric models in Sect. 7. Regression models are considered in Sect. 8. The various approaches are compared in Sect. 9.

Further reading on interval censoring are Sun (2006) and Hougaard (2014). In particular, the latter includes a chapter that gives more details on the issues discussed in this paper. Further reading on multivariate survival data is Hougaard (2000).

2 Univariate Interval-Censored Data

For each subject one or more examinations are made over time to find out if/when the subject gets the disease, or, more generally, experiences the event. It is assumed that the event studied (like outbreak of a disease) induces a permanent change that can be measured without error. For example, an infectious disease leads to antibodies, and in the interval censoring frame, it is assumed that these are detectable at any time thereafter.

If all subjects are studied at the same times, the data are grouped and can easily be analysed. So, we will consider the more general case of individual inspection times. The inspection times are supposed to be chosen independently of the response process and not informative of the parameters governing the response process. The likelihood then has the following form

$$\prod_i \{S_i(L_i) - S_i(R_i)\}, \tag{1}$$

where $S_i(\cdot)$ is the survivor function for the time to the event, for subject i. Strictly speaking, this function is only the probability of the observations, when the inspection times are fixed beforehand. If, instead the inspection times are chosen randomly, but independent of the failure time process, the density of this distribution enters as a factor. However, as this factor does not influence the maximization, we may omit that term. That is, Eq. (1) can still be used as the likelihood of the observations.

However, the inspection times could easily depend on the failure time process, for example, if we study patients coming to a general practitioner. The chance that a person will go to a doctor must in general be higher when the subject suffers from a disease than for a completely healthy subject. This case is not treated in the present paper.

A parametric model is easily handled just by inserting the relevant expression for $S_i(\cdot)$ into Eq. (1). If there are many different potential inspection times, and the model is reasonable, the distribution is identifiable, and the estimated parameters can be found by Newton-Raphson iteration and one can derive asymptotic results in the usual way, that is, using the observed information (minus the second derivative of the log likelihood function), which, *inter alia*, implies that the asymptotic distribution has an asymptotic order of $\sqrt{n}$, where n is the number of observations.

A non-parametric model is somewhat more complicated. If the inspection times are chosen from a finite set of times, say the birthdays of the subjects, we can only identify period probabilities, in the birthday case, 1-year probabilities. The asymptotic calculations will still follow standard principles. If on the other hand, the inspection times are chosen randomly from a continuous distribution, we can asymptotically identify the survivor function at all times (within the range of the inspection time distribution). However, the estimated survivor function will follow a slower than standard asymptotic order, namely $n^{1/3}$. This result has been proven under either an assumption of only one measurement for each subject (current status data) or under an assumption of several measurements per subject with the requirement that two measurements on the same subject cannot happen arbitrarily close (that is, the interval between measurements must be larger than some $\epsilon > 0$).

For a given data set, we cannot determine the full distribution. Indeed, the resolution cannot exceed the intervals generated by the left and right endpoints (L and R). That is, all that can be determined are the masses of these intervals. These interval probabilities are uniquely estimated. Actually, most of the intervals will have estimate 0. Peto (1973) suggested a simple procedure that could identify some of the intervals with estimate 0 and thus simplify the estimation problem to find the probabilities of the remaining intervals. Various software can be used to find these estimates. For the parametric models, SAS includes the procedure lifereg to cover selected models, and the procedure nlmixed, which can handle more general models. In the latter case, it is necessary to code the survivor functions, but no derivatives (neither with respect to time, nor with respect to the parameters) are needed. For the non-parametric case, SAS has a macro called ICE that covers the one-sample case.

The subscript i on the survivor function is introduced in order to allow for regression models, either parametric or semi-parametric. In the semi-parametric case, the models have to be hazard-based, which could either be a proportional hazards model, or a more complex model, like a frailty model. Accelerated failure time models are markedly more complicated in the semi-parametric case and not covered by the present paper. Regression models are considered in more detail in Sect. 8.

3 Multivariate Data

Multivariate data can either be family data, or multivariate data for a single subject. A common example of the second type is the age at eruption of teeth. All teeth are then checked at visits to a dentist at one or more times. Indeed, most of the examples in the literature have been of the second type. An example of the first type of data could be pairs of twins studied for the time to outbreak of a disease that could only be detected by some sort of bioanalytical measurement.

Due to the complexity, this paper will be formulated for bivariate data rather than general multivariate data. A bivariate distribution can be formulated in several different ways. The most general is just to formulate the bivariate survivor function, that is, $S(t_1, t_2) = Pr\{T_1 > t_1, T_2 > t_2\}$. Here, the subscript i has been neglected. However, in some cases, it is an advantage to parametrize the model by means of the marginal distributions $S_1(t)$, respectively, $S_2(t)$, and then use a copula model to obtain the joint distribution as $S(t_1, t_2) = C(S_1(t_1), S_2(t_2))$. The copula $C(\cdot, \cdot)$ is a bivariate distribution on the unit square, which is used to model the dependence. When studying a single bivariate distribution, this is just another way to express the distribution. Indeed, for continuous distributions, there is a unique relationship between these quantities. However, when we consider a family of distributions in a statistical model, for example, a regression model, the two formulations can lead to different models. Frailty models are of the copula type.

Some methods will require the survivor function to be known, whereas other methods may work with less explicit expressions, like an integral.

3.1 Purpose

The purpose of studying multivariate data could be to study the dependence (as was the case in the dental application). As a consequence to this dependence, we may use the information available at some time point for predicting later events. For example, if one twin is found to suffer from an inherited disease, we may suspect that the partner either has or will develop the same disease. This risk can be quantified by calculating the conditional distribution given information on the first twin or by a more symmetric bivariate measure, like Kendall's τ or Spearman's ρ. Of course, we could also be interested in the dependence just for understanding the underlying processes.

Another purpose could be to study the effect of some covariates. For this purpose, it is important whether the regression coefficients are shared, because if they are not shared, it may be sufficient (and certainly simpler) to study the marginal distributions separately. When the coefficients are shared for the various components, we may gain precision by considering them simultaneously, and the multivariate approach is necessary in order to evaluate the precision correctly. Also for a comparison within groups, a multivariate approach is necessary. To be slightly more precise, a multivariate approach is not always necessary for a comparison within groups. A classical example of this is the paired t-test. However, there is no analogue of this test for interval censoring, so in practice, it is difficult to handle such a comparison without modelling the full bivariate distribution. When the aim is to study the effect of covariates, it might not be necessary to quantify the dependence.

3.2 Frailty Models

One way to obtain a model for multivariate data is to use a frailty model. This is basically a random effects model, where the frailty refers to the shared random effect. The conditional hazard formulated with the hazard of T_{ij} conditional on the frailty Y_i as

$$Y_i \mu_{ij}(t),$$

so that the frailty Y_i is common for the i-th group and the hazard $\mu_{ij}(t)$ may be a parametrized function of i, j and t. In the non-parametric case, the function may depend only on t or only on j and t. Furthermore, it is assumed that the times are independent given the frailty, or in other words, it is the frailty that creates the dependence. A frailty model may offer simple expressions for the survivor function, because it is simple to integrate the frailty out. In general, the survival function (neglecting the subscript i) is found as

$$S(t_1, t_2) = \int_0^\infty g(y) \exp[-y\{M_1(t_1) + M_2(t_2)\}]dy = L(M_1(t_1) + M_2(t_2)), \quad (2)$$

where $g(y)$ is the density of Y and $L(s) = E \exp(-sY)$ is the Laplace transform of the frailty. Finally $M_j(t) = \int_0^t \mu_j(u)du$ is the integrated conditional hazard.

As a specific example, consider a gamma frailty model, which has Laplace transform $L(s) = (s + \theta)^\delta / \theta^\delta$. We may restrict the scale parameter by letting $\theta = \delta$, which secures the mean frailty is 1. With Weibull conditional hazards, the survivor function is

$$S(t_1, t_2) = 1/\{1 + (\lambda_1 t_1^\gamma + \lambda_2 t_2^\gamma)/\delta\}^\delta.$$

The value of Kendall's τ is $1/(1 + 2\delta)$. The Spearman correlation depends only on δ, and is most naturally derived by numerical integration. So it is relatively simple to quantify the dependence as it does not depend on the hazard function.

Describing the gamma frailty model is enough to illustrate the idea, but there are other possibilities, where the most interesting are distributions with 1–2 parameters having an explicit Laplace transform.

4 Multivariate Interval-Censored Data

Based on examinations at various time points, which may be common or individual for the components, we derive interval observations. The observations will be of the form $(L_{ij}, R_{ij}]$, where i refers to the group and j to the individual within the group.

Handling probabilities is more complicated in the bivariate case than in the univariate. In the univariate case, the probability of an interval $(a, b]$, that is, $Pr(T \in (a, b])$, is found as $S(b) - S(a)$, but in the bivariate case, the corresponding formula is

$$Pr(T_1 \in (a_1, b_1], T_2 \in (a_2, b_2]) = S(b_1, b_2) - S(a_1, b_2) - S(b_1, a_2) + S(a_1, a_2).$$
(3)

This formula is easily generalized to higher dimensions, but the number of terms quickly increases, being 2^k for k-dimensional data, and therefore, it may be preferable to keep the dimension low.

For setting up the likelihood, we then have to insert the L and R values in Eq. (3) and multiply over subjects. We may also have covariates, which in general will depend on both i and j, and thus be formulated as vectors z_{ij}.

4.1 Inspection Pattern

The inspection pattern becomes even more important in the multivariate case than it was in the univariate case. In simple cases, like the dental example, all teeth of a subject are considered simultaneously and the time of examination is determined by external factors like a whole school being examined each year at the same time. This is also called univariate monitoring times.

When there is only one such inspection for each subject, this is called multivariate current status data (Jewell et al. 2005). In the case of multivariate current status data, it is not in the non-parametric case possible to identify the full bivariate distribution even asymptotically. More precisely, it is asymptotically possible to identify the two marginal distributions $S(t, 0)$ and $S(0, t)$ and the diagonal $S(t, t)$, see Jewell et al. (2005). So, in this case, one should be cautious with a non-parametric model. One can either be satisfied with this limited identifiability, or use more restricted models, like those presented in Sects. 5 or 7. More generally, we can say the inspection process needs to be sufficiently rich in order to be able to determine the whole distribution.

Also in this case, non-independent inspection is possible. For example, if one subject in a couple is found to have an infectious disease, one would immediately examine the other and due to the dependence this would not be independent inspection. This case is not treated in the present paper.

5   Parametric Models

Here we consider a parametric model for the multivariate set of times to events, and it is then assumed that we have interval-censored observations from this distribution.

One standard multivariate model is the normal distribution (for the logarithm to the times). It is, however, more difficult to argue for its relevance to survival data, and therefore, it has not been used much for such data. Besides, an explicit expression for the survivor function is not available.

As we are considering survival times, a better alternative might be a frailty model as described in Sect. 3.2. We will then have a range of choices for the hazard function, like Weibull, Gompertz, piecewise constant hazards, or other standard or non-standard distributions with a preference for distributions, which have explicit hazard functions as well as explicit integrated hazard functions. There is also a range of choices for the frailty distributions, with a preference for distributions with an explicit Laplace transform. Above, only the gamma distribution has been described, but there are other possibilities.

When the dimension is above two, the normal distribution is more flexible with respect to dependence as the correlations can vary freely, whereas the standard (shared) frailty models will have only a single dependence parameter; that is, in spirit like the compound symmetry model for normally distributed data.

Estimation can follow two lines. One approach is to work directly with the bivariate distribution, that is, the estimation is based on inserting the relevant expressions in Eq. (3), with insertion of the right hand expression in Eq. (2). After taking the logarithm, summing over subjects and differentiating, one can use the Newton-Raphson method to find the estimate. Another approach, which is useful, when the multivariate model is formulated by means of conditional independence, like, for example, the frailty model, is to set up the likelihood as a product of individual (univariate) contributions conditional on the frailty and then integrating out over the frailty. This corresponds to using the middle expression in Eq. (2). In some cases, this integration can be done automatically by the software. In particular, it may be sensible, when the dimension of the data is high (in which case, the generalization of Eq. (3) has too many terms), or when the Laplace transform is not explicitly known (in which case the bivariate survivor function is not explicitly known). An example of the latter type is a frailty model, where the frailty follows a lognormal distribution. SAS proc nlmixed can accommodate both lines of estimation.

6   Non-parametric Models

This approach assumes a completely general multivariate distribution. This is the
natural generalization of the non-parametric approach from the univariate case. This
implies, for example, that no covariates are accounted for. The purpose of using
this method is to avoid any parametric assumptions, which may be an advantage,
when we want to evaluate the goodness-of-fit of a specific parametric or semi-
parametric model. That is, the results of a parametric model can be compared to
the non-parametric estimate. It turns out that in this case, there are many difficulties
compared to the univariate case. From a practical point of view, it is difficult to
handle a multivariate non-parametric survivor function, and the practical problems
become worse with the dimension of the data.

Compared to the univariate case, the estimation method runs with exactly the
same steps. However, all of these steps are more complicated than in the univariate
case. First, one must select the intervals, where there can be positive mass. This
is possible, but it is more complicated than in the univariate case. For finding the
intervals, there is no longer a simple explicit approach, like the Peto approach.

Second, one must optimise the probabilities, and the likelihood in Eq. (1) should
be modified to account for Eq. (3). The likelihood still includes sums of interval
probabilities and thus the estimation procedure is formally the same as in the
univariate case. However, it is not in all cases possible to determine the interval
probabilities uniquely. This is a new problem compared to the univariate case,
where the interval probabilities are uniquely estimable. An example is shown in
Fig. 1, where there are four bivariate observations, $(2, 3] \times (1, 6]$, $(4, 5] \times (1, 6]$,
$(1, 6] \times (2, 3]$, and $(1, 6] \times (4, 5]$. The interval selection procedure leads to the
following four intervals that potentially can have mass, $(2, 3] \times (2, 3]$, $(2, 3] \times (4, 5]$,
$(4, 5] \times (2, 3]$, and $(4, 5] \times (4, 5]$, say they have probabilities p_1, p_2, p_3, p_4. The
likelihood becomes $(p_1 + p_2)(p_3 + p_4)(p_1 + p_3)(p_2 + p_4)$. So even though these
are sums of interval probabilities, the terms are more complicated than for the
likelihood functions seen in the univariate case, because the subscripts to p are not
necessarily consecutive. For example, a term like $(p_1 + p_3)$ would not be possible
in the univariate case. This implies that the likelihood is not guaranteed to offer
a unique solution. The example illustrates the problem. The maximum likelihood
is obtained when $p_1 = p_4 \in [0, 0.5]$ and $p_2 = p_3 = 0.5 - p_1$. This will give
each observation a likelihood contribution of 1/2 and thus the likelihood value is
2^{-4}. If for some data, this problem occurs, it is easily detected because the matrix
of second derivatives is no longer negative definite. Yu et al. (2000) present the
example described above and suggest a procedure to select one of the parameter
values among those with maximal likelihood. They also show that asymptotically
any choice is satisfactory. That is, even though the problem is present also for large
samples, the probability that might be moved between sets becomes smaller.

Third, it can be difficult to illustrate the survivor function estimate graphically.
Even in the bivariate case, it is difficult to report the estimate in a table or figure,
and this makes the approach less attractive in many cases. This is a problem already

Fig. 1 Artificial data on four
bivariate observations,
illustrating non-identifiability.
Observations (*dashed*):
$(1,6] \times (2,3]$, $(1,6] \times (4,5]$,
$(2,3] \times (1,6]$, and $(4,5] \times (1,6]$.
Sets with possible mass
shown in *solid*

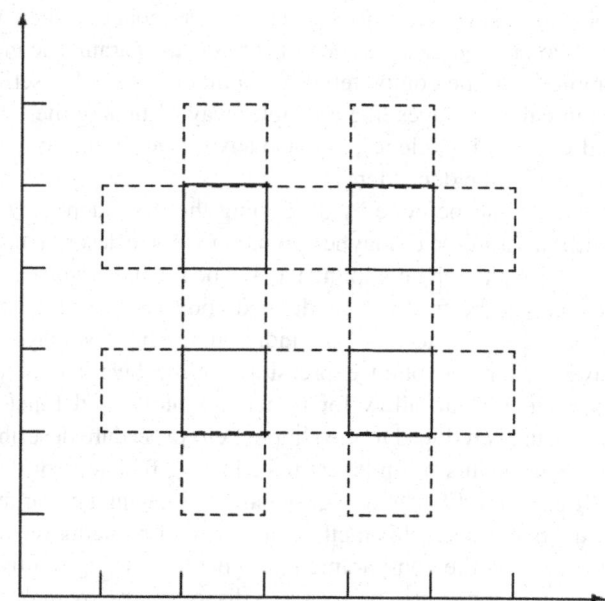

in the right-censored case, as illustrated in Hougaard (2000, Chap. 14), which also
compares the various graphical approaches to illustrate a non-parametric bivariate
survivor function. The interval probabilities estimates could be reported in a (long)
table, but reporting it as a bivariate survivor function would be very difficult. The
problem is that the survivor function cannot be determined in all points, because we
need the probability of sets of the form $\{T_1 \geq t_1, T_2 \geq t_2\}$, and when these sets cut
through a bivariate interval, which has positive estimate, we cannot determine the
probability of the set.

Furthermore, the completely non-parametric model does not give a quantifiable
expression for the dependence in terms of Kendall's τ and Spearman's ρ, for
example, and for the marginal distribution, there might be large sets, where it is
not identifiable.

Due to these problems and the technical problems, it may in many cases be
preferable to select another approach, like fitting a parametric or semi-parametric
model.

7 Semi-parametric Models

Semi-parametric modelling implies that some quantities are considered in a parametric way, whereas other are considered in a non-parametric way. This section
considers a non-parametric model for the hazard as function of time, but a
parametric model for the dependence between the coordinates. Thus, the section

does not allow for covariates. This model could be seen as a compromise between the two previous suggestions. It extends the parametric models of Sect. 5 and it is a submodel of the completely non-parametric model described in Sect. 6. This offers technical advantages like a simpler way of finding the intervals with positive mass and improved efficiency, but also advantages in interpretation, as it becomes easier to quantify the dependence.

This could be done by describing the dependence by means of a frailty model (with just a single or maybe two parameters to describe the dependence), and letting the non-parametric component describe the univariate distributions. In practice, this means that the frailty Y as defined above is shared between the family members, respectively the teeth of an individual. The advantage of this model is that we have a simple explicit expression for the bivariate survivor function and at the same time it can allow for rather flexible hazard functions. The interval finding procedure is reduced to the simple Peto procedure described above and Kendall's τ and Spearman's ρ can be estimated being functions of the frailty distribution. This will also simplify the model in case of including covariates in a regression model. Thus, one can see this method as a way of reducing the dimension of the problem, as it reduces the non-parametric aspect from being multivariate to being univariate. Of course, it can also be seen as a disadvantage, by making the model less flexible.

The purpose of such a study could be to study the dependence or to find the marginal distribution accounting for dependence. To be more specific, the semi-parametric model has the advantage that the dependence is easily quantifiable, at least for some models. It is easy to reduce the problem to the intervals with potentially positive mass. It is also easier to report the estimate as the non-parametric component is only one-dimensional. However, we do not completely avoid the problem of non-uniqueness of the estimate, but the problem will occur less frequently.

The model will still suffer from the slow convergence (asymptotic order $n^{1/3}$) for the survival time distribution, but the dependence parameter will show standard results (asymptotic order $n^{1/2}$), see Wang and Ding (2000).

8 Regression Models

The advantage of using a regression model is that the dependence on some covariates is described in a simple and interpretable way that allows for testing of the effect on the one hand, and on the other hand, if there is a significant effect, it gives a quantifiable expression for the effect. Indeed, the purpose of such a study is often to find these regression coefficients and to test whether a specified covariate has an influence. The covariates are given as a vector, denoted z.

This paper will mention three types of regression models, which are first described for the univariate case. The *accelerated failure time model*, which assumes $S_z(t) = S_0(t / \exp(\eta'z))$, where $S_0(\cdot)$ denotes the survivor function for a subject with 0 value of all covariates, and η is the vector of regression coefficients. This model is very easy to apply for parametric models. However, it is much more complicated when the hazard is described non-parametrically, both for right-censored and interval-censored data, and therefore not applied in practice. The *proportional hazards model* assumes $S_z(t) = S_0(t)^{\exp(\beta'z)}$, where we have used a different symbol for the regression coefficients, in order not to confuse the two models. This model is very easy to apply both for parametric models and non-parametric models for the hazard. Indeed, it is the standard model in the non-parametric case. The final model is the *conditional proportional hazards model*, which assumes that conditional on the frailty, $S_z(t \mid Y) = S_0(t)^{Y \exp(\beta'z)}$. When Y is gamma distributed, this makes an extension of the proportional hazards model, so that the hazards in the marginal distribution (when Y is integrated out) are non-proportional. The case of proportional hazards occurs on a boundary of the parameter set. The Weibull model is both an accelerated failure time model and a proportional hazards model, and it is the only model, where the two regression models coincide.

In the multivariate parametric case, we have a choice between these models, with the first two models always applicable and the third model applicable, when the dependence is given by a frailty model.

In the multivariate non-parametric case, the bivariate survivor function is not defined without a description of the dependence structure. Without covariates, we could let it be arbitrary, but with a covariate, we need to specify the relation between the covariate and the dependence. An assumption of the dependence being of the copula type would be sufficient to make the model well defined. Alternatively, one could use a GEE (generalized estimating equation) type model, where the dependence structure is not explicitly formulated.

In the multivariate semi-parametric case, we have a non-parametric model for the hazard as function of time, but a parametric model for the dependence between the coordinates and for the effect of covariates. Again, this model is well defined for the first two regression models, whereas the last model is only defined when the dependence is created by a frailty model. To make these considerations practical, we assume that the dependence is indeed created by a frailty model. However, the accelerated failure time model is not easy to fit with right-censored or interval-censored data, so it is less useful in practice. For the other two models, where we assume either proportional hazards in the marginal distributions, or proportional hazards conditional on the frailty, fitting is possible, also with interval-censored data. The probability will be concentrated on a set of intervals, which can be found by the simple Peto procedure applied separately on each coordinate (if the hazards are not shared over coordinates) or the combination of all marginal data (if the hazards are shared). Furthermore, the dependence can be quantified by Kendall's τ or Spearman's ρ, which are both functions of the frailty distribution. All in all, this is quite operational.

The purpose of such a study could be to find the effect of covariates accounting for dependence, or to evaluate the dependence accounting for the effect of selected covariates. When the aim is to find the effect of a covariate, one should always consider whether the same research question could be considered by means of univariate data, because it will make it technically so much easier to handle.

9   Comparison and Discussion

First, we note that in the univariate case, the combination of interval censoring and a non-parametric model is much more complicated than either alone (that is, a parametric model for interval-censored data; or a non-parametric model for right-censored data). These complexities carry over to the multivariate case.

A parametric model for multivariate interval-censored data is easy to handle, when the dimension is low. When the dimension is high, it becomes more complicated, because the number of terms in the generalization of Eq. (3) grows. Such models will have the usual disadvantages of parametric models, namely that we need to specify a sensible model, and the results might be more or less misleading, in the case when the model is not satisfied. The assumptions for the parametric models will have two directions, the (marginal) distributions for the times, and the dependence.

A non-parametric model for multivariate interval-censored data suffers from a number of technical issues, finding intervals, handling intervals, potential parameter non-uniqueness and difficulties in reporting the estimates. The latter problem includes both reporting the survivor function and quantifying the dependence. Overall, this makes it intrinsically more complicated than non-parametric models for univariate interval-censored data. Therefore, this model is less attractive.

A compromise between these models is a semi-parametric model for multivariate interval-censored data, where the dependence is generated by a frailty model (with 1–2 parameters for the dependence). This will be more complicated than the univariate non-parametric model for interval-censored data, but it will not be *intrinsically* more complicated, and therefore tractable. In popular terms, the non-parametric issues are reduced to dimension one. On the other hand, this model is more flexible than parametric models, by allowing for non-parametric hazards. We will still have to formulate models for the dependence, so the non-parametric component only refers to assuming a general hazard over time.

All types of regression models are easily introduced into parametric models. For the semi-parametric model, it is easy to handle the hazard-based models, whereas the accelerated failure time model is complicated. The non-parametric model does not allow for introducing regression effects, without restricting the dependence structure (which implies that it is no longer a non-parametric model).

Weighing all the evidence above, the practical conclusion is that when we insist on using the accelerated failure time model, only a parametric model makes sense, whereas without this restriction, the semi-parametric approach is overall the most attractive.

Finally, it should be said that interval censoring for multivariate data is so complicated that we should always consider whether the conclusion can be drawn based on univariate data only rather than using multivariate data.

References

Hougaard, P. (2000). *Analysis of multivariate survival data*. New York: Springer.

Hougaard, P. (2014). *Analysis of interval-censored survival data*. Book manuscript (in preparation).

Jewell, N., Van der Laan, M., & Lei, X. (2005). Bivariate current state data with univariate monitoring times. *Biometrika, 92*, 847–862.

Peto, R. (1973). Experimental survival curves for interval-censored data. *Applied Statistics, 22*, 86–91.

Sun, J. (2006). *The statistical analysis of interval-censored failure time data*. New York: Springer.

Wang, W., & Ding, A. (2000). On assessing the association for bivariate current status data. *Biometrika, 87*, 879–883.

Yu, Q., Wong, G., & He, Q. (2000). Estimation of a joint distribution function with multivariate interval-censored data when the nonparametric mle is not unique. *Biometrical Journal, 42*, 747–763.

Multivariate Survival Models Based on the GTDL

Gilbert MacKenzie and Il Do Ha

Abstract Correlated survival times may be modelled by introducing a random effect, or frailty component, into the hazard function. For multivariate survival data we extend a non-PH model, the generalized time-dependent logistic (GTDL) survival model (MacKenzie, J R Stat Soc 45:21–34, 1996; MacKenzie, Stat Med 16:1831–1843, 1997), to include random effects. The extension leads to two different, but related, non-PH models according to the method of incorporating the random effects in the hazard function. The h-likelihood procedures of Ha et al. (Biometrika 88:233–243, 2001) and Ha and Lee (J Comput Graph Stat 12:663–681, 2003), which obviate the need for marginalization (over the random effect distribution) are derived for these extended models and their properties discussed. The new models are used to analyze two practical examples in the survival literature and the results are compared with those obtained from fitting PH and PH frailty models.

Keywords Frailty models • Generalized time-dependent logistic • h-likelihood • Non-PH model • Random effect

1 Introduction

Proportion hazards (PH) models (Cox 1972), extended to incorporate a frailty component, are frequently used to analyze multivariate survival data which may arise when recurrent or multiple event times are observed on the same subject. However, the assumption of proportionality of the basic hazard function can sometimes be untenable.

G. MacKenzie (✉)
The Centre for Biostatistics, University of Limerick, Limerick, Ireland
e-mail: gilbert.mackenzie@ul.ie

G. MacKenzie and D. Peng (eds.), *Statistical Modelling in Biostatistics and Bioinformatics*, Contributions to Statistics, DOI 10.1007/978-3-319-04579-5_3, © Springer International Publishing Switzerland 2014

Accordingly, we investigate the utility of two flexible non-PH random-effect models based on the generalized time-dependent logistic (GTDL) survival model, MacKenzie (1996). The GTDL generalizes the relative risk (RR) in Cox's semi-parametric PH model to time-dependent form. The model, a wholly parametric competitor for the PH model, has several interesting properties including a mixture interpretation. In particular, by retaining Cox's constant of proportionality as the leading term in the time-dependent relative risk, the model is not only capable of representing data which conform to the PH assumption, but can also accommodate a wider class of survival data in which the assumption of proportionality does not hold.

We thus extend the GTDL model to the multivariate survival data setting in two ways, adopting the hierarchical-likelihood (h-likelihood) method of Ha et al. (2001) and Ha and Lee (2003) for inference. In general, the h-likelihood approach provides a unified inferential framework and a numerically efficient fitting algorithm for various random-effect models (Lee and Nelder 1996, 2001) and, novelly, allows us to consider time-dependent frailties. We use the new models to analyze two well-known practical data sets from the literature and compare the results with those obtained by fitting PH and PH frailty models.

The paper is organized as follows. In Sect. 2 we review the GTDL model briefly, while in Sect. 3 we formulate the two extended models based on the GTDL. The h-likelihood approach to inference is developed in Sect. 4, and in Sect. 5 the models are used to analyze two well-known data sets which have appeared in the survival literature, the results being compared with those obtained from the corresponding PH models. Finally, some further discussion is given in Sect. 6.

2   The GTDL Regression Models

A non-PH model, the GTDL regression model (MacKenzie 1996) is defined by the hazard function:

$$\lambda(t; x) = \lambda_0 p(t; x), \tag{1}$$

where $\lambda_0 > 0$ is a scalar, $p(t; x) = \exp(t\alpha + x^T \beta)/\{1 + \exp(t\alpha + x^T \beta)\}$ is a linear logistic function in time, α is a scalar measuring the effect of time and β is a $p \times 1$ vector of regression parameters associated with fixed covariates $x = (x_1, \ldots, x_p)^T$. The time-dependent relative risk, RR(t), the ratio of hazard rates for two subjects with different covariate vectors, x_1 and x_2, is given by

$$\rho(t; x_1, x_2) = \lambda(t; x_1)/\lambda(t; x_2) = \exp\{(x_1 - x_2)^T \beta\}\psi(t; x_1, x_2), \tag{2}$$

where

$$\psi(t; x_1, x_2) = \frac{\{1 + \exp(t\alpha + x_2^T \beta)\}}{\{1 + \exp(t\alpha + x_1^T \beta)\}}.$$

The leading term on the right hand side of (2) is Cox's constant of proportionality (the RR in a PH model) and thus in the GTDL model this constant is moderated by $\psi(\cdot)$, a function of both time and covariates, demonstrating, unequivocally, that the model is non-PH. Moreover, it should be noted that (2) does not depend on the parameter λ_0. When $\alpha = 0$ the relative risk does not depend on time and from (1) the resulting model is PH—an Exponential with $\lambda(t; x) = \lambda_0 p(x)$, i.e., a multiple of the usual multiple logistic function (Cox 1970).

From (1), the cumulative hazard function is given by

$$\Lambda(t; x) = \int_0^t \lambda(s; x)ds = \frac{\lambda_0}{\alpha} \log \left\{ \frac{1 + \exp(t\alpha + x^T \beta)}{1 + \exp(x^T \beta)} \right\}. \tag{3}$$

Under non-informative censoring the ordinary censored-data likelihood, which depends on (1) and (3), is constructed and the maximum likelihood estimators for the parameters can be obtained using numerical methods such as Newton–Raphson: for more details see MacKenzie (1996, 1997).

It is often convenient to take $\lambda_0 = 1$. MacKenzie (1996, 1997) has shown that this model is satisfactory in a variety of applications and leads to a formulation in which the covariates act linearly on the log-odds hazard scale, rather than on the log hazard scale, as in the PH model. For more details, including the role of this model in the analysis of strata, see MacKenzie (1996).

3 Extended GTDL Models

The correlation between survival times, which arises in recurrent or multiple event times on the same subject, may be modelled by introducing a frailty, or random effect. We thus extend the non-PH model (1) to include random effects in two different ways.

First we define the multivariate data structures as follows. Let T_{ij} ($i = 1, \ldots, q$, $j = 1, \ldots, n_i$, $n = \sum_i n_i$) be the survival time for jth observation of the ith subject and C_{ij} be the corresponding censoring time. Let the observable random variables be $Y_{ij} = \min(T_{ij}, C_{ij})$ and $\delta_{ij} = I(T_{ij} \leq C_{ij})$, where $I(\cdot)$ is the indicator function. Denote by U_i the continuous random variable denoting the unobserved frailty (or random effect) for the ith subject, with density $g(.|\theta)$.

3.1 Non-PH Frailty Model

Our first extension includes a frailty term acting multiplicatively on the individual hazard rate of (1). The GTDL non-PH frailty model is then defined as follows. Given $U_i = u_i$, the conditional hazard function of T_{ij} takes the form

$$\lambda_{ij}(t|u_i) = \lambda_{ij}(t)u_i, \tag{4}$$

where $\lambda_{ij}(t) = \lambda_0[\exp(t_{ij}\alpha + x_{ij}^T\beta)/\{1 + \exp(t_{ij}\alpha + x_{ij}^T\beta)\}]$ is given in (1) and $x_{ij} = (x_{ij1}, \ldots, x_{ijp})^T$. The frailties U_i are assumed to be independent and identically distributed random variables with a density function depending on the frailty parameter θ. Note that if in the model (4) $\lambda_{ij}(t) = \lambda_0(t)\exp(x_{ij}^T\beta)$ with unspecified baseline hazard function $\lambda_0(t)$, it becomes a semiparametric PH frailty model, an extension of Cox's model to allow frailty: see, for example, McGilchrist and Aisbett (1991) and Ha et al. (2001).

3.2 Non-PH Random Effects Model

Secondly, we consider another natural extension of model (1), by including a random component in the linear predictor, $t\alpha + x^T\beta$, of (1). Let $V_i = \log U_i$. The GTDL non-PH random effect model is then defined as follows. Given $V_i = v_i$, the conditional hazard function of T_{ij} is then of the form

$$\lambda_{ij}(t|v_i) = \lambda_0 \frac{\exp(t_{ij}\alpha + x_{ij}^T\beta + v_i)}{1 + \exp(t_{ij}\alpha + x_{ij}^T\beta + v_i)}. \tag{5}$$

The V_i are assumed to be independent and identically distributed random variables with a density function depending on the frailty parameter θ.

Models (4) and (5) are similar, but the manner in which the random effect is allowed to influence the basic GTDL hazard function differs in each case. That is, (4) assumes that the random effects $v_i = \log_e(u_i)$ act additively on the log hazard scale while (5) assumes they are additive on a generalized $\log_e$-odds hazard scale, which is the usual $\log_e$-odds hazard scale when $\lambda_0 = 1$. Note that model (4) is a conventional frailty model, but (5) is not since the random effect does not operate multiplicatively on the GTDL hazard function.

It may be observed that in model (5) the conditional log-odds hazard given v_i is linear in t. In general we have:

$$\log\left\{\frac{\lambda(t|v)}{1 - \lambda(t|v)}\right\} = t\alpha + x^T\beta + v$$

which is a direct generalization of model (1) when $\lambda_0 = 1$. Thus, we note that in (5) the quantity $\exp(t\alpha + x^T\beta + v)$ has a conditional odds ratio interpretation whereas in the PH model it is a relative risk. However, in model (4) $\exp(t\alpha + x^T\beta + v)$ may be shown to have a generalized conditional odds-ratio interpretation.

In practice, the choice of $g(.|\theta)$ may be important. For h-likelihood inference, the choice of parametric forms is wide and testable, since marginalization is not required. In this paper we shall adopt the log-Normal distribution for h-likelihood inference—a choice to which inference on β is robust (Ha et al. 2001; Ha and Lee 2003). An alternative choice for model (4) is the Gamma distribution, see Blagojevic et al. (2003) for a marginal likelihood approach in this scenario. For the use of other frailty distributions see Hougaard (2000) (Chap. 7). Alternatively, one may adopt a non-parametric mixture model.

Because of the convenience mentioned in Sect. 2, hereafter we adopt $\lambda_0 = 1$ in (4) and (5), which gives a reduced form of each model.

4   H-Likelihood Estimation

4.1   Estimation of Non-PH Frailty Model

Estimation in the Non-PH GTDL family has been considered in detail by Ha and MacKenzie (2010). However, for the sake of self-sufficiency and because we consider two different parametrizations of the Non-PH GTDL, we reproduce the main line below.

From Lee and Nelder (1996) and Ha et al. (2001), the h-likelihood for model (4), denoted by h, is defined by

$$h = h(\alpha, \beta, \theta) = \sum_{ij} \ell_{1ij} + \sum_{i} \ell_{2i}, \qquad (6)$$

where

$$\ell_{1ij} = \ell_{1ij}(\alpha, \beta; y_{ij}, \delta_{ij}|u_i)$$
$$= \delta_{ij} \log \lambda(y_{ij}|u_i) - \Lambda(y_{ij}|u_i)$$
$$= \delta_{ij}(\log p_{ij} + v_i) + u_i \alpha^{-1} \log(q_{ij} g_{ij})$$

is the logarithm of the conditional density function for Y_{ij} and δ_{ij} given $U_i = u_i$, and $\ell_{2i} = \ell_{2i}(\theta; v_i)$ is the logarithm of the density function for $V_i = \log U_i$ with parameter θ. For many models this device places the random effect, exactly (or approximately) on the same scale as the linear predictor—see Lee and Nelder (1996) for further details. With these arrangements the conditional hazard becomes $\lambda(y_{ij}|u_i) = p_{ij}u_i$ where

$$p_{ij} = p_{ij}(\alpha, \beta) = \exp(y_{ij}\alpha + x_{ij}^T\beta)/\{1 + \exp(y_{ij}\alpha + x_{ij}^T\beta)\}$$

and the conditional cumulative hazard $\Lambda(y_{ij}|u_i) = -u_i\alpha^{-1}\log(q_{ij}g_{ij})$ with $q_{ij} = 1 - p_{ij}$ and $g_{ij} = g_{ij}(\beta) = 1 + \exp(x_{ij}^T\beta)$.

The maximum h-likelihood (MHL) joint estimating equations of $\tau = (\alpha, \beta^T, v^T)^T$ with $v = (v_1, \ldots, v_q)^T$ are given by

$$\partial h/\partial \tau = 0.$$

The score equations are then:

$$\partial h/\partial \alpha = \sum_{ij}\{\delta_{ij}q_{ij}y_{ij} - (u_i/\alpha)p_{ij}y_{ij} - (u_i/\alpha^2)\log(q_{ij}g_{ij})\},$$

$$\partial h/\partial \beta_k = \sum_{ij}\{\delta_{ij}q_{ij} + (u_i/\alpha)(r_{ij} - p_{ij})\}x_{ijk}(k = 1, \ldots, p), \qquad (7)$$

$$\partial h/\partial v_i = \sum_{j}\{\delta_{ij} + (u_i/\alpha)\log(q_{ij}g_{ij})\} + \partial\ell_{2i}/\partial v_i (i = 1, \ldots, q),$$

where $u_i = \exp(v_i)$ and $r_{ij} = r_{ij}(\beta) = \exp(x_{ij}^T\beta)/\{1 + \exp(x_{ij}^T\beta)\}$. The first two equations depend on θ only through $v = (v_1, \ldots, v_q)^T$ as does the first member of the third equation. However, the second member of the third equation is, in general, a function of the frailty parameter θ. Given θ, the estimating equations (7) are easily solved using the Newton–Raphson method and Lee and Nelder (1996, 2001) and Ha et al. (2001) have shown that the asymptotic covariance matrix for $\hat{\tau} - \tau$ is given by the inverse of $H = -\partial^2 h/\partial \tau^2$.

In order to estimate the frailty parameter, θ, we adopt the restricted likelihood (Lee and Nelder 1996, 2001) (or adjusted profile h-likelihood) approach which yields a likelihood $h_P(\theta)$ for θ, after eliminating τ, defined by

$$h_P(\theta) = h_A|_{\tau=\hat{\tau}}, \qquad (8)$$

where $h_A = h + \frac{1}{2}\log\{\det(2\pi H^{-1})\}$ and $\hat{\tau} = \hat{\tau}(\theta)$. Given estimates of τ, Lee and Nelder (2001) REML (restricted maximum likelihood) estimating equation for θ, maximizing h_P, is given by

$$\partial h_A/\partial \theta|_{\tau=\hat{\tau}} = 0. \qquad (9)$$

4.2 Estimation of Non-PH Random Effect Model

The corresponding h-likelihood for the model (5) is given by

$$h = h(\alpha, \beta, \theta) = \sum_{ij}\ell_{1ij} + \sum_{i}\ell_{2i}, \qquad (10)$$

where

$$\ell_{1ij} = \ell_{1ij}(\alpha, \beta; y_{ij}, \delta_{ij}|v_i)$$

$$= \delta_{ij} \log \lambda(y_{ij}|v_i) - \Lambda(y_{ij}|v_i)$$

$$= \delta_{ij} \log p'_{ij} + \alpha^{-1} \log(q'_{ij} g'_{ij})$$

is the logarithm of the conditional density function for Y_{ij} and δ_{ij} given $V_i = v_i$, and $\ell_{2i} = \ell_{2i}(\theta; v_i)$ is the logarithm of the density function for V_i with parameter θ. Here, the conditional hazard is $\lambda(y_{ij}|v_i) = p'_{ij}$ where

$$p'_{ij} = p'_{ij}(\alpha, \beta, v_i) = \exp(y_{ij}\alpha + x_{ij}^T \beta + v_i)/\{1 + \exp(y_{ij}\alpha + x_{ij}^T \beta + v_i)\}$$

and the conditional cumulative hazard $\Lambda(y_{ij}|v_i) = -\alpha^{-1} \log(q'_{ij} g'_{ij})$ with $q'_{ij} = 1 - p'_{ij}$ and $g'_{ij} = g'_{ij}(\beta, v_i) = 1 + \exp(x_{ij}^T \beta + v_i)$. In this case the score equations for $\tau = (\alpha, \beta^T, v^T)^T$ are given by

$$\partial h/\partial \alpha = \sum_{ij} \{\delta_{ij} q'_{ij} y_{ij} - (1/\alpha) p'_{ij} y_{ij} - (1/\alpha^2) \log(q'_{ij} g'_{ij})\},$$

$$\partial h/\partial \beta_k = \sum_{ij} \{\delta_{ij} q'_{ij} + (1/\alpha)(r'_{ij} - p'_{ij})\} x_{ijk} (k = 1, \dots, p),$$

$$\partial h/\partial v_i = \sum_{j} \{\delta_{ij} q'_{ij} + (1/\alpha)(r'_{ij} - p'_{ij})\} + \partial \ell_{2i}/\partial v_i (i = 1, \dots, q),$$

where $r'_{ij} = r'_{ij}(\beta, v_i) = \exp(x_{ij}^T \beta + v_i)/\{1 + \exp(x_{ij}^T \beta + v_i)\}$.

With the h-likelihood (10) and the score equations given above, the fitting procedure outlined in the previous section can be applied directly to model (5).

5 Examples

We illustrate the use of the proposed models by analyzing two well-known multivariate survival data sets. For the purposes of comparison, we include two classical PH models—Cox's PH and PH frailty model. For the reasons given above, we have chosen the distribution of the random effect to be log-Normal. Accordingly, we consider the following five models:

- M1 (PH): Cox's PH model without frailty component.
- M2 (PHF): Cox's PH model with frailty component.
- M3 (NPH): GTDL non-PH model without frailty component.
- M4 (NPHF): GTDL non-PH with frailty component.
- M5 (NPHR): GTDL non-PH with random-effect component.

Here M1 and M2 are PH models, whereas M3, M4 and M5 are non-PH models.

Table 1 Analyses from various models for the kidney infection data

	M1(PH)		M1(PHF)		M3(NPH)		M4(NPHF)		M5(NPHR)	
Variable	Est.	SE	Est.	SE	Est.	SE	Est.	SE	Est.	SE
Intercept					−3.069	0.527	−2.065	0.783	−2.099	0.773
Sex	−0.830	0.297	−1.368	0.427	−0.940	0.288	−1.542	0.445	−1.521	0.438
Time (α)					−0.001	0.001	0.002	0.001	0.002	0.001
θ			0.509				0.656		0.663	
$-2h_P$	370.0		364.7		688.0		679.9		680.0	

Est., estimate; SE, standard error; θ, variance of random-effect distribution; M1(PH), Cox's PH model without frailty component; M2(PHF), Cox's PH model with frailty component; M3(NPH), GTDL non-PH model without frailty component; M4(NPHF), GTDL non-PH with frailty component; M5(NPHR), GTDL non-PH with random-effect component; h_P, the restricted likelihood, given in (8)

5.1   Kidney Infection Data

McGilchrist and Aisbett (1991) presented a small data set, which describes times to the first and second recurrences of infection in 38 kidney patients being treated by portable dialysis. Infections may occur at the location where the catheter is inserted. The catheter is removed if infection occurs and can be removed for other reasons, in which case, the observation is censored. Thus, survival time is defined as the time from insertion of the catheter to infection. Survival times measured on the same patient may be correlated because they share the same patient characteristics. For the purpose of illustration, we consider fitting a single fixed covariate—sex of the patient, coded as 1 for female and as 0 for male. The results of fitting the five models are summarized in Table 1.

Overall, the results from models M1 and M3, which do not contain random components, are similar, as are the results from models M2, M4 and M5, in which random components have been incorporated. In particular, the non-PH random-effect models M4 and M5 lead to similar results, despite the fact that in model M4 the random effect is not quite on the same scale as the linear predictor. Overall, this is reassuring given the similarity of the functional forms involved in their formulation.

For testing the absence of a random component (i.e. $H_0 : \theta = 0$), we use the deviance ($-2h_P$ in Table 1) based upon the restricted likelihood h_P (Lee and Nelder 2001). Because such a hypothesis is on the boundary of the parameter space, the critical value is $\chi^2_{2\lambda}$ for a size λ test. This value results from the fact that the asymptotic distribution of likelihood ratio test is a 50:50 mixture of χ^2_0 and χ^2_1 distributions (Chernoff 1954; Self and Liang 1987): for application to random-effect models, see Stram and Lee (1994) and Vu and Knuiman (2002) and Ha and Lee (2005).

Firstly, for the PH models, M1 and M2, testing $H_0 : \theta = 0$ yields a difference in deviances of 5.28, indicating that the frailty component is necessary, i.e. $\theta > 0$. In other words, the correlation between survival times is significant at the 5 % level ($\chi^2_{1,0.10} = 2.71$). Moreover, we conclude that M2 with frailty is superior to

M1 without it. Secondly, for the three non-PH models (M3, M4 and M5), testing $H_0 : \theta = 0$ yields differences 8.09 and 7.96, from M3 and M4 and M3 and M5, respectively. Thus, models M4 and M5 also explain the correlation and are to be preferred to M3. In particular, when comparing M4 and M5 with M3, the sign of the time coefficient α changes, from negative to positive, suggesting that the frailty has been taken into account successfully, i.e., the decreasing time-trend in hazard has been abolished. A similar finding is sometimes observed in M3 when important missing covariates are added—see MacKenzie (1996) for further details.

In all five models the sex effect is highly statistically significant indicating that the female patients are at lower risk of infection compared with males. However, the absolute magnitude of the fixed effect (and its SE) in both M1 and M3 is smaller than in M2, M4 and M5, presumably, because the former models fail to account for the correlation between survival times on the same patient—see Ha et al. (2001) for more detail. In relation to models M2, M4 and M5 the results are similar, both with respect to the magnitude of the fixed effect, $\hat{\beta}$ (and its SE) and with respect to $\hat{\theta}$, the estimate of the frailty parameter.

Table 1 suggests that models M2, M4 and M5, all of which incorporate random components, provide reasonable explanations for the correlated survival data. However, models M4 and M5 cannot be formally justified, on this occasion, since $\hat{\alpha}$ is not significantly different from zero.

5.2 CGD Data

Fleming and Harrington (1991) provide more extensive multivariate survival data on a placebo-controlled randomized trial of gamma interferon (γ-IFN) in chronic granulomatous disease (CGD). The aim of the trial was to investigate the effectiveness of the γ-IFN in reducing the rate of serious infections in CGD patients. In this study, 128 patients were followed for approximately 1 year. Out of the 63 patients in the treatment group, 14 patients experienced at least one infection and a total of 20 infections were recorded. In the placebo group, 30 out of 65 patients experienced at least one infection, with a total of 56 infections being recorded. Here, the survival times are the times between repeated CGD infections on each patient (i.e., gap times). Censoring occurred at the last observation on all patients, except one, who experienced a serious infection on the date he left the study. The recurrent infection times for each patient are likely to be correlated as in the kidney infection data study.

We fitted the same set of fixed covariates considered by Yau and McGilchrist (1998), namely: treatment ($0 = placebo$, $1 = \gamma$-IFN), pattern of inheritance ($0 =$ autosomal recessive, $1 =$ X-linked); age (in years); height (in cm); weight (in kg); using corticosteroids at time of study entry ($0 =$ no, $1 =$ yes); using prophylactic antibiotics at time of study entry ($0 =$ no, $1 =$ yes); sex ($0 =$ male, $1 =$ female), hospital region ($0 =$ U.S., $1 =$ Europe), and a longitudinal variable representing the accumulated time from the first infection in years. The rationale

Table 2 Analyses from various models for the CGD data

	M1(PH)		M1(PHF)		M3(NPH)		M4(NPHF)		M5(NPHR)	
Variable	Est.	SE	Est.	SE	Est.	SE	Est.	SE	Est.	SE
Intercept					−5.551	1.080	−5.706	1.298	−5.707	1.299
Inheritance	−0.634	0.287	−0.650	0.358	−0.666	0.288	−0.684	0.359	−0.684	0.359
Age	−0.082	0.037	−0.085	0.043	−0.084	0.037	−0.087	0.043	−0.087	0.043
Height	0.007	0.010	0.008	0.013	0.007	0.010	0.008	0.013	0.008	0.013
Weight	0.012	0.016	0.010	0.020	0.012	0.016	0.011	0.020	0.011	0.020
Corticosteroids	1.793	0.594	1.962	0.795	1.851	0.593	2.039	0.801	2.034	0.797
Prophylactic	−0.542	0.324	−0.662	0.421	−0.550	0.325	−0.660	0.422	−0.660	0.421
Sex	−0.709	0.394	−0.751	0.496	−0.752	0.394	−0.796	0.498	−0.795	0.497
Hospital region	−0.636	0.318	−0.688	0.377	−0.655	0.318	−0.712	0.377	−0.711	0.377
Longitudinal	1.442	0.467	0.914	0.505	1.605	0.459	1.062	0.500	1.067	0.501
T (α)					0.003	0.001	0.004	0.002	0.004	0.002
θ			0.508				0.511		0.513	
$-2h_P$	694.6		690.5		1,074.2		1,069.9		1,069.8	

Est., estimate; SE, standard error; θ, variance of random-effect distribution; M1(PH), Cox's PH model without frailty component; M2(PHF), Cox's PH model with frailty component; M3(NPH), GTDL non-PH model without frailty component; M4(NPHF), GTDL non-PH with frailty component; M5(NPHR), GTDL non-PH with random-effect component; h_P, the restricted likelihood, given in (8)

under-pinning this variable is that the infection rate may increase over time following the first infection (Yau and McGilchrist 1998). The results pertaining to the five models are given in Table 2.

Overall, the results are similar to those for the kidney infection data, except for the findings in relation to time-dependent effects. In particular, the interpretation of the beneficial effect of treatment is unequivocal in all models. The results for models M4 and M5 are very similar in these data, the time parameter $\hat{\alpha}$ is statistically significant in each, showing that the PH-class is formally inappropriate. However, the magnitude of the dependence of the hazard on time is so small as to be almost immaterial in this case. However, the non-PH random-effect models M4 and M5 suggest that the longitudinal effect is on the borderline of statistical significance. Models M1 and M3 also support the existence of the effect, but rather exaggerate its significance, especially M3. On the other hand, further evidence for its existence, may be adduced from the analysis by Yau and McGilchrist (1998), which identified a longitudinal effect using a more complicated PH model with time-dependent AR(1) frailties. This analysis highlights the advantages of fitting a variety of different models to the same dataset, rather than drawing conclusions from a single model class (typically PH).

6 Discussion

The Cox model with frailty is based on a conditional PH hazard function. In general, the marginal survival model, obtained by integrating out the frailty from the conditional model, will be non-PH (Hougaard 2000). Exactly how the marginal model deviates from proportionality is unknown for many frailty distributions, including the log-Normal distribution adopted in this paper. Accordingly, there is considerable scope for expanding the class of non-PH models available in this setting. This consideration led us to two new non-PH models based on the GTDL. Both models were easily implemented in the h-likelihood framework and have proved flexible tools for analyzing PH or non-PH correlated data. An interesting point is that the similarity of the conclusions suggests that the use of the canonical scale (Lee et al. 2006) for random effects and fixed effects is not strictly necessary, thereby extending the envelope within which h-likelihood methods work.

It remains to be seen which of the two models proves the more successful in practice. Overall, the findings suggest that the models are capable of representing data which are more non-PH than the datasets analyzed in this paper (i.e., when $\alpha \not\approx 0$).

It should be noted that both of these models, are wholly parametric competitors for the PH frailty model, and are more convenient computationally, as all of the time-dependent quantities of interest (hazard trend, odds-ratios and relative risks) may be readily derived.

From Tables 1 and 2 we have observed that the values of deviance $(-2h_P)$ in PH models (M1 and M2) are very different from those in non-PH models (M3, M4 and M5). The reason is that the former models are semiparametric with nonparametric baseline hazard, while the latter models are wholly parametric. Thus, developing a suitable measure for model selection among these PH and non-PH models would be an interesting piece of future work.

Acknowledgements The work in this paper was supported by the Science Foundation Ireland's (SFI, www.sfi.ie) project grant number 07/MI/012 (BIO-SI project, www3.ul.ie/bio-si) and by KOSEF, Daejeon, South Korea.

References

Blagojevic, M., MacKenzie, G., & Ha, I. (2003). A comparison of non-ph and ph gamma frailty models. In *Proceedings of the 18th International Workshop on Statistical Modelling*, Leuven, Belgium (pp. 39–44).

Chernoff, H. (1954). On the distribution of the likelihood ratio. *The Annals of Mathematical Statistics, 25*, 573–578.

Cox, D. R. (1970). *The analysis of binary data*. London: Methuen.

Cox, D. R. (1972). Regression models and life-tables (with discussion). *Journal of the Royal Statistical Society, 34*, 187–220.

Fleming, T. R., & Harrington, D. P. (1991). *Counting processes and survival analysis*. New York: Wiley.

Ha, I. D., & Lee, Y. (2003). Estimating frailty models via poisson hierarchical generalized linear models. *Journal of Computational and Graphical Statistics, 12*, 663–681.

Ha, I. D., & Lee, Y. (2005). Multilevel mixed linear models for survival data. *Lifetime Data Analysis, 11*, 131–142.

Ha, I. D., Lee, Y., & Song, J. (2001). Hierarchical likelihood approach for frailty models. *Biometrika, 88*, 233–243.

Ha, I. D., & MacKenzie, G. (2010). Robust frailty modelling using non-proportional hazards models. *Statistical Modelling, 10*(3), 315–332.

Hougaard, P. (2000). *Analysis of multivariate survival Data*. New York: Springer.

Lee, Y., Nelder, J. A. (1996). Hierarchical generalized linear models (with discussion). *Journal of the Royal Statistical Society, 58*, 619–678.

Lee, Y., & Nelder, J. A. (2001). Hierarchical generalised linear models: A synthesis of generalised linear models, random-effect models and structured dispersions. *Biometrika, 88*, 987–1006.

Lee, Y., Nelder, J. A., & Pawitan, Y. (2006). Generalised linear models with random effects: Unified analysis via h-likelihood. London: Chapman and Hall.

MacKenzie, G. (1996). Regression models for survival data: The generalised time dependent logistic family. *Journal of the Royal Statistical Society, 45*, 21–34.

MacKenzie, G. (1997). On a non-proportional hazards regression model for repeated medical random counts. *Statistics in Medicine, 16*, 1831–1843.

McGilchrist, C. A., & Aisbett, C. W. (1991). Regression with frailty in survival analysis. *Biometrics, 47*, 461–466.

Self, S. G., & Liang, K. Y. (1987). Asymptotic properties of maximum likelihood estimators and likelihood ratio tests under nonstandard conditions. *Journal of the American Statistical Association, 82*, 605–610.

Stram, D. O., & Lee, J. W. (1994). Variance components testing in the longitudinal mixed effects model. *Biometrics, 50*, 1171–1177.

Vu, H. T. V., & Knuiman, M. W. (2002). A hybrid ml-em algorithm for calculation of maximum likelihood estimates in semiparametric shared frailty models. *Computational Statistics and Data Analysis, 40*, 173–187.

Yau, K. K. W., & McGilchrist, C. A. (1998). Ml and reml estimation in survival analysis with time dependent correlated frailty. *Statistics in Medicine, 17*, 1201–1213.

Frailty Models with Structural Dispersion

Joseph Lynch and Gilbert MacKenzie

Abstract In observational survival studies unmeasured covariates are the norm. In univariate survival data we allow for their influence by means of frailty models. Below we develop two Gamma frailty models with parametric basic hazard functions: one with a proportional basic hazard function and the other with a non-proportional basic hazard function. It transpires that both of the resulting marginal frailty models have non-proportional hazard functions. We use these models to analyse survival from breast cancer in the local health authorities in the West Midlands of England in the UK and show that North Staffordshire is at, or near to, the bottom of the resulting league tables, confirming the findings of other workers who analysed earlier data at a National level. We also introduce and explain the notion of structural dispersion which generalises the frailty variance to a regression-based, subject-specific form and show that the fit of the structural dispersion models is superior to the classical Gamma frailty models, but that the applied results are unchanged.

Keywords Frailty models • Generalized time-dependent logistic • Non-PH model • Random effect • Structural dispersion • Weibull

1 Introduction

The proportional hazards (PH) model implies that the hazard function is fully determined by the observed fixed-effect covariates. Because we are all biologically different, the natural course of a given disease and the effect of its treatment vary from person to person. When modelling survival, some of this heterogeneity

J. Lynch (✉)
The Centre for Biostatistics, University of Limerick, Limerick, Ireland
e-mail: joseph.lynch@ul.ie

G. MacKenzie and D. Peng (eds.), *Statistical Modelling in Biostatistics and Bioinformatics*, Contributions to Statistics, DOI 10.1007/978-3-319-04579-5__4,
© Springer International Publishing Switzerland 2014

may be explained in terms of the fixed-effects, i.e., the covariates. However, in many settings not all of the relevant covariates may be measured. Indeed, from a scientific perspective, the set of relevant covariates may not even be known. This provides an intrinsic justification for always making allowance for unmeasured covariates. One approach is by using the concept of *frailty* whereby an unobservable, non-negative, random effect is introduced which multiplies on the usual basic hazard function, as in

$$\lambda(t|x, u) = u.\lambda(t|x),$$

where u is the multiplicative random effect and $\lambda(t|x)$ is the basic hazard function. A convenient choice for u is the Gamma distribution which we adopt below.

When the data are univariate, as in the time to a single event, the frailty, describes the effect of unobserved covariates in the model for each individual. Thus, the survival of an individual with $u = 1$ follows the basic hazard function, while for individuals with $u > 1$, the basic hazard is increased and early failure is then more likely. In multivariate settings with recurrent events, u is common to several individuals and generates the correlation between the survival times.

In this short paper only univariate data are studied and we have elected to present results for two wholly parametric frailty models with different basic hazard functions, PH and non-PH. We generalise the parametric PH Weibull model to a Gamma frailty model in order to illustrate our methods. However, not all survival data are PH and a flexible non-PH model is the Generalised Time-Dependent Logistic (GTDL) described by MacKenzie (1996). Accordingly, we generalise this model to frailty form by using a multiplicative frailty term. Here, too, we assume the random effect follows a Gamma distribution, whence both the resulting frailty models studied have closed forms after marginalisation and are non-PH (Hougaard 2000).

Finally, we generalise both frailty models to have structural dispersion (Lee and Nelder 2001) and investigate the performance of the models when analysing survival in a large study of incident cases of breast cancer in the West Midlands of the UK.

2 Regression Models with Frailty

The failure time density $f(t|\theta, \beta)$ is the product of the hazard function $\lambda(t|.)$ and the survivor function $S(t|.)$ where θ is a vector valued parameter and β is a $p \times 1$ vector of regression parameters. Frailty is represented by the random variable U with density $g(\mu, \sigma^2)$, such that $E(U) = 1$ and $Var(U) = \sigma^2$.

The marginal density is found by integrating out the random effects and the marginal likelihood function L_f is obtained from the joint probability of this marginal density for $i = 1, \ldots, n$ subjects with individual survival times t_i, covariates x_i, censoring indicators δ_i and frailty components u_i,

$$L_f(\theta, \beta, \sigma^2) = \prod_{i=1}^{n} \int_0^\infty \lambda(t_i|u_i, \theta, \beta)^{\delta_i} (t_i|u_i, \theta, \beta) g(u_i|\sigma^2) du_i$$

and this forms a natural vehicle for inference since it retains the properties of a conventional (Fisherian) likelihood.

2.1 Weibull Model

The Weibull model has a hazard function given by

$$\lambda(t|x) = \lambda\rho(t\lambda)^{\rho-1}\exp(x'\beta),$$

where $0 \leq t < \infty$. β is a $p \times 1$ vector of regression parameters associated with fixed covariates $x' = (x_1, \ldots, x_p)$. The scale parameter λ and the shape parameter ρ are both > 0. The censored log-likelihood is

$$l(\lambda, \rho, \beta) = \sum_{i=1}^{n} \left[\delta_i (\log_e \rho + \rho\log_e \lambda + (\rho-1)\log_e t_i + x_i'\beta) - (\lambda t_i)^\rho \exp(x_i'\beta) \right].$$

For the Weibull-gamma frailty model, we assume the random component U has a multiplicative effect on the hazard, such that $\lambda(t, x, u) = u\lambda(t, x)$. $\Gamma(1, \sigma^2)$ distribution, then

$$g(u|\sigma^2) = \frac{u^{\frac{1}{\sigma^2}-1}\exp(\frac{-u}{\sigma^2})}{\Gamma(\frac{1}{\sigma^2})\sigma^{2\frac{-1}{\sigma^2}}}.$$

Integrating out the random effect, we get the frailty survival distribution,

$$S_f(t|x) = [1 + \sigma^2(t\lambda)^\rho \exp(x_i'\beta)]^{\frac{-1}{\sigma^2}}.$$

The marginal hazard is

$$\lambda_f(t|x) = \frac{\lambda(t\lambda)^{\rho-1}\rho\exp(x_i'\beta)}{1 + \sigma^2(t\lambda)^\rho \exp(x_i'\beta)}.$$

The log likelihood is

$$l(\lambda, \rho, \beta, \sigma^2) = \sum_{i=1}^{n} \left[\delta_i \log_e (\lambda^\rho t_i^{\rho-1}\rho\exp(x_i'\beta)) - (\delta_i + \sigma^2)\log_e (\sigma^2(t_i\lambda)^\rho \exp(x_i'\beta) + 1) \right].$$

2.2 GTDL Model

The GTDL model has a hazard function given by

$$\lambda(t|x) = \lambda \frac{\exp(t\alpha + x'\beta)}{1 + \exp(t\alpha + x'\beta)},$$

where α is a time parameter, β is a $p \times 1$ vector of regression parameters associated with fixed covariates, $x' = (x_1, \ldots, x_p)$ and $\lambda > 0$ is a scalar.

The corresponding survival function is:

$$S(t|x) = \left[\frac{1 + \exp(t\alpha + x'\beta)}{1 + \exp(x'\beta)} \right]^{\frac{-\lambda}{\alpha}}.$$

The censored log-likelihood is

$$l(\lambda, \alpha, \beta) = \sum_{i=1}^{n} [\delta_i \log_e \lambda + \delta_i \log_e \left(\frac{\exp(t_i\alpha + x'\beta)}{1 + \exp(t_i\alpha + x'_i\beta)} \right) + \frac{\lambda}{\alpha} (\log_e g_i + \log_e q_i)],$$

where

$$q_i = \frac{1}{1 + \exp(t_i\alpha + x'_i\beta)},$$

$$g_i = 1 + \exp(x'_i\beta).$$

Using similar techniques as for the Weibull model, the log likelihood for the frailty distribution is

$$l(\lambda, \rho, \beta, \sigma^2) = \sum_{i=1}^{n} \left[\delta_i \log_e(p_i\lambda) - (\delta_i + \sigma^2)\log_e(1 - \frac{\lambda\sigma^2}{\alpha} \log_e(q_i g_i)) \right].$$

In evaluating the marginal frailty distribution for the GTDL model, we again assume the frailty component U has a $\Gamma(1, \sigma^2)$ distribution. The marginal survival distribution is

$$S_f(t|x) = \left[1 - \frac{\lambda\sigma^2}{\alpha} \log_e(q_i g_i) \right]^{\frac{-1}{\sigma^2}}$$

and the marginal hazard is

$$\lambda_f = \frac{\lambda p_i}{1 - \frac{\lambda\sigma^2}{\alpha} \log_e(q_i g_i)}.$$

See also Blagojevic et al. (2003) and Blagojevic and MacKenzie (2004) for other details.

2.3 Goodness-of-Fit Measures

We compared the fit of the Weibull and GTDL models, without frailty, with frailty and with structural dispersion using a range of techniques, i.e., AIC, BIC and a modified χ^2 measure of goodness-of-fit. The latter test statistic is the sum of the squared difference between the Kaplan Meier (KM) and the model survivor functions estimates for each subject, divided by the subject's model survivor function estimates

$$\chi_v^2 = \sum_{i=1}^{n} \frac{\{S_{KM}(t_i) - S_{Model}(t_i)\}^2}{S_{Model}(t_i)},$$

for $i = 1, \ldots, n = 15,516$ subjects, where v is unknown. This corresponds to a quasi Chi-squared goodness-of-fit statistic in which the role of the observed values is played by the KM survivor estimates and the role of the expected values are played by the model survivor estimates. The statistic can be presented in graphical form as the partial sum (y-axis) plotted against time (x-axis) enabling one to see where any lack of fit emerges.

3 The Concept of Structural Dispersion

In many regression models we are used to modelling the mean structure in a relatively sophisticated way, and, in survival analysis, the same is true for the hazard function. This is very natural as the hazard function is the defining component of the survival distribution.

On the other hand, MacKenzie and Pan (2007) have highlighted the importance of joint mean-covariance modelling in longitudinal data setting. These ideas spill-over to joint hazard-dispersion modelling in the frailty survival modelling context, especially in multi-component frailty models. Moreover, they extend further into the arena of model selection, e.g., Ha et al. (2007).

Meanwhile, let us consider why it is important to model the dispersion jointly with the hazard. In many physical problems additional random components are often required to accommodate departures from standard models (e.g., over-dispersion in the Poisson model, random trajectories over time in longitudinal studies, etc.). Put another way, these components account in some sense for variation which is unexplained in the standard model. However, we may enquire where this variation comes from and how it is structured in terms of intrinsic factors, such as baseline covariates, in the original physical problem. Taking this view is more likely to be persuasive, since "plucking" multiple random effects from the ether to improve the fit of models often seems unrealistic in scientific terms. On the other hand, if it can be shown that the random effects are required and that their variance is controlled by factors intrinsic to the physical problem, the model gains additional scientific credence. Thus, viewing the variance of the random effect as being controlled by fixed effects may sometimes make sense and contribute to a greater scientific understanding.

If we consider the simplest univariate frailty case, covariates which influence the hazard function via the regression $x'\beta$, may or may not, also influence the frailty variance, σ^2. Thus, just as we can assess the influence of factors on the hazard, we can also assess the influence of the same or other factors, on the amount of unexplained variation, via another regression, $x'\beta^*$. We can estimate β and β^* by their joint MLE $(\hat{\beta}, \hat{\beta}^*)$ and hence obtain $\text{cov}(\hat{\beta}, \hat{\beta}^*)$ by standard methods. Accordingly, the univariate frailty models can be generalised by replacing σ^2 by σ_i^2, where

$$\sigma_i^2 = \exp(x_i'\beta^*).$$

Thus, in general, the frailty variance is not constant, as in the classical case, but is subject-specific. The additional linear predictor, $x_i'\beta^*$, always contains an intercept term, $x_{0i} = 1$, $\forall i$, so that when the frailty variance does not depend on the variable components in x_i we automatically recover the classical model. On the other hand, the larger any particular component, the more that particular variable contributes to the unexplained variation. Thus, when there is significant structure we can assess the independent contribution of the individual components. It should be noted that the structural dispersion model is *not* a random coefficient model.

4 Analysis

Using a relative survival approach, Coleman (1998) reported that North Stafford-shire Local Health Authority (LHA) was ranked last of 99 LHAs in England & Wales with respect to breast cancer survival. The method makes no allowance for case-mix. Accordingly, we re-analyse an augmented dataset from the West Midlands of England, including North Staffordshire, by more traditional methods and report on the resulting case-mix adjusted league tables.

4.1 Data for Analysis

The data set obtained from the West Midlands Cancer Intelligence Unit, comprised 15,516 women diagnosed with incident breast cancer between 1991 and 1995

Table 1 Five-year adjusted survival league tables

LHA	$\hat{S}_G$	LHA	$\hat{S}_{G+GF}$	LHA	$\hat{S}_W$	LHA	$\hat{S}_{W+GF}$	LHA	$\hat{S}_{G+SD}$	LHA	$\hat{S}_{W+SD}$
Unknown	0.79	Unk	0.85	Unk	0.78	Unk	0.79	Unk	0.88	Unk	0.83
Birm'ham	0.74	Cov	0.76	Bir	0.75	Bir	0.74	Bir	0.71	Bir	0.71
Coventry	0.73	Bir	0.76	Her	0.74	Her	0.73	Cov	0.71	Her	0.71
Hereford	0.72	Her	0.75	Cov	0.74	Cov	0.72	Her	0.71	Cov	0.70
Solihull	0.72	Wolv	0.73	Warw	0.72	Wolv	0.67	Wolv	0.69	Sand	0.69
Shropsh	0.71	Sol	0.73	Sol	0.72	Sand	0.67	Shrop	0.69	Wolv	0.68
Warwick	0.71	Sand	0.73	Sand	0.72	Sol	0.67	Warw	0.69	Warw	0.68
Sandwell	0.70	Warw	0.73	Shrop	0.71	Worc	0.66	Sol	0.68	Shrop	0.68
Wolverhm	0.70	Shrop	0.72	Wolv	0.71	Warw	0.65	Sand	0.68	Sol	0.67
Worcester	0.69	Dudl	0.72	Worc	0.71	Shrop	0.65	Worc	0.68	Worc	0.67
Dudley	0.69	Worc	0.72	Dudl	0.70	Dudl	0.65	Dudl	0.68	Dudl	0.66
Walsall	0.68	Wals	0.70	Wals	0.70	Wals	0.6	Wals	0.66	NSt	0.66
NStaff	0.67	SSt	0.69	NSt	0.69	SSt	0.62	NSt	0.65	Wals	0.65
SStaff	0.67	NSt	0.69	SSt	0.68	NSt	0.62	SSt	0.64	SSt	0.64

G = GTDL, W = Weibull, GF = Gamma frailty, SD = structural dispersion

in the West Midlands. They were followed up over a 10-year period from 1991 to 2001. Nine categorical covariates were initially studied in each patient. They were age, diagnosis basis, stage, morphology, screening, Townsend score, year of diagnosis, LHA and treatment. Age refers to age at diagnosis. Diagnosis basis refers to whether the diagnosis of breast cancer was made on clinical, histological or cytological grounds. Stage refers to how far the tumour has spread from its site of origin at the time of diagnosis. Morphology refers to the histological tissue type of tumour. Screening detection refers to whether or not the patient had her breast screened prior to referral. Townsend score is a social deprivation index. Years of diagnosis range from 1991 to 1995, so earlier years had a longer follow up. There were 13 different LHAs and one unknown category to which 94 patients were allocated. Treatment includes the various combinations of surgery, chemotherapy, radiotherapy and hormone therapy which each patient received during the course of the study.

4.2 League Tables

Initial analysis using the Cox model showed that the PH assumption did not hold up for some of the covariates studied. Accordingly, the survivor functions for each model, with and without frailty, were computed at the mean of the baseline covariates in all 14 LHAs and the 5-year survival figures were ranked (Table 1). The results are broadly similar from model to model. Goldstein and Spiegelhalter (1996) caution that league tables based on the rank of Health Authorities should be interpreted with caution as small quantitative differences may result in large changes in rank. However, it seems that, overall, Coleman's National findings are

Table 2 Goodness-of-fit measures for the six models fitted

Model	$\ell(\hat{\theta})$	Parameters	AIC	BIC
Weibull	−21,427.95	62	42,979.90	43,456.18
GTDL	−21,430.64	62	42,985.28	43,459.56
Weibull Frailty	−21,627.42	63	43,380.84	43,862.77
GTDL Frailty	−21,300.73	63	42,727.46	43,209.39
Weibull SD	−21,058.83	123	42,363.66	43,304.56
GTDL SD	−20,977.94	123	42,201.88	43,142.78

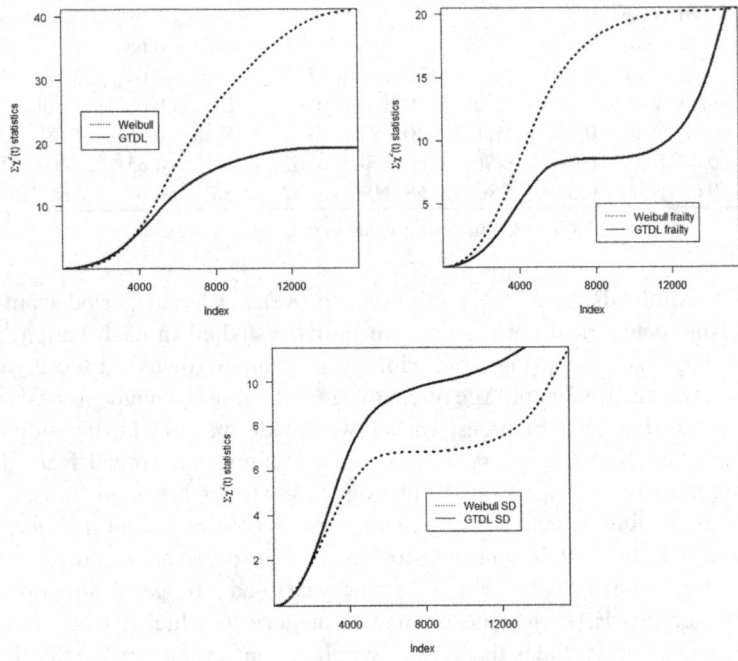

Fig. 1 Comparison of χ^2 goodness-of-fit estimates for the six fitted models. Panels: *left*—basic survival curves, *right*—frailty models and *centre*—frailty with structural dispersion. Weibull (*dashed*), GTDL (*solid*) and Index = ordered time

corroborated by our more detailed regional analysis. Survival in North Staffordshire is poor even after taking the effect of the measured and unmeasured covariates into account by means of frailty. It should be noted that Birmingham, which is a regional centre, dealing with the most difficult cases, comes top after adjusting for case-mix variables.

On the whole, structural dispersion models fitted better than frailty models, which, in turn were better fitting than the models without frailty (Table 2). The cumulative quasi chi-squared measures of fit are presented in Fig. 1 which also shows that the structural dispersion models fit best. However, these goodness-of-fit measures are not concordant with the AIC and BIC information criteria in

Table 2 when comparing Weibull and GTDL models. For example, in relation to the structural dispersion models, Table 2 suggests that the GTDL model fits best but Fig. 1 (centre panel) suggests that the Weibull model fits best. These inconsistencies require further research pending which we prefer to rely on the classical information criteria.

5 Discussion

The applied findings of this study largely confirm Coleman's original conclusions and will disappoint clinicians working on breast cancer care in North Staffordshire in the West Midlands of the United Kingdom. In 1999, these clinicians were skeptical about Coleman's finding arguing that they were already out of date and that, in the interim, many improvements to the service in North Staffordshire had been made. However, it seems that our more sophisticated analysis of the local cancer registry data over a longer period of time shows that survival in North Staffordshire remains poor and that this LHA is at, or is near, the bottom of the regional league table in terms of 5-year survival rates.

Our analyses take nine major covariates into account as well as allowing for the non-PH nature of some of the covariates. We have also allowed for the effect of unmeasured covariates by generalising the basic models to incorporate Gamma frailty extensions. Usually, these models provide a better fit to the data than the more basic models. Moreover, we have shown the value of extending the Gamma frailty models to incorporate structural dispersion. It seems that there are real gains to be made in the standard model selection criteria using this method. While this is an interesting technical improvement, it seems that the applied findings are unchanged.

There are several additional analyses which remain to be carried out, but at the time of writing, further studies aimed at improving survival in North Staffordshire need to be designed and undertaken.

Acknowledgements The work in this paper was supported by IRCSET, Ireland, and by the Science Foundation Ireland's (SFI, www.sfi.ie) project grant number 07/MI/012 (BIO-SI project, www3.ul.ie/bio-si).

References

Blagojevic, M., & MacKenzie, G. (2004). A comparison of ph and non-ph frailty models. In *Correlated data modelling* (pp. 239–249). Milano: Franco Angeli.

Blagojevic, M., MacKenzie, G., & Ha, I. (2003). A comparison of non-ph and ph gamma frailty models. In *Proceedings of the 18th International Workshop on Statistical Modelling* (pp. 39–44). Statistical, Modelling Society, Leuven.

Coleman, M. (1998). Cancer survival in the health authorities of England up to 1998. A report prepared for the national health services executive.

Goldstein, H., & Spiegelhalter, D. (1996). League tables and their limitations. *Journal of the Royal Statistical Society, 59*, 385–343.

Ha, I., Lee, Y., & MacKenzie, G. (2007). Model selection for multi-component frailty models. *Statistics in Medicine, 26*(26), 4790–4807.

Hougaard, P. (2000). *Analysis of multivariate survival data*. New York: Springer.

Lee, Y., & Nelder, J. A. (2001). Hierarchical generalised linear models: A synthesis of generalised linear models, random-effect models and structured dispersions. *Biometrika, 88*, 987–1006.

MacKenzie, G. (1996). Regression models for survival data: The generalised time dependent logistic family. *Journal of the Royal Statistical Society, 45*, 21–34.

MacKenzie, G., & Pan, J. (2007). Optimal covariance modelling. In *Correlated data modelling*. Milano: Franco Angeli.

Random Effects Ordinal Time Models for Grouped Toxicological Data from a Biological Control Assay

Marie-José Martinez and John P. Hinde

Abstract Discrete survival times can be viewed as ordered multicategorical data. Here a continuation-ratio model is considered, which is particularly appropriate when the ordered categories represent a progression through different stages, such as survival through various times. This particular model has the advantage of being a simple decomposition of a multinomial distribution into a succession of hierarchical binomial models. In a clustered data context, random effects are incorporated into the linear predictor of the model to account for uncontrolled experimental variation. Assuming a normal distribution for the random effects, an EM algorithm with adaptive Gaussian quadrature is used to estimate the model parameters. This approach is applied to the analysis of grouped toxicological data obtained from a biological control assay. In this assay, different isolates of the fungus *Beauveria bassiana* were used as a microbial control for the *Heterotermes tenuis* termite, which causes considerable damage to sugarcane fields in Brazil. The aim is to study the pathogenicity and the virulence of the fungus in order to determine effective isolates for the control of this pest population.

Keywords Adaptive quadrature • Clustered data • Multicategorical data • Ordinal regression • Random effects

1 Introduction

Discrete survival times can be viewed as ordered multicategorical data. In the ordinal data modelling context, a variety of multinomial regression models can be used, including the baseline-category logit model, the cumulative logit model, the

John P. Hinde (✉)
School of Mathematics, Statistics and Applied Mathematics, National University of Ireland, Galway, University Road, Galway, Ireland
e-mail: john.hinde@nuigalway.ie

G. MacKenzie and D. Peng (eds.), *Statistical Modelling in Biostatistics and Bioinformatics*, Contributions to Statistics, DOI 10.1007/978-3-319-04579-5_5,
© Springer International Publishing Switzerland 2014

adjacent-category logit model or the continuation-ratio logit model. This last model has been given some attention in the literature (Agresti 2002). Such a model form is useful when the ordered categories represent a progression through different stages, such as survival through various times. This particular model has the advantage of being a simple decomposition of a multinomial distribution into a succession of hierarchical binomial models. The property of conditional independence enables us to fit it by adapting the methods available for binary response data (Agresti 2002).

When one has ordered replicated data, random effects can be incorporated into the linear predictor to account for uncontrolled experimental variation (this may be apparent through overdispersion of multinomial responses across the replicates). An increasing number of papers are concerned with random effects models for ordered categorical responses. For example, Stram et al. (1988) fit a cumulative model separately for each time in a repeated measures context. In a psychological study, Ten Have and Uttal (1994) present subject-specific and population-averaged continuation ratio logit models for multivariate discrete time survival data. In their paper, they consider a modified Gibbs sampling algorithm to estimate the parameters of the subject-specific model. Tutz and Hennevogl (1996) consider the general case of an ordinal cumulative model including random effects and develop three alternative estimation procedures based on the EM-algorithm.

Here, we focus on random effects continuation-ratio models. We consider a continuation-ratio model and include a random intercept into the linear predictor in order to analyse grouped toxicological data with overdispersion. More specifically, the data considered here have been obtained from a biological control assay carried out by the Insect Pathology Laboratory of ESALQ-USP, Sao Paulo, Brazil (De Freitas 2001). In this assay, different isolates of the fungus *Beauveria bassiana* are used as a microbial control for the *Heterotermes tenuis* termite which causes much damage to sugarcane fields in Brazil. In this context, experiments have been carried out to study the pathogenicity and the virulence of the fungus in order to determine effective isolates for the control of this pest population. The full data set compares 142 separate isolates of the fungus. A solution of each isolate was applied to groups of 30 termites, with five independent replicates for each isolate, and the cumulative mortality in each group is measured daily during an eight-day period after the application of the fungus. Figure 1 displays the cumulative proportions of dead termites for 30 different isolates showing the five replicates. It clearly shows different isolate efficacies and different degrees of variability among the replicates within the different isolates. The aim of this study is to determine effective isolates for use in the field taking into account the replicated data structure.

To fit the proposed random effects models, we consider here different approaches to maximum likelihood estimation. As in the general case of generalized linear mixed models, the likelihood of the observed data is obtained by integrating out the random effects. Unfortunately, this marginal likelihood does not generally have a closed form expression and some form of approximation is needed for parameter estimation. Classical methods commonly used include penalized quasi-likelihood (PQL) or Gaussian quadrature (GQ) methods. The first method is based on a decomposition of the data into the mean and an appropriate error term using a linear

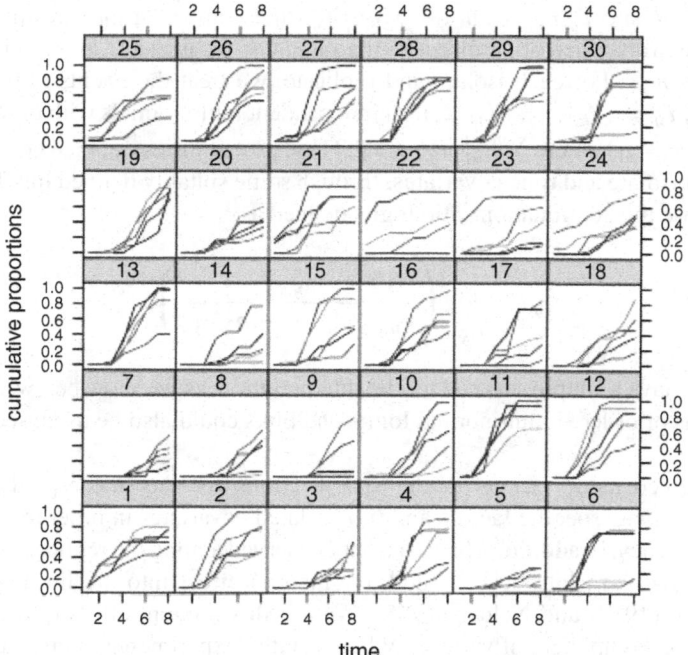

Fig. 1 Cumulative proportions of dead termites for 30 isolates with five replicates of each

Taylor expansion of the mean around current estimates of the fixed and random effects. We refer to Breslow and Clayton (1993) for more details. The second method is a standard approach that evaluates the likelihood numerically using Gauss-Hermite quadrature. An improvement on Gaussian quadrature is adaptive Gaussian quadrature (AGQ), which essentially consists of shifting and scaling the quadrature locations to adapt them to the integrand. Assuming normal distributions for the random effects, we propose here to use AGQ methods combined with an EM-algorithm to estimate the model parameters.

The paper is organized as follows. The random effects continuation-ratio models proposed to fit the grouped toxicological data set are developed in Sect. 2. The procedure considered to estimate the model parameters is given in Sect. 3. The results of fitting the different proposed mixed models are presented in Sect. 4, while Sect. 5 discusses the advantages and the limits of this methodology.

2 Model Specification

Suppose the cumulative mortality is measured over d consecutive days. For the jth replicate of isolate i, $j = 1, \ldots, r$ and $i = 1, \ldots, n$, we denote the initial number of insects by m_{ij}. Let $Y_{ij,k}$ denote the number of dead insects on day k,

$k = 1, \ldots, d$ and $Y_{ij,d+1} = m_{ij} - \sum_{k=1}^{d} Y_{ij,k}$ the number of insects still alive on day d. The probability of an insect dying on day k for isolate i and replicate j is denoted by $\pi_{ij,k}$. For each isolate and replicate, we treat the counts in the $d + 1$ categories, $Y_{ij} = (Y_{ij,1}, \ldots, Y_{ij,d+1})$, as independent multinomials with probabilities $(\pi_{ij,1}, \ldots, \pi_{ij,d+1})$ where $\sum_{k=1}^{d+1} \pi_{ij,k} = 1$. These probabilities can then be modelled, in terms of isolate and time covariates, through some suitably defined link function. Here, we use the continuation-ratio logits defined as

$$\eta_{ij,k} = \log \left(\frac{\pi_{ij,k}}{\pi_{ij,k+1} + \cdots + \pi_{ij,d+1}} \right),$$

since these have a simple survival model interpretation, as we show below. Note that other forms of ordered multinomial logits and links could also be used, see Agresti (2002).

We now consider various model specifications for the linear predictor $\eta_{ij,k}$ containing isolate specific factors and time-related covariates in order to model the time dependency. In addition, the variability observed among the replicates for some isolates leads us to introduce an additive random effect into the linear predictor as in Hinde (1982) and Nelder (1985). We use this random effect to account for an additional component of variability between the experimental units, namely the replicates for each isolate.

We first consider a model with a common arbitrary day effect, giving a baseline cumulative mortality pattern, an isolate effect and a random effect with a linear predictor defined by

Model I: $\eta_{ij,k} = \alpha_i + \beta_k + \sigma \, \xi_{ij}, i = 1, \ldots, n, \; j = 1, \ldots, r, \; k = 1, \ldots, d.$

Here α_i is the effect of isolate i, β_k the time effect of day k, σ is the random effect scale parameter, $\xi_{ij} \sim \mathcal{N}(0, 1)$ and the ξ_{ij}'s are assumed independent. Note that we could also have formulated the random effect term as $u_{ij} \sim \mathcal{N}(0, \sigma^2)$ as in Brillinger and Preisler (1983), however, the above formulation has the advantage of passing the random effect parameter into the linear predictor and having a completely specified (parameter-free) distribution for the unobserved variable ξ_{ij}. The two formulations in fact lead to different EM algorithms with different convergence rates, see Hinde (1997), although the basic computational approaches are the same.

Next we consider a second model in which we add an isolate specific time trend to the previous linear predictor leading to

Model II: $\eta_{ij,k} = \alpha_i + \beta_k + \gamma_i \, t_k + \sigma \, \xi_{ij},$

where $t_k = k$ is a quantitative variable giving a linear trend over days, and γ_i is the linear time effect for isolate i allowing variation from the common baseline cumulative mortality pattern.

The third model considered is a simplification that attempts to model the time dependency purely in terms of an isolate specific linear time trend and excludes the arbitrary common baseline pattern.

$$\text{Model III:} \qquad \eta_{ij,k} = \alpha_i + \gamma_i\, t_k + \sigma\, \xi_{ij}.$$

Finally, two additional models will be considered using quadratic rather than linear isolate specific time trends. This is an attempt to capture the overall variation in the response patterns over time.

$$\text{Model IV:} \qquad \eta_{ij,k} = \alpha_i + \beta_k + \gamma_i\, t_k + \delta_i\, t_k^2 + \sigma\, \xi_{ij},$$

$$\text{Model V:} \qquad \eta_{ij,k} = \alpha_i + \gamma_i\, t_k + \delta_i\, t_k^2 + \sigma\, \xi_{ij}.$$

Note that all coefficients α_i, β_k, γ_i and δ_i, $i = 1, \ldots, n$ and $k = 1, \ldots, d$, in the five models are assumed to be constant over replicates.

These five models are all random intercept models in which the introduction of an additive random effect allows a random location shift in the linear predictor for each replicate of each isolate in an attempt to capture the appreciable within isolate replicate variability. In this work, we consider a logit link leading to random effects continuation-ratio logit models. Other link functions can also be used and another common choice is the complementary log–log link yielding the so-called proportional hazards model.

An advantage of the continuation ratio model is that it can be viewed as a sequence of binomial models by considering the conditional probability, $w_{ij,k}$, that an insect dies on day k given that it has survived up to this day, for isolate i and replicate j. This conditional probability is defined by

$$w_{ij,k} = \frac{\pi_{ij,k}}{\sum_{k'=k}^{d+1} \pi_{ij,k'}}.$$

Let $b(m; y; w)$ denote the binomial probability of obtaining y successes out of m trials with probability w for each trial. The multinomial probability for $(y_{ij,1}, \ldots, y_{ij,d+1})$ can be expressed in the form

$$b(m_{ij}; y_{ij,1}; w_{ij,1}) \times b(m_{ij} - y_{ij,1}; y_{ij,2}; w_{ij,2}) \times \cdots \times b(m_{ij} - y_{ij,1} - \ldots - y_{ij,d-1}; y_{ij,d}; w_{ij,d}).$$

Thus, the multinomial model can be expressed as a succession of hierarchical binomial models, see McCullagh and Nelder (1989). The continuation-ratio logits are then defined as

$$\eta_{ij,k} = \log\left(\frac{\pi_{ij,k}}{\pi_{ij,k+1} + \cdots + \pi_{ij,d+1}}\right) = \log\left(\frac{w_{ij,k}}{1 - w_{ij,k}}\right) = \mathrm{logit}(w_{ij,k}),$$

Table 1 Rearrangement of the data for the jth replicate of the ith isolate

Day	No. at risk	No. of deaths	Prob(death)
1	m_{ij}	$y_{ij,1}$	$\pi_{ij,1}$
2	$m_{ij} - y_{ij,1}$	$y_{ij,2}$	$w_{ij,2} = \frac{\pi_{ij,2}}{1-\pi_{ij,1}}$
3	$m_{ij} - y_{ij,1} - y_{ij,2}$	$y_{ij,3}$	$w_{ij,3} = \frac{\pi_{ij,3}}{1-\pi_{ij,1}-\pi_{ij,2}}$
$\vdots$			
d	$m_{ij} - y_{ij,1} - \cdots - y_{ij,d-1}$	$y_{ij,d}$	$w_{ij,d} = \frac{\pi_{ij,d}}{1-\sum_{k'=1}^{d-1}\pi_{ij,k'}}$

and are ordinary logits of the conditional probabilities $w_{ij,k}$. Clearly, a main advantage of the continuation-ratio model is that it can be fitted using methods for binomial logit models merely by a rearrangement of the data. Thus, to fit the different logit models, we require a derived data structure as presented in Table 1, a binomial model specification and appropriately defined linear predictors.

3 Parameter Estimation

In this section, parameter estimation for the random effects continuation-ratio models defined previously is considered based on the EM algorithm. This algorithm is a powerful computational technique for maximizing likelihoods including unobserved variables. However, as with the binary model, the non-conjugate normal distribution for ξ means that the marginal likelihood cannot be obtained analytically. Indeed, assuming that $\varphi(.)$ denotes the standard normal density function, the likelihood of the kth replicate of the ith isolate is given by

$$L_{ij}(\theta, \sigma) = \int_{-\infty}^{+\infty} \prod_{k=1}^{d} f(y_{ij,k}|\theta, \sigma, \xi_{ij})\, \varphi(\xi_{ij}; 0, 1)\, d\xi_{ij}$$

$$= \int_{-\infty}^{+\infty} \prod_{k=1}^{d} w_{ij,k}^{y_{ij,k}}\, (1 - w_{ij,k})^{m_{ij}-\sum_{k'=1}^{k-1} y_{ij,k'}}\, \varphi(\xi_{ij}; 0, 1)\, d\xi_{ij}$$

$$= \int_{-\infty}^{+\infty} \prod_{k=1}^{d} \left[\frac{\exp(\eta_{ij,k})}{1 + \exp(\eta_{ij,k})}\right]^{y_{ij,k}}$$

$$\times \left[\frac{1}{1 + \exp(\eta_{ij,k})}\right]^{m_{ij}-\sum_{k'=1}^{k-1} y_{ij,k'}} \varphi(\xi_{ij}; 0, 1)\, d\xi_{ij}.$$

Clearly, this likelihood function has no closed form and has to be evaluated numerically before being maximized as a function of the fixed effect parameters θ and the random effect parameter σ. Note that, for model IV for instance, θ is the vector of $(\alpha_i, \beta_k, \gamma_i, \delta_i)$ for all i and k. In this section, we consider two integration methods for approximating the likelihood which will be then combined with an EM algorithm for the maximization step.

First, we consider classical Gaussian quadrature to evaluate numerically this likelihood integral. Gauss-Hermite quadrature methods have already been used in the important case of ordered categorical data. For instance, they have been considered by Jansen (1990) for the case of shifted thresholds and by Hinde (1982) or Anderson and Hinde (1988) for the binary case. The dimension of the integral determining the likelihood function depends on the random effect structure. When the random effects are assumed normally distributed and the dimension is small, as in the integral defined above, Gaussian-Hermite quadrature methods can approximate the likelihood function. In fact, Gauss-Hermite quadrature approximates the integral of a function $f(.)$ multiplied by another function having the shape of a normal density by a finite weighted sum of the function evaluated at a set of points called the quadrature points. Thus, the likelihood is approximated by

$$L_{ij}(\theta, \sigma) \approx \sum_{q=1}^{Q} v_q \left\{ \prod_{k=1}^{d} f(y_{ij,k}|\theta, \sigma, z_q) \right\},$$

with weights v_q and quadrature points z_q that are tabulated. Note that the approximation improves as the number Q of quadrature points increases. However, in practice, a large number of quadrature points is often required to approximate correctly the likelihood. Moreover, the approximation can be poor for large random effect variances or can fail for small cluster sizes. We refer to Crouch and Spiegelman (1990); Lesaffre and Spiessens (2001) or Albert and Follmann (2000), who point out some of these problems.

To solve these problems associated with ordinary quadrature, we then consider AGQ methods. An adaptive version of the Gauss-Hermite quadrature shifts and scales the quadrature points to place them under the peak of integrand. Note that after normalization with respect to ξ_{ij}, the integrand is the posterior density of ξ_{ij} given the response and can be approximated for large sample sizes by a normal density $\varphi(\xi_{ij}; \mu_{ij}, \tau_{ij}^2)$ with mean μ_{ij} and variance τ_{ij}^2. In this version, the normal density $\varphi(\xi_{ij}; \mu_{ij}, \tau_{ij}^2)$ approximating the posterior density is treated as the weight function. The integral is now written as

$$L_{ij}(\theta, \sigma) = \int_{-\infty}^{+\infty} \varphi(\xi_{ij}; \mu_{ij}, \tau_{ij}^2) \frac{\prod_{k=1}^{d} f(y_{ij,k}|\theta, \sigma, \xi_{ij}) \, \varphi(\xi_{ij}; 0, 1)}{\varphi(\xi_{ij}; \mu_{ij}, \tau_{ij}^2)} \, d\xi_{ij},$$

and applying the standard quadrature rules, the integral is now approximated by

$$L_{ij}(\theta, \sigma) \approx \sum_{q=1}^{Q} v_{ij,q} \left\{ \prod_{k=1}^{d} f(y_{ij,k}|\theta, \sigma, z_{ij,q}) \right\}.$$

Hence, the adaptive quadrature points are given by $z_{ij,q} = \tau_{ij} z_q + \mu_{ij}$ with corresponding weights $v_{ij,q} = \sqrt{2\pi} \tau_{ij} \exp(\frac{z_q^2}{2}) \varphi(z_{ij,q}) v_q$.

Essentially, the posterior density is here approximated by a normal density with the same mean and variance. However, the posterior mean and variance required in this approach are not known and have to be computed. As in Rabe-Hesketh et al. (2005), we obtain these posterior moments using adaptive quadrature leading to an iterative integration. This approach is similar to the method described in Naylor and Smith (1988) in a different context. Note that an alternative way to approximate the posterior moments μ_{ij} and τ_{ij}^2 is proposed by Liu and Pierce (1994) by using the mode and the curvature at the mode. More precisely, this approach centers the quadrature points with respect to the mode of the integrand and scales them according to the estimated curvature at the mode.

In this work, quadrature methods are thus used to evaluate numerically the integral in calculating the marginal likelihood. In general, the higher the order Q, the better the approximation is. Typically, AGQ needs less quadrature points than classical quadrature. On the other hand, AGQ is more time consuming since the quadrature points and weights used in this approach depend on the unknown parameters and hence will need to be updated in each step of the iterative estimation procedure. The differences between ordinary and adaptive quadrature are discussed in particular in Lesaffre and Spiessens (2001) or Rabe-Hesketh et al. (2002).

Finally, once the marginal likelihood is evaluated numerically for given parameter values, it has to be maximized with respect to θ and σ. Several methods for maximizing the likelihood can be considered and combined with the two integration methods presented above. Rabe-Hesketh et al. (2005) use, for instance, a Newton–Raphson algorithm where the Hessian matrix is obtained by numerical differentiation. In this work, we consider an EM-algorithm which is easy to implement compared to other optimization methods (Anderson and Hinde 1988).

4 Results

We now consider the analysis of the data of interest presented previously. The results of fitting the models described in Sect. 2 are presented here. For simplicity, we only consider a subset of 30 isolates. Obviously, results for all 142 isolates can be obtained in the same way. Table 2 shows disparity and σ values for models I, II, III, IV, and V using ordinary Gaussian quadrature with 3, 5, 10, 20, 40, and 60 quadrature points and AGQ using 3, 5, and 10 quadrature points. For each of these models, we also fit the associated fixed model obtained by dropping the random effect ξ_i.

As expected, the different results show that those obtained by AGQ are the same from using 10 quadrature points and more. For as few as 3 quadrature points, only very small differences can be observed. On the other hand, the results, in particular the variance estimates, change considerably using ordinary Gaussian quadrature.

Table 2 Disparity and σ values for models I, II, III, IV and V using ordinary and adaptive quadrature methods

		GQ(3)	GQ(5)	GQ(10)	GQ(20)	GQ(40)	GQ(60)
Model I	$-2\log L$	4,937.8	4,899.9	4,924.4	4,933.6	4,940.0	4,940.2
	σ	0.972	0.976	1.084	0.971	0.839	0.836
Model II	$-2\log L$	4,269.2	4,269.7	4,274.7	4,287.8	4,294.8	4,294.9
	σ	0.931	1.014	1.143	1.027	0.852	0.850
Model III	$-2\log L$	5,202.6	5,197.8	5,189.2	5,195.0	5,204.8	5,205.0
	σ	0.930	1.012	1.066	1.077	0.908	0.893
Model IV	$-2\log L$	3,991.88	3,988.96	3,988.70	4,006.33	4,011.36	4,011.44
	σ	0.910	0.984	1.162	0.990	0.840	0.837
Model V	$-2\log L$	4,069.82	4,065.57	4,068.77	4,082.00	4,087.36	4,087.44
	σ	0.913	0.989	1.112	1.007	0.844	0.841
		AGQ(3)	AGQ(5)	AGQ(10)		Fixed model	
Model I	$-2\log L$	4,941.0	4,940.2	4,940.2		5,651.8	
	σ	0.831	0.836	0.836		–	
Model II	$-2\log L$	4,295.7	4,294.9	4,294.9		5,014.5	
	σ	0.846	0.850	0.850		–	
Model III	$-2\log L$	5,206.0	5,205.1	5,205.1		6,029.7	
	σ	0.887	0.893	0.893		–	
Model IV	$-2\log L$	4,012.2	4,011.4	4,011.4		4,697.5	
	σ	0.833	0.837	0.837		–	
Model V	$-2\log L$	4,088.2	4,087.4	4,087.4		4,783.1	
	σ	0.837	0.841	0.841		–	

Clearly, we need to increase the number of quadrature points to 40 for ordinary quadrature in order to get similar results. Therefore, it is clear that we may be able to achieve good accuracy with a smaller number of quadrature points using AGQ instead of ordinary Gaussian quadrature for the different models I, II, III, IV or V.

Table 3 displays deviance, AIC and BIC values for models I, II, III, IV and V using AGQ with 10 quadrature points. Deviance, AIC and BIC values for the associated simple GLMs are also displayed. These fixed effect models led to an AIC value of 5,725.8, 5,146.5, 6,149.7, 4,887.5 and 4,963.1 for models I, II, III, IV and V, respectively. Introducing a random effect into the linear predictors of these models improved these results, yielding, respectively, AIC values of 5,016.2, 4,430.9, 5,327.1, 4,207.4 and 4,269.4. Thus, the large variability in the data has been captured by these random effects models.

As noted previously, fitting random effects models yields the AIC value 5,016.2 for Model I, 4,430.9 for Model II, and 5,327.1 for Model III. Model III which imposes more structure on the linear predictor and implies a more specific form of the response over time appears not convincing in this particular case. Clearly, this linear trend model does not seem to capture all of the structure in the data. Adding the time factor effect β_j into the linear predictor makes the structure over time more flexible reproducing an overall common baseline response pattern and allowing

Table 3 Deviance, AIC and BIC values for Models I, II, III, IV, V and their associated fixed models

	Model I	Model II	Model III	Model IV	Model V
Deviance	3,329.9	2,684.6	3,594.8	2,401.2	2,477.2
AIC	5,016.2	4,430.9	5,327.1	4,207.4	4,269.4
BIC	5,209.6	4,777.0	5,637.6	4,706.3	4,732.6
	Fixed I	Fixed II	Fixed III	Fixed IV	Fixed V
Deviance	4,041.6	3,404.2	4,419.4	3,087.2	3,172.8
AIC	5,725.8	5,146.5	6,149.7	4,887.5	4,963.1
BIC	5,914.2	5,482.4	6,455.1	5,371.1	5,421.2

isolate-specific effects to capture departures from this in terms of the location and steepness of the response. In comparison with Model I, the AIC value of Model II which is defined by adding a time trend into the linear predictor decreases by 585.3 on 30 df.

Concerning Model IV and Model V, it seems that adding a quadratic term in time allows us to get near to reproducing the general overall pattern over all isolates and all replicates. The AIC value is 4,207.4 for Model IV and 4,269.4 for Model V. Thus, Model IV with the smallest AIC value seems to be the model among the five continuation-ratio random effects logit models considered in this paper that best fits the data. From now, all results presented are obtained from Model IV.

For each isolate, Fig. 2 shows the fitted replicate-specific evolutions and the marginal average evolution implied by Model IV. The posterior quantities of interest are the random effects and the corresponding model random linear predictors. As noted by Aitkin (1996), one nice feature of using numerical integration via the EM-algorithm is that we can easily calculate these quantities from the estimated posterior distribution of the random effects. For example, using ordinary Gaussian quadrature methods, the posterior distribution of ξ_{ij} is provided by

$$f(z_q|y_{ij}) = \frac{v_q \prod_{k=1}^{d} f(y_{ij,k}|\theta, \sigma, z_q)}{\sum_{l=1}^{Q} v_l \prod_{k=1}^{d} f(y_{ij,k}|\theta, \sigma, z_l)} = p_{ij,q}, \qquad q = 1, \dots, Q.$$

These posterior probabilities p_{ijq} that the unobserved ξ_{ij} takes the value z_q correspond to the weights at the final iteration of the EM-algorithm, and they provide the posterior distribution of the ξ_{ij} in the empirical Bayes sense by replacing the unknown parameters by their ML estimates. In Model IV, for instance, the linear predictors are defined as

$$\log\left(\frac{w_{ij,k}}{1 - w_{ij,k}}\right) = \eta_{ij,k} = \alpha_i + \beta_k + \gamma_i t_k + \delta_i t_k^2 + \sigma \xi_{ij},$$

and the corresponding means as $w_{ij,k} = \dfrac{\exp(\eta_{ij,k})}{1 + \exp(\eta_{ij,k})}.$

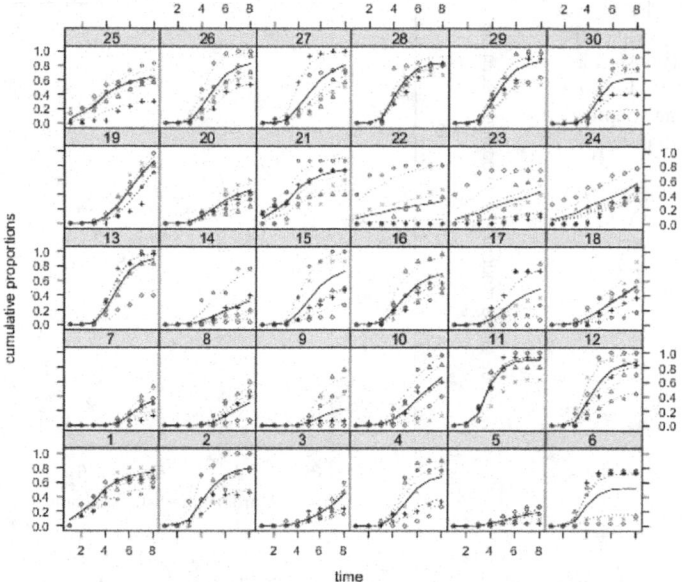

Fig. 2 Graphical representation of the predicted replicate-specific evolutions (*dotted lines*) and the marginal average evolution (*solid line*) obtained from Model IV using adaptive Gaussian quadrature

In this case, the empirical Bayes predictions are calculated by:

$$\hat{p}_{ij,q} = \frac{v_q \prod_{k=1}^{d} f(y_{ij,k}|\hat{\boldsymbol{\theta}}, \hat{\sigma}, z_q)}{\sum_{l=1}^{Q} v_l \prod_{k=1}^{d} f(y_{ij,k}|\hat{\boldsymbol{\theta}}, \hat{\sigma}, z_l)},$$

$$\hat{\xi}_{ij} = \sum_{q=1}^{Q} \hat{p}_{ij,q} z_q,$$

$$\hat{\eta}_{ij,k} = \sum_{q=1}^{Q} \hat{p}_{ij,q} \hat{\eta}_{ij,k,q} \quad \text{with} \quad \hat{\eta}_{ij,k,q} = \hat{\alpha}_i + \hat{\beta}_k + \hat{\gamma}_i t_k + \hat{\delta}_i t_k^2 + \hat{\sigma} z_q,$$

$$\hat{w}_{ij,k} = \frac{\exp(\hat{\eta}_{ij,k})}{1 + \exp(\hat{\eta}_{ij,k})}.$$

Note that a similar approach is used when using AGQ. Finally, the fitted probabilities of real interest $\hat{\pi}_{ij,k}$ are directly obtained from the empirical Bayes predictions $\hat{w}_{ij,k}$.

Concerning the marginal average evolution, note that it can be derived from averaging the conditional means over the random effects ξ_{ij}. Again, this can be done using numerical integration methods or based on numerical averaging by sampling a large number of random effects from their fitted distribution (Molenberghs and

Fig. 3 Marginal LT_{50}
against the variance of the
random effects posterior
estimates obtained from
Model IV using adaptive
Gaussian quadrature

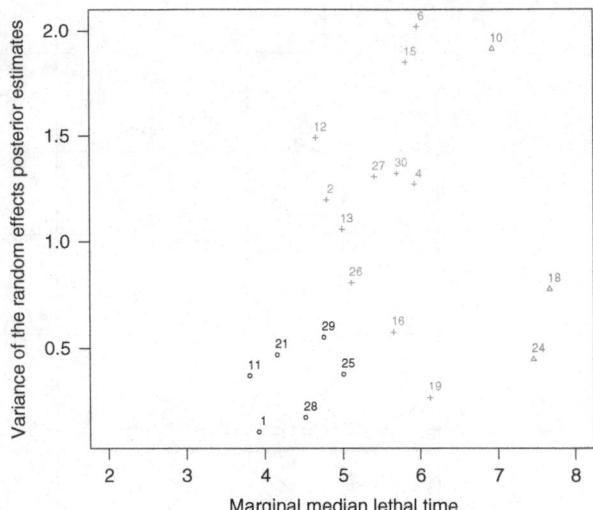

Verbeke 2005). In this work, we derive the marginal average evolution based on the second method by sampling 1,000 random effects ξ_{ij} from their fitted distribution. Note that the approach which consists of plotting the profile for an "average" replicate, i.e., a replicate with random intercept $\xi_{ij} = 0$ rather than the marginal average usually results in different fitted average trends (Molenberghs and Verbeke 2005).

Finally, one of the aims of this study is to determine the effective isolates. In this context, one quantity commonly used is the lethal time LT_p which is the time required to obtain $p\%$ mortality. This quantity can be easily used to summarize and to rank the different isolate effectiveness. For the 30 isolates, Fig. 3 shows the marginal median lethal time (LT_{50}) over the replicates obtained from Model IV using AGQ. More precisely, for each isolate, we plot the marginal LT_{50} when it is smaller than 8 against the variance of the posterior estimates of the random effect to account for variability among the replicates. Clearly, effective isolates are those with both low lethal time and low replicate variability. Using the K-means clustering method on the two-dimensional data matrix formed by the marginal median lethal times and the variances of the posterior estimates of the random effect, the different isolates are grouped here into three clusters: strongly, intermediate and weakly virulent. This provides some indication of which isolates to use in the field.

5   Discussion

In this paper, we have proposed to use random effects continuation-ratio models to model discrete survival times by considering them as ordered multicategorical data. We have seen that this particular model can be easily fitted using the methods available for binary response data by a rearrangement of the data. The use of this specific model also makes possible the generalization of these approaches to replicate measures. In this work, we have introduced a random intercept into the linear predictor to model the variability observed among the replicates within the different isolates. A possible extension of this work is to include both a random intercept and a random slope. By including a random coefficient into the linear predictor, we allow the time effect to vary between the replicates of each isolate. In this case, the random effects could be assumed to have a bivariate normal distribution with unknown covariance matrix.

In the different models considered in this work, the random effects are assumed to be sampled from a normal distribution. This assumption reflects the prior belief that the random effects are drawn from one homogeneous population. However, if we look in detail at the results obtained using ordinary Gaussian quadrature in Table 2, we can observe that the disparity does not decrease monotonically as we increase the number of quadrature points. In other words, bad approximations can give better fits. This behaviour, observed for instance in Lesaffre and Spiessens (2001), suggests that maybe the normality assumption is not really convincing in this case. To relax this assumption, it would be interesting in future work to use heterogeneity models as defined by Molenberghs and Verbeke (2005). This extension consists of replacing the normality assumption by a mixture of normal distributions. Thus, the model will reflect the prior belief of the presence of unobserved heterogeneity among the replicates. The use of this particular model would be an interesting extension since it relaxes the classical normality assumption and is also perfectly suitable for classification purposes.

Acknowledgements This work was part-funded under Science Foundation Ireland's Research Frontiers Programme (07/RFP-MATF448) and Science Foundation Ireland's BIO-SI project, grant number 07/MI/012.

References

Agresti, A. (2002). *Categorical data analysis* (2nd ed.). New York: Wiley.

Albert, P., & Follmann, D. (2000). Modeling repeated count data subject to informative dropout. *Biometrics, 56*, 667–677.

Anderson, D., & Hinde, J. (1988). Random effects in generalized linear models and the EM algorithm. *Communications in Statistics—Theory and Methods, 17*, 3847–3856.

Aitkin, M. (1996). Empirical Bayes shrinkage using posterior random effect means from non-parametric maximum likelihood estimation in general random effect models. In *Proceedings of the 11th International Workshop on Statistical Modelling* (pp. 87–94). Orvieto: Statistical Modelling Society.

Breslow, N., & Clayton, D. (1993). Approximate inference in generalized linear mixed model. *Journal of the American Statistical Association, 88*, 9–25.

Brillinger, D., & Preisler, M. (1983). Maximum likelihood estimation in a latent variable problem. In S. Karlin, T. Amemiya, & L. Goodman (Eds.), *Studies in econometrics, time series and multivariate statistics* (pp. 31–35). New York: Academic.

Crouch, E., & Spiegelman, D. (1990). The evaluation of integrals of the form $\int f(t)\exp(-t^2)dt$: Application to logistic-normal models. *Journal of the American Statistical Association, 85*, 464–469.

De Freitas, S. (2001). *Modelos para Proporções com Superdispersão proveniente de Ensaios Toxicológicos no Tempo* (Ph.D. thesis). ESALQ, Universidade de São Paulo.

Hinde, J. (1982). Compound Poisson regression models. In R. Gilchrist (Ed.), *GLIM 82*. New York: Springer.

Hinde, J. (1997). Contribution to discussion of The EM algorithm - An old folk-song to a fast new tune by Meng, X-L. and Van Dyk, D. *Journal of the Royal Statistical Society, Series B, 59*, 549–550.

Jansen, J. (1990). On the statistical analysis of ordinal data when extravariation is present. *Applied Statistics, 39*, 74–85.

Lesaffre, E., & Spiessens, B. (2001). On the effect of the number of quadrature points in a logistic random-effects model: An example. *Applied Statistics, 50*, 325–335.

Liu, Q., & Pierce, D. (1994). A note on Gauss-Hermite quadrature. *Biometrika, 81*, 624–629.

McCullagh, P., & Nelder, J. (1989). *Generalized linear models*. London: Chapman & Hall.

Molenberghs, G., & Verbeke, G. (2005). *Models for discrete longitudinal data*. New York: Springer.

Naylor, J., & Smith, A. (1988). Econometric illustrations of novel numerical integration strategies for Bayesian inference. *Journal of Econometrics, 38*, 103–125.

Nelder, J. (1985). Quasi-likelihood and GLIM. In R. Gilchrist, B. Francis, & J. Whittaker (Eds.), *Generalized linear models: Proceedings of the GLIM 85 conference*. New York: Springer.

Rabe-Hesketh, S., Skrondal, A., & Pickles, A. (2002). Reliable estimation of generalized linear mixed models using adaptive quadrature. *The Stata Journal, 2*, 1–21.

Rabe-Hesketh, S., Skrondal, A., & Pickles, A. (2005). Maximum likelihood estimation of limited and discrete dependent variable models with nested random effects. *Journal of Econometrics, 128*, 301–323.

Stram, D., Wei, L., & Ware, J. (1988). Analysis of repeated categorical outcomes with possibly missing observations and time-dependent covariates. *Journal of the American Statistical Association, 83*, 631–637.

Ten Have, T., & Uttal, D. (1994). Subject-specific and population-averaged continuation ratio logit models for multiple discrete time survival profiles. *Applied Statistics, 43*, 371–384.

Tutz, G., & Hennevogl, W. (1996). Random effects in ordinal regression models. *Computational Statistics and Data Analysis, 22*, 537–557.

Part II
Longitudinal Modelling and Time Series

Modelling Seasonality and Structural Breaks: Visitors to NZ and 9/11

John Haywood and John Randal

Abstract We demonstrate the poor performance, with seasonal data, of existing methods for endogenously dating multiple structural breaks. Motivated by iterative nonparametric techniques, we present a new approach for estimating parametric structural break models that perform well. We suggest that iterative estimation methods are a simple but important feature of this approach when modelling seasonal data. The methodology is illustrated by simulation and then used for an analysis of monthly short-term visitor arrival time series to New Zealand, to assess the effect of the 9/11 terrorist attacks. While some historical events had a marked structural effect on trends in those arrivals, we show that 9/11 did not.

Keywords Break dates • Endogenous dating of structural changes • Iterative fitting • Multiple breaks • Trend extraction

1 Introduction

The economic importance of tourism to New Zealand is high and has increased considerably in recent years. As Pearce (2001) noted in his review article, international visitor arrivals increased by 65 % over the period 1990–1999, and foreign exchange earnings increased by 120 % (in current terms). More recently, for the year ended March 2004 tourism expenditure was $17.2 billion (Statistics New Zealand 2005). In that year, the tourism industry made a value-added contribution to GDP of 9.4 %, while 5.9 % of the total employed workforce had work directly engaged in tourism. Further, tourism's 18.5 % contribution to exports was greater than that of all other

J. Haywood (✉)
School of Mathematics, Statistics and Operations Research, Victoria University of Wellington,
PO Box 600, Wellington, New Zealand
e-mail: john.haywood@vuw.ac.nz

G. MacKenzie and D. Peng (eds.), *Statistical Modelling in Biostatistics and Bioinformatics*, Contributions to Statistics, DOI 10.1007/978-3-319-04579-5__6,
© Springer International Publishing Switzerland 2014

industries including dairy products, which in turn was greater than the contributions from meat and meat products, wood and wood products, and seafood.

The time series of monthly short-term visitor arrivals to New Zealand is one direct and easily recorded measurement of the international tourist contribution to the New Zealand economy. A useful precursor to development of tourism policy or business strategy is an understanding of the dynamic behaviour of these seasonal data. A classical time series decomposition includes unobserved components representing an evolving trend, a seasonal encapsulating regular deviation from the trend on a within-year basis, and an irregular, which is the residual or unexplained variation in the data. There are various ways to estimate these components, using both parametric and nonparametric approaches; see for example Harvey (1989), Hamilton (1994), Findley et al. (1998), Franses (1998) and Makridakis et al. (1998). Such a decomposition then allows an interpretation of the dynamic behaviour of visitor arrivals in terms of the estimated components.

There seems little doubt that the terrorist attacks of 11 September 2001 have had a pronounced influence on world events since that time. For example, see US Department of State (2004), for a summary of 100 editorial opinions from media in 57 countries around the world, commenting on the 3 years following September 2001. Those terrorist events and their subsequent effects have been used to explain apparent movements in many time series, and in this paper we concentrate on a particular example: the number of short-term visitor arrivals to New Zealand.

Our focus is to detect any longer term, or structural, changes in trend or seasonal components of the arrivals as a result of the 9/11 events. We also wish to compare the magnitude of any 9/11 effects with those due to other causes. Consequently we do not wish to specify the dates of any structural changes, but rather estimate the number and position of these endogenously. To achieve this we use Bai and Perron's (1998, 2003) procedures for estimating multiple structural changes in a linear model. Their approach permits periods of stable dynamic behaviour between relatively infrequent but significant changes to the parameters of the model. However, there is clearly no empirical requirement that changes in the trend and seasonal components occur simultaneously. As we demonstrate, for the visitor arrivals data changes typically occur more frequently in the trend. In contrast, direct application of Bai and Perron's (1998, 2003) methodology fits components simultaneously and yields a relatively poor decomposition, as we show via a simulation study and analysis of the visitor arrivals. We propose a new iterative fitting procedure for seasonal data, based on Bai and Perron (1998, 2003) and using existing R packages (R Development Core Team 2007), which gives much improved performance in terms of flexibility of fitted trends (via more appropriate placement of breaks) and lack of residual serial correlation.

Throughout the paper the term "trend" (or trend component) is used to describe the evolving, underlying behaviour of a time series. That underlying behaviour reflects both long-term movements and medium-term cyclical fluctuations, where long term and medium term are in relation to the (shorter) period of the evolving seasonal component that we also consider explicitly. This notion of trend agrees with that used by many national statistical offices; e.g., see Australian Bureau of

Statistics (2003, Sect. 2.1). Certainly we agree with Busetti and Harvey (2008), that the strong but common assumption in the econometrics literature of a constant underlying slope when testing for a trend is often implausible. Since our focus is on breaks in the structure of the trend and seasonal components, we choose to model those components as piecewise linear, with endogenously estimated changes in the trend slope and/or seasonal pattern corresponding to identified structural changes.

We find there is actually little to suggest that the September 11 incidents had much effect on New Zealand visitor arrivals, when viewed in the context of "normal" historically observed movements. In contrast, we identify some other historical events which do appear to have affected visitor arrivals to New Zealand quite markedly. We make no attempt to forecast the arrivals data using structural break models; we suggest other approaches, such as ARIMA modelling (Box and Jenkins 1976), would be more suitable if prediction was the aim. In fact Haywood and Randal (2004) used that approach to demonstrate that the 9/11 events did not significantly affect New Zealand visitor arrivals, by showing that the observations post-9/11 were contained within out of sample prediction intervals computed using a seasonal ARIMA ("airline") model, fitted to arrivals data up to 9/11. In this paper though, the focus is explicitly on identifying structural changes if they exist in the arrivals data, in trend and/or seasonal components.

In Sect. 2 we present an exploratory data analysis (EDA) of New Zealand visitor arrivals and a discussion of some apparent sources of variability in the data. Section 3 motivates and presents the iterative estimation of a parametric model that allows separate structural changes in the trend and seasonal components. Simulated data is used to illustrate the good performance of the new methodology. In Sect. 4 we use our iterative approach to model the arrivals data and in Sect. 5 we give some concluding comments.

2 EDA of Short-Term Visitor Arrivals to New Zealand

We consider 25 complete years of monthly short-term visitor arrival series from January 1980 to December 2004. The arrivals are from the seven most important countries of origin, ranked by current proportion of the total: Australia, UK, USA, Japan, Korea, China, Germany, as well as a residual series from "Other" origins. We analyse these series individually along with their aggregate, denoted "Total" (Fig. 1).

As seen in Fig. 1 a "U"-shaped seasonal pattern is common, with visitor numbers reaching a local maximum in the summer months December to February, and a local minimum in the winter months June and July. Further, it is apparent that the amplitude of the seasonal variation tends to increase with the level of the series, indicating a multiplicative relationship between trend and seasonal components. Australian and UK arrivals appear to be growing at a relatively steady rate. In contrast, a large downturn in arrivals from the USA is evident in the late 1980s, a period which immediately followed the stock market crash of October 1987. The

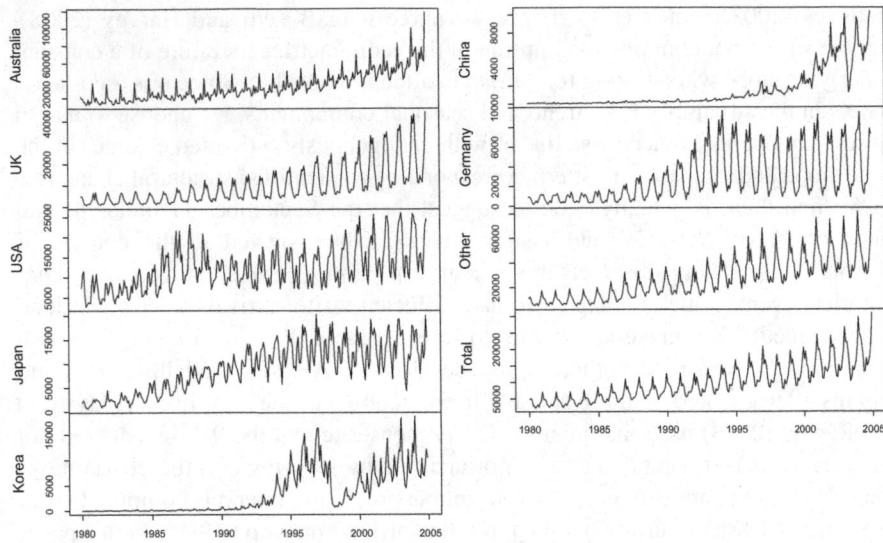

Fig. 1 Monthly short-term visitor arrivals to New Zealand, by origin, from January 1980 to December 2004. The vertical scales are not equal

trend in Japanese arrivals levels off over the last 15 years. The effect of the Asian financial crisis of 1997 is evident especially in the Korean data, with visitor numbers dramatically reduced just after this event. Arrivals from China contain perhaps the most visible short-term effect in these series, which is due to the SARS epidemic that virtually eliminated international travel by Chinese nationals during May and June 2003. German arrivals show a clear change from exponential growth prior to the early 1990s to a more stable pattern in recent times. The Other arrivals show a SARS effect much less prominent than that seen in the Chinese arrivals, as do some further series including Total arrivals. One of the more obvious shifts in the aggregate Total series appears to be linked to the Korean downturn, which can be attributed to the Asian financial crisis.

The Asian financial crisis of 1997–1998 markedly affected stock markets and exchange rates in several Asian countries and regions, including: Hong Kong, Indonesia, Japan, Korea, Malaysia, Philippines, Singapore, Taiwan and Thailand. See Kaminsky and Schmukler (1999) for a chronology of the crisis in those locations, from the official onset marked by the devaluation of the Thai baht on 2 July, 1997 up to the resignation of Indonesian President Suharto in May 1998. Kaminsky and Schmukler (1999) suggest the presence of important contagion effects in those markets, based on an analysis of identified market jitters. More recent analysis by Dungey et al. (2004) suggests, however, that increased exchange rate volatility observed in Australia and New Zealand around that time was not due to contagion from Asian countries, or unanticipated factors, but rather to common (anticipated) world factors such as trade linkages. This is one context in which

Table 1 Summary statistics for the monthly proportion of visitors to New Zealand, by origin

	Min	LQ	Median	UQ	Max	80–04	80–84	00–04
Australia	21.8	30.0	35.9	41.6	58.8	33.8	44.9	33.3
UK	3.4	6.3	8.0	10.6	18.3	9.8	7.6	11.8
USA	6.3	10.3	13.0	16.3	29.4	12.4	16.7	10.0
Japan	2.8	7.1	9.1	11.0	17.8	9.2	5.9	7.8
Korea	0.0	0.2	1.0	4.3	10.5	3.4	0.2	4.8
China	0.0	0.2	0.4	1.2	4.7	1.4	0.1	3.1
Germany	0.8	1.5	2.2	3.4	7.5	2.9	1.8	2.6
Other	17.9	23.4	26.1	28.6	34.3	27.0	22.8	26.7

The final three columns give proportions of the Total for the entire 25 year sample period, and the 5-year periods 1980–1984 and 2000–2004, respectively

changes in short-term visitor arrivals to New Zealand from Asian countries around 1997–1998 can be viewed, since tourism has become such an important sector of the New Zealand economy, as noted above. In particular, Korea is one of the five source countries with the largest recent (2000–2004) proportion of visitors to New Zealand (Table 1).

Table 1 shows that Australia is by far the biggest single source of visitors to New Zealand, accounting for almost exactly one-third of visitors in the 2000–2004 5-year period and slightly more over the entire data period. The maximum proportion in a month from Australia was 58.8 % in June 1985, and the minimum was 21.8 % in February 1997. An Australian influence is notable in the Total arrivals, because as the nearest neighbour to a geographically isolated country, arrivals from Australia exhibit variation not seen in the remaining data. As seen in Fig. 1, the Australian data has a regular seasonal pattern which is quite different from that of any other country. A closer examination indicates three peaks per year before 1987 and four thereafter; we discuss this further in Sect. 4.

One way of estimating unobserved trend and seasonal components is to use a robust, nonparametric technique such as STL (Cleveland et al. 1990); here we use STL as implemented in R (R Development Core Team 2007). This procedure consists of an iterated cycle in which the data is detrended, then the seasonal is updated from the resulting detrended seasonal subseries, after which the trend estimate is updated. At each iteration, robustness weights are formed based on the estimated irregular component and these are used to down-weight outlying observations in subsequent calculations. A typical STL decomposition is shown in Fig. 2 for the natural logarithm of the Total arrivals. The log transformation is commonly used to stabilise a seasonal pattern which increases with the level of the series, and effectively transforms a multiplicative decomposition into an additive one.

Figure 2 shows an evolving seasonal pattern, an upward trend with several changes in slope, and a relatively small irregular component. A vertical line is added to indicate September 2001. There is no obvious (structural) change in the trend at or about this month, although there is a reduction in the slope of the trend nearer

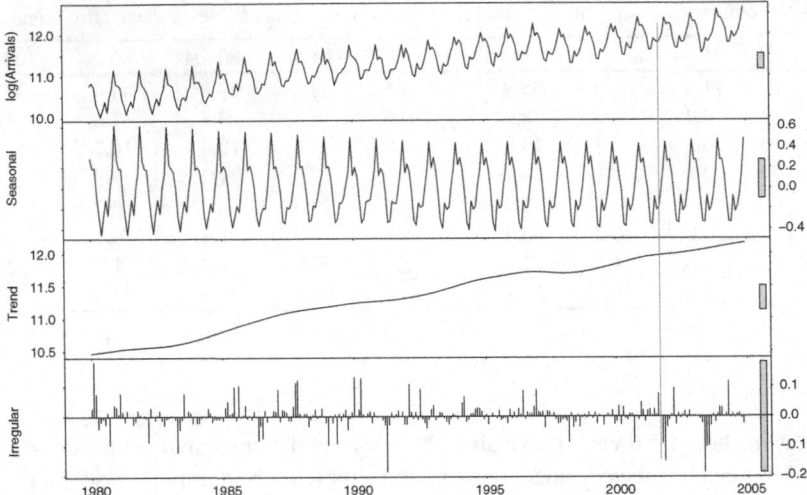

Fig. 2 The STL decomposition of the log aggregate monthly visitor arrivals to New Zealand from January 1980 to December 2004. The *vertical grey line* is at September 2001, and the *solid bars* on the right hand side of the plot are all the same height, to aid comparisons

the start of 2001, which we discuss further in Sect. 5. More prominent is a cluster of negative irregulars immediately following 9/11, the largest of which is the third largest negative irregular in the sample period. Jointly though, these irregulars are smaller and less persistent than those occurring at the time of the SARS outbreak in 2003. Our exploratory analysis with STL thus suggests that while the events of 9/11 may have had a moderate short-term (irregular) effect, there is nothing to suggest that a longer term (structural) effect occurred. We investigate this hypothesis more formally in Sect. 4.

3 Iterative Break Estimation for Seasonal Data

Bai and Perron (1998, 2003) present a methodology for fitting a linear model with structural breaks, in which the break points, i.e. the times at which the parameters change, are determined optimally. The optimal positions of m break points are determined by minimising the residual sum of squares, for each positive integer $m \leq m_{max}$. The optimal number of break points ($0 \leq m^* \leq m_{max}$) may then be determined by, for example, minimising an information criterion such as BIC (Schwarz 1978). Given a sample of T observations, the selected break points are estimated consistently, with rate T convergence of the estimated break fractions (that is, the proportions of the data between consecutive breaks).

The maximum number of break points, m_{max}, is determined by the number of observations relative to the number of parameters in the model. In general, for a model with m breaks and q parameters, at least q observations are needed between each pair of break points, requiring at least $T \geq (m + 1)q$ observations in total. Clearly if the model has many parameters, fewer break points can be estimated from a given sequence of observations.

We consider implementing this approach for a time series of the form

$$Y_t = T_t + S_t + I_t, \qquad t = 1, \ldots, T,$$

where Y_t are the observed data (transformed if necessary), T_t is an unobserved trend component, S_t is an unobserved seasonal component with seasonal period s, and I_t is an unobserved irregular component. Many observed time series do not follow an additive decomposition, including the NZ visitor arrivals as noted in Sect. 2; however, we assume a suitable stabilizing transformation can be applied (e.g., see Sect. 4). In the following model, the evolution of trend and seasonal components is explicitly modelled as structural changes occurring at endogenously identified break points. Short-term, random changes may also occur, but these are modelled by the irregular component I_t. We assume that between two break points t^*_{j-1} and t^*_j ($j = 1, \ldots, m + 1$), the trend T_t is linear,

$$T_t = \alpha_j + \beta_j t, \qquad t = t^*_{j-1} + 1, \ldots, t^*_j$$

and, again between break points, the seasonal component is fixed,

$$S_t = \sum_{i=1}^{s-1} \delta_{i,j} D_{i,t}, \qquad t = t^*_{j-1} + 1, \ldots, t^*_j,$$

where $D_{i,t}$ are seasonal dummies. We use the convention that $t^*_0 = 0$ and $t^*_{m+1} = T$ (Bai and Perron 1998). Under these assumptions, we note that for daily or monthly data (with $s = 7$ and $s = 12$ respectively), and for quarterly data (with $s = 4$) to a lesser extent, the trend component will be parsimonious relative to the seasonal component.

Bai and Perron's (1998, 2003) methodology offers two alternatives for estimating the unknown break points, t^*_j ($j = 1, \ldots, m$), in such a model. The first is that the coefficients of one component are fixed over the entire sample period (a partial structural change model); the second is that parameters in both components should have the same break points (a pure structural change model). We demonstrate below that neither of these options is satisfactory for the type of data examined in this paper, i.e. seasonal time series with evolving trends, and large s (in this case, $s = 12$).

When considering trend extraction and assuming that structural breaks will be required, in general we wish to allow break points in the seasonal component, which is inconsistent with a partial structural change model. Conversely, we would not necessarily wish to constrain any seasonal break points to occur at the same places as the trend break points, as required in a pure structural change model. On the face of it, this requirement is not necessarily restrictive, since the parameter estimates of one component are not forced to change from one segment of the data to the next. However, when selecting the optimal number of break points using a penalised likelihood criterion, e.g. BIC, this compromises the ability to detect break points in the data, i.e. the selected number of breaks may be too low. One example of where these issues may be important is in arrivals from Australia. As noted in Sect. 2, the Australian arrivals seem to have a seasonal break point in 1987 (changing from three peaks to four), with no apparent change in trend.

To address this concern we estimate the trend and seasonal components separately, using a new iterative approach motivated by the Macaulay cycle seasonal decomposition method (Macaulay 1931) and the iterative technique of STL. This allows more flexible structural break estimation than fitting both components simultaneously. As above, we assume that the time series can be decomposed into a piecewise linear time trend and a piecewise constant seasonal pattern. Each component is then estimated using the methodology of Bai and Perron (1998, 2003), implemented in R (R Development Core Team 2007) using the strucchange package of Zeileis et al. (2002). We employ the default method of selecting the number of breaks, which uses BIC.

The trend of the data Y_t is estimated using a piecewise linear model for the seasonally adjusted time series $V_t = Y_t - \hat{S}_t$, i.e.,

$$V_t = \alpha_j + \beta_j t + \epsilon_t, \qquad t = t_{j-1}^* + 1, \ldots, t_j^*$$

for $j = 1, \ldots, m + 1$, where ϵ_t is a zero-mean disturbance and t_j^*, $j = 1, \ldots, m$, are the unknown trend break points. For the first iteration, we set $\hat{S}_t = 0$ for all t.

Once the trend has been estimated, we estimate the seasonal component of Y_t using a piecewise seasonal dummy model for the detrended data $W_t = Y_t - \hat{T}_t$, i.e.,

$$W_t = \delta_{0,j} + \sum_{i=1}^{s-1} \delta_{i,j} D_{i,t} + v_t, \qquad t = t_{j-1}' + 1, \ldots, t_j'$$

for $j = 1, \ldots, m' + 1$, where $D_{i,t}$ are the seasonal dummies, v_t is a zero-mean disturbance and t_j', $j = 1, \ldots, m'$, are the unknown seasonal break points. As before, we take $t_0' = 0$ and $t_{m'+1}' = T$. The estimates $\hat{\delta}_{i,j}$ are adjusted at the end of each iteration so that they add to zero within each full seasonal cycle (between seasonal breaks), to prevent any change in trend appearing as a result of a seasonal break happening "mid-year". That is,

$$\sum_{i=0}^{s-1} \hat{\delta}_{i,j} = 0 \qquad \text{for all } j.$$

This estimation process is then iterated to convergence of the estimated break points.

We are thus able to estimate a trend which, due to its parsimonious representation, is able to react to obvious shifts in the general movement of the

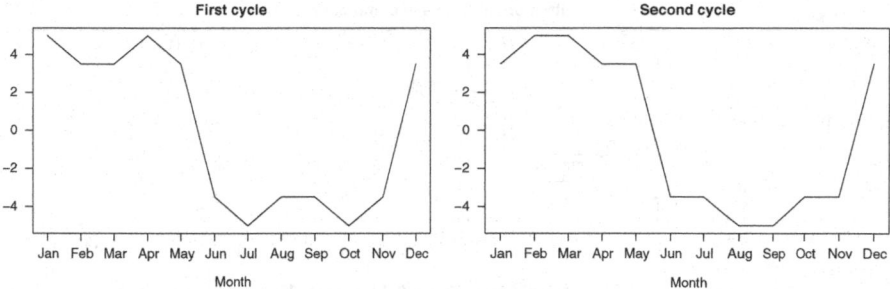

Fig. 3 The two seasonal cycles used for the seasonal component in the illustrative simulation

data. If required, we are able to identify important changes in the seasonal pattern separately. Since the trend and seasonal break points, t_j^* and t_j' respectively, are estimated independently, they are not constrained to occur concurrently. Of course, this does not preclude (some) trend and seasonal break points coinciding if appropriate. In all data analysis and simulations we have followed the recommendations of Bai and Perron (2003) and Zeileis et al. (2003), concerning the fraction of data needed between breaks. For monthly seasonal data, we used 3 full years (36 observations) as a minimum, corresponding to 12 % of a 25-year data span. However, a further consequence of the iterative estimation of trend and seasonal breaks is that while any two breaks of the same type must have a minimum separation (3 years here), the distance between a trend break and a seasonal break has no constraints. This feature is of practical importance, e.g. as shown for the arrivals data in Sect. 4, and is another desirable feature of the new iterative approach.

The importance of this method is now illustrated using simulated data. Consider a time series with piecewise linear trend given by

$$T_t = \begin{cases} 20 + 0.05t, & t = 1, \ldots, 78 \\ 23.9, & t = 79, \ldots, 234 \\ 23.9 + 0.05(t - 234), & t = 235, \ldots, 312 \end{cases}$$

and piecewise fixed seasonal component with a break point at $t = 156$. The two seasonal cycles are shown in Fig. 3, and are identical except for the ordering of the Jan/Feb, Mar/Apr, Jul/Aug and Sep/Oct values. The data are given by

$$Y_t = T_t + S_t + I_t, \qquad I_t \sim \text{i.i.d. } N(0, 1)$$

and thus have three break points: two associated solely with the trend, and one associated only with the seasonal component.

We simulated 500 independent series as above, and for each of them estimated the trend and seasonal components simultaneously using the Bai and Perron (1998, 2003) approach. In particular, we restricted the parameters in both the trend and

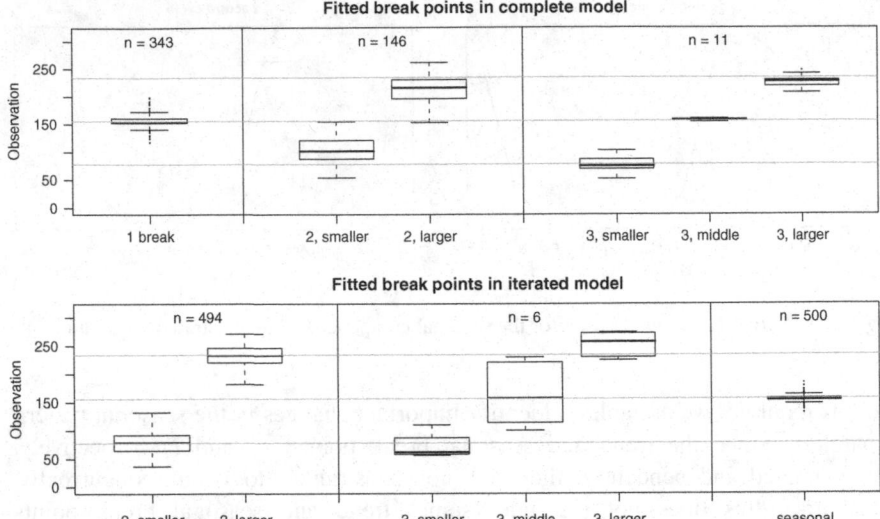

Fig. 4 The estimated break points for 500 simulated series. True break dates are at the *horizontal grey lines*. Results in the *upper panel* are for the Bai and Perron methodology, with the new iterated methodology in the *lower panel*. The number of cases is shown above each boxplot, while the total number of estimated breaks is given below. In the iterated panel, trend break points are shown on the *left* and the (single) seasonal break point on the *right*

seasonal components to change simultaneously; i.e., a pure structural change model. Between breaks, the constant term in the estimated trend was corrected so that the seasonal component added to zero. We also applied the iterated methodology to the same series, fitting the trend and seasonal components separately. Figure 4 shows the estimated break points for the 500 series using the two competing methodologies. In both panels are boxplots of the estimated break points for the series, and these have been grouped depending on how many break points were estimated.

The estimated break points obtained fitting both components simultaneously are in the upper panel of Fig. 4. In 343 series (68.6 %) only one break point was estimated, and the sample distribution of these is summarised in the extreme left boxplot. The estimates appear to be unbiased for the central (seasonal) break point. In the middle of the upper panel are the sample distributions of the two break points, as estimated in 146 series (29.2 %). These appear to be biased estimates of the true trend break points, with each being closer to the seasonal break point than to the nearest end of the series. On the right, the sample distributions of the three break points are displayed, estimated in 11 of the series (2.2 %). These appear unbiased, although the sample size is very small. In conclusion, fitting the two components simultaneously has allowed us to correctly identify the true break points in only 2.2 % of the series. Despite correctly dating the breaks in these 11 series, this approach does not attribute the change to any one component of the structural

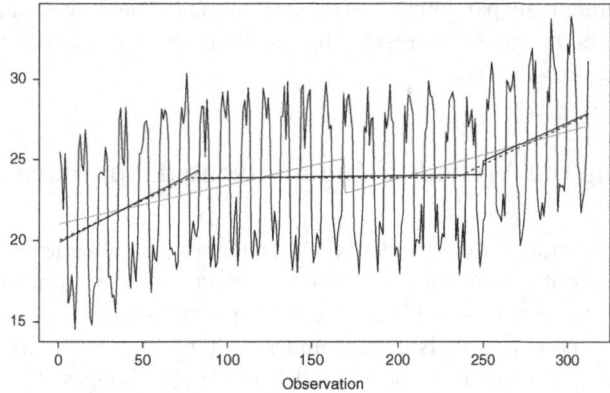

Fig. 5 Simulated data (*solid*) with true piecewise linear trend (*dashed*). Estimated piecewise linear trends using the Bai and Perron methodology (*grey*) and the iterated methodology (*black*)

model. Clearly though, each true change affects only one of the trend or seasonal components.

In the lower panel of Fig. 4 are comparable results for the new iterated approach. All series have at least two estimated trend break points and a single seasonal break. Two trend breaks are estimated in 494 series (98.8 %) and are displayed on the left; they appear to be unbiased estimates of the true trend break points. In the remaining six series (1.2 %), a third trend break is estimated. The estimated seasonal break points for all 500 series are shown on the right; these are clearly unbiased, and estimated relatively precisely. In conclusion, fitting the two components iteratively allowed us to correctly identify and attribute the trend and seasonal break points in 98.8 % of the series; a dramatic improvement over the simultaneous approach. The use of sequential F-tests instead of BIC to select the number of breaks in the simultaneous approach does not substantially change the number of series with the correct number of estimated breaks.

Figure 5 shows a single example series that results in typical estimation behaviour, with the true trend and both estimated trends also plotted. For the complete model, BIC selects only one break point at $t = 168$. Applying the iterated methodology to the data, two trend break points are estimated at $t = 83$ and $t = 249$, and a single seasonal break point is estimated at $t = 157$. Note that the complete model induces a "quadratic" trend in the residuals on either side of the single break, which is expected after viewing the estimated and true trends together as in Fig. 5. That (local) trending behaviour is reflected by significant residual sample autocorrelations at low lags; clear evidence that the model is misspecified. In contrast, the residuals from the iterative approach show no significant autocorrelations at low lags, reflecting the more appropriate modelling of the true trend component.

This simulation shows the undesirable consequences of fitting two components simultaneously when a parameter-rich seasonal component breaks at times other than those of a relatively parsimonious trend component. Our new iterated approach to fitting such components addresses this concern. Next we apply this iterated technique to the arrivals data.

4   Modelling the Arrivals Using an Iterated Approach

The seasonal variation of the arrivals typically increases with the level of the series (Fig. 1). Applying the new iterated approach directly to the untransformed data would certainly require seasonal breaks to account for the changes in amplitude of the seasonal component. This is clearly undesirable because such changes usually evolve smoothly, so should not be modelled as abrupt changes. Consequently a stabilising transformation is needed.

A log transformation is one obvious possibility, but this does not yield an optimal stabilising transformation for all these series and instead we estimate a power transformation, identified using the robust spread-vs-level plots described in Hoaglin et al. (1983). For each individual series we calculate the median and interquartile range (IQR) of the monthly arrivals for each of the 25 calendar years, then regress log IQR on log median. The appropriate stabilising transformation is $x^{1-\text{slope}}$, and the transformed series are shown in Fig. 6, with the estimated powers.

Confidence intervals for the slopes in these spread-vs-level regressions support the use of logs only in the case of the UK, USA and Total arrivals (i.e. a power of zero, or a slope of one). In the case of Germany the estimated power is negative, so $-x^{1-\text{slope}}$ is used to preserve order in the transformed arrivals. All further analysis is conducted on the transformed data.

In the case of the transformed arrivals data, each linear time trend requires two parameters, and each dummy seasonal an additional $s - 1 = 11$. Figure 6 indicates that for most series a linear time trend would need breaks. Further, while the seasonal patterns generally have constant variation over the length of the series due to the power transformations, we do not wish to preclude seasonal changes during the data period. As the simulation study demonstrated, the parameter-rich trend-plus-seasonal (complete) model would severely limit our ability to appropriately fit the data, since the large number of seasonal dummies would reduce the possible number of breaks, especially when selected by BIC.

As with the simulated data, we use a minimum period between breaks of 36 observations for estimation of both trend and seasonal components. In fact, when estimating the trend and seasonal components iteratively, there is scope to reduce that minimum period for estimation of the trend component, since it only requires two parameters between breaks. This possibility further increases the flexibility of trends estimated using our new iterated approach. However, to simplify comparisons we have not pursued this option here. For the iterative approach, three iterations were sufficient to ensure convergence of the estimated break points in all cases but Other and Total, which each required four.

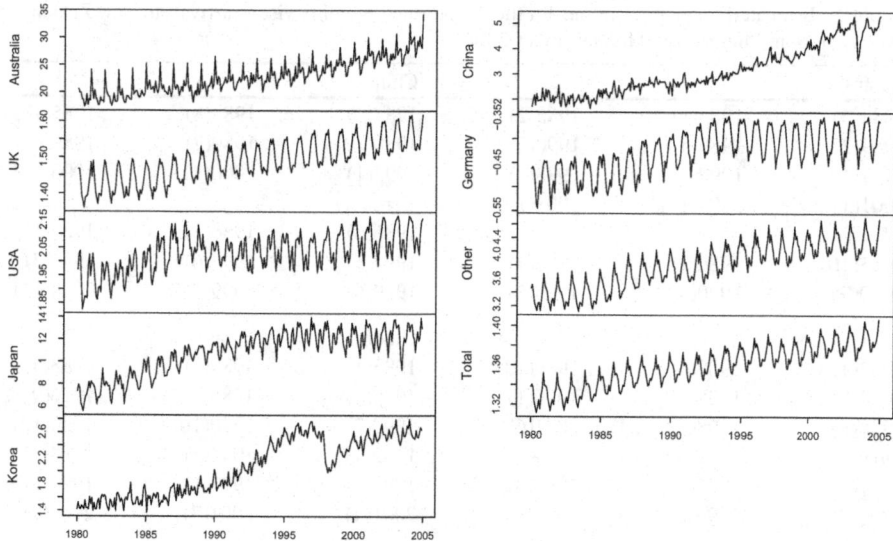

Fig. 6 Power transformed monthly short-term visitor arrivals to New Zealand, by origin, from January 1980 to December 2004. The power transformations are: Australia 0.3, UK 0.05, USA 0.08, Japan 0.27, Korea 0.11, China 0.18, Germany −0.11, Other 0.13, and Total 0.03

The estimated trend break points are shown in Table 2 along with estimated 95 % confidence intervals. The confidence intervals have been formed with heteroscedasticity and autocorrelation consistent (HAC) estimates of the covariance matrix (Andrews 1991). These confidence intervals are computed and displayed as standard output using the R package sandwich; they make use of a quadratic spectral kernel with vector autoregressive prewhitening, as recommended by Andrews and Monahan (1992). Details of the R implementation are given in Zeileis (2004, 2006). Figure 7 displays the estimated parametric trends and break points (with confidence intervals), along with nonparametric trends estimated by STL. September 2001 is included in only two confidence intervals, indicating the possibility that the terrorist events of 9/11 may be linked to a structural break in the trend of arrivals for those two origins: Australia and Other. Other is difficult to interpret given its composite nature, although it is plausible that the 9/11 events did have an effect on tourist behaviour in some of these countries. An alternative (or perhaps complementary) explanation is discussed in Sect. 5.

In the case of Australia, a break is estimated in the month following 9/11, which results in an increased trend slope but a decreased intercept. A relevant confounding effect is the collapse of Ansett Australia, which occurred just 3 days after the terrorist attacks of 9/11; hence it is impossible to separate these two effects with monthly data. The termination of flights by Ansett Australia and Ansett International on 14 September 2001 certainly affected capacity and timing of arrivals to New Zealand. In addition, in the following week, strike action targeted at Air New Zealand occurred at Melbourne and Perth airports (Air New Zealand

Table 2 Estimated trend break points for the transformed monthly visitor arrivals to New Zealand, by origin, from January 1980 to December 2004

Australia			China		
1984(5)	1985(1)	1985(2)	1984(7)	1984(8)	1985(1)
1989(3)	1989(4)	1990(5)	1988(10)	1989(7)	1989(9)
1997(10)	1997(12)	1998(1)	1997(1)	2000(11)	2000(12)
2001(1)	2001(10)	2001(11)	Germany		
UK			1986(6)	1986(7)	1986(11)
1985(10)	1986(1)	1986(4)	1994(5)	1994(6)	1994(7)
1990(7)	1990(8)	1996(5)	1999(6)	1999(8)	2000(11)
USA			Other		
1982(12)	1983(3)	1986(12)	1983(1)	1983(3)	1983(4)
1988(9)	1988(10)	1990(1)	1985(6)	1986(8)	1986(9)
1998(6)	1998(8)	2001(6)	1990(7)	1990(10)	1990(12)
Japan			1992(11)	1994(1)	1994(3)
1987(3)	1987(6)	1987(8)	1997(3)	1997(6)	1997(8)
1996(2)	1996(8)	1996(10)	2001(4)	2001(7)	2001(9)
Korea			Total		
1982(8)	1983(12)	1984(4)	1982(12)	1983(1)	1983(3)
1990(9)	1990(10)	1990(11)	1987(10)	1987(12)	1988(4)
1994(9)	1994(11)	1994(12)	1989(8)	1990(12)	1991(4)
1997(10)	1997(11)	1997(12)	1997(1)	1997(3)	1997(6)
2000(10)	2000(11)	2001(1)			

The middle column gives the estimated break points, while the first and third columns give the lower and upper 95 % confidence limits respectively, estimated using a HAC estimate of the covariance matrix

had acquired control of Ansett Australia during the year preceding its collapse). Those strikes required the cancellation of all Air New Zealand trans-Tasman flights operating from Melbourne and Perth. These physical constraints on passenger numbers are a plausible explanation for a decrease in intercept, while the subsequent increase in the rate of arrivals from New Zealand's nearest neighbour is unlikely to have any causal links from the terrorist events of September 2001.

Focusing on Fig. 7 more generally, we note that it is often difficult to distinguish between the two alternative trend estimates; i.e. those from our iterated approach and STL. In particular, the iterative parametric method achieves similar flexibility in its trend estimate to the nonparametric technique, with the latter essentially fitting linear time trends at each point in the series using only a local window of observations to estimate parameters. The break point technology allows instantaneous changes in the trend, however, unlike the STL technique. In effect, STL requires an "innovational outlier" approach to any structural changes in the data, while our parametric procedure models the changes directly and permits an "additive outlier" approach. (In a series of papers, Perron and coauthors popularised the use of these "outlier" terms, to describe an approach which is attributed to the intervention analysis work of Box and Tiao 1975.) An obvious contrast between

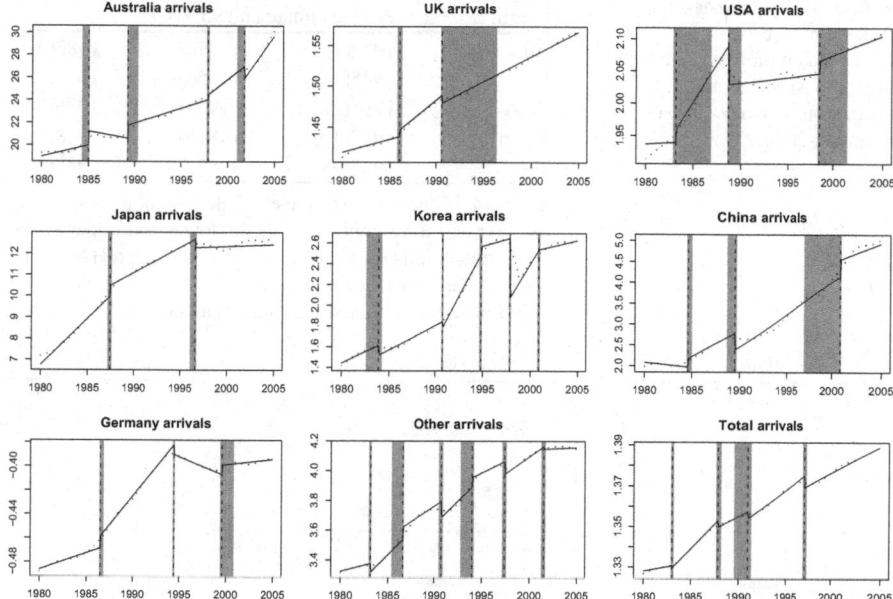

Fig. 7 Estimated trends and trend break points for the transformed monthly visitor arrivals to New Zealand, by origin, from January 1980 to December 2004. The *solid line* is the piecewise linear time trend, while the *dotted line* is the estimated STL trend. The *vertical dashed lines* and *grey regions* respectively indicate the fitted break points and their 95 % confidence intervals, estimated using a HAC estimate of the covariance matrix

the two approaches is seen in the Korean data at the time of the Asian financial crisis. The parametric break point is dated at November 1997 (with a narrow 95 % confidence interval of October to December), which corresponds exactly to the month that the financial crisis first affected Korea (Kaminsky and Schmukler 1999). However, STL spreads the downward impact of the crisis over a number of months, in contrast to the observed behaviour.

Table 3 gives the estimated seasonal break points for the transformed arrivals, with the estimated seasonal components shown in Fig. 8. Korea, China, Germany and Other have no estimated seasonal break points. As the power transformations have effectively stabilised the seasonal variation, any changes in the seasonal patterns more likely reflect behavioural changes in the time of year when visitors arrive. For example, in Australia's seasonal pattern the "middle" peak has moved and one extra peak has been added, reflecting a shift from a three-term school year to a four-term year in New South Wales in 1987 (NSW Department of Education 1985). The placement of the seasonal break point coincides exactly with the final month under the old three-term system, with the first holiday in the new sequence occurring in July 1987. The UK data show a shift in arrivals from the second half of the year to the first and a shift in the peak arrivals from December to February. The USA and Japanese arrivals have had relatively complex changes, while the Total

Table 3 Estimated seasonal break points for the transformed monthly visitor arrivals to New Zealand, by origin, from January 1980 to December 2004

Origin	Point estimate and 95 % CI		
Australia	1987(1)	1987(6)	1987(9)
UK	1985(11)	1986(6)	1987(9)
USA	1995(1)	1995(4)	1995(12)
Japan	1987(10)	1988(6)	1988(12)
Total	1987(3)	1987(7)	1988(1)

The middle column gives the estimated break points, while the first and third columns give the lower and upper 95 % confidence limits respectively, estimated using a HAC estimate of the covariance matrix. Korea, China, Germany and Other have no estimated seasonal break points

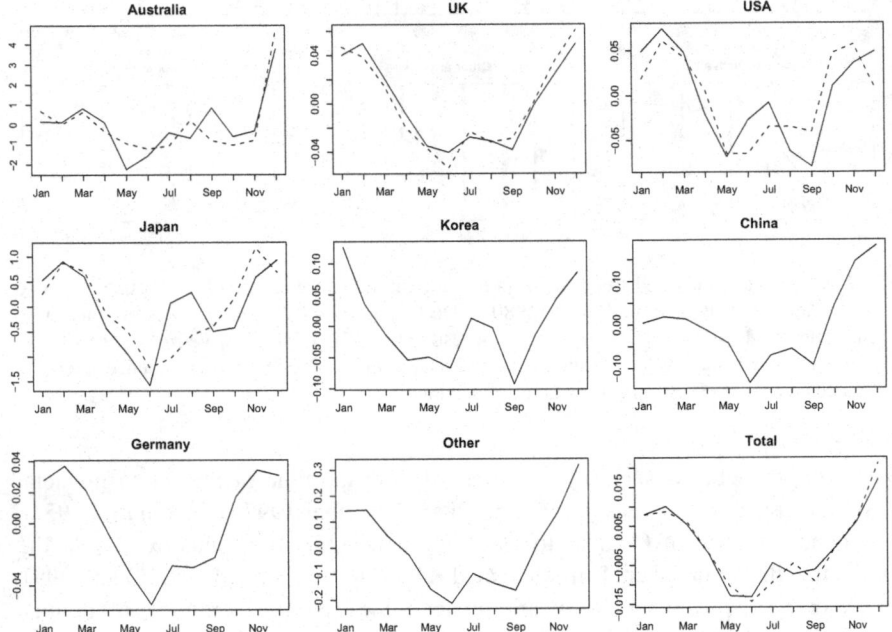

Fig. 8 The estimated seasonal components for visitors to New Zealand by origin. The *solid line* is the final estimated seasonal component; it is the only estimate in four of the nine cases, where no seasonal breaks were detected. The *five dashed lines* are the seasonal components prior to the seasonal break points listed in Table 3

series has seen most change in the winter months. Note here the practical relevance of allowing breaks in the seasonal component of any given series to be independent of those in the trend, with no minimum separation between them: four of these five seasonal breaks (all except USA) are less than 3 years away from at least one corresponding trend break (see Tables 2 and 3). However, none of the dates for trend and seasonal breaks coincide in any given series, which reinforces the need to allow the components to break separately for additional flexibility in the fitted model.

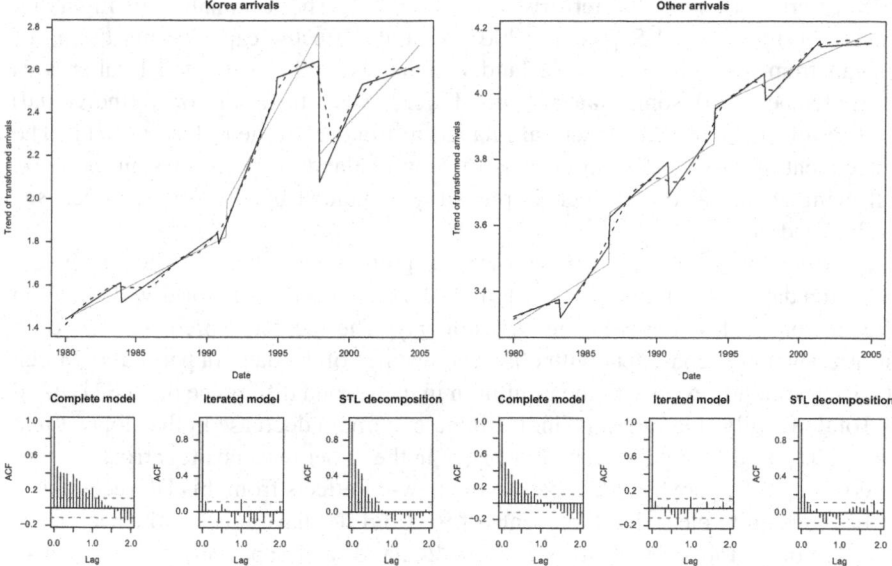

Fig. 9 Trend estimates for the Korean arrivals and those from Other origins. The trend estimates are based on the complete model (*grey*), the new iterated approach (*black*) and STL (*dashed*). Also shown are sample autocorrelation functions for the residuals from the three methods

To conclude this section, we compare the trend estimates obtained from our new iterated approach to the trends obtained fitting a complete structural break model (with 13 parameters between breaks), and using STL. In Fig. 9 we present trends for the Korean arrivals and those from Other origins. We also show sample autocorrelation functions for the three sets of residuals from each series. The trends are all similar, but the agreement is closest for the iterated approach and STL. Some differences are evident particularly at the end of the series though, which would be important for prediction. For Other arrivals, the number of parameters required for the complete model clearly restricts the estimated number of breaks, leading to greater departures from the STL trend than achieved by iteration. The irregular components also favour the iterated approach over STL and the complete model, as the residuals for the latter are highly autocorrelated, especially at low lags. In contrast, the residuals of the iterated method exhibit far less autocorrelation, indicating a better overall decomposition (see Fig. 9).

5 Discussion

The growth in the number of visitor arrivals to New Zealand was lower than expected in late 2001 (e.g., by the New Zealand Ministry of Tourism, as noted in Haywood and Randal 2004), yet there is no conclusive evidence to attribute this forecast error solely to the terrorist events of 9/11. The termination of flights by Ansett Australia on 14 September 2001 certainly affected capacity and timing of arrivals from Australia to New Zealand, and that would have affected Total arrivals in September 2001 somewhat as well. Indeed Australia is the only (individual) country of origin with a structural change in trend identified close to 9/11. The subsequent rate of Australian arrivals to New Zealand in fact shows an *increase*, following an initial drop which is plausibly explained by the Ansett effect; see Table 2 and Fig. 7.

A further plausible cause for the lower than forecast number of visitors is the US recession dated March 2001 (Hall et al. 2001), along with the world-wide flow-on effects from a slow down in the US economy. The recession predates 9/11 by 6 months but that is consistent with observed features of the data. In particular, March 2001 corresponds exactly to the minimum in the second difference of an STL trend of Total monthly (log) arrivals, indicating a maximum decrease in the slope at that time. It is possible that the slow down seen in the Other (composite) arrivals series, dated July 2001, may be due in part to the flow-on effects from this US recession.

It seems quite clear that the events of 9/11 did not have much influence on the longer term numbers of visitors to New Zealand, and especially not a negative influence. In contrast our analysis identifies other events which have had marked structural effects on the trends in these data, especially from certain countries of origin. In particular, the stock market crash of October 1987 preceded a dramatic decline in arrivals from the USA, followed by a sustained period of only moderate growth. In turn, both the intercept and slope of Total arrivals decreased in December 1987. Similarly, the Asian financial crisis of 1997–1998 precipitated a massive drop in arrivals from Korea, with the intercept and slope of Total arrivals again both decreasing in 1997. The SARS epidemic affected arrivals from China in a different way, with a very short-lived but large reduction, which we class as temporary and not structural. The overall effects of 9/11 might also be seen as temporary and negative, but of a smaller magnitude than those associated with SARS.

Estimation of structural breaks was facilitated by a new implementation of Bai and Perron (1998, 2003) work that is recommended for seasonal data. Specifically, use of an iterative approach to estimate the trend and seasonal components separately enabled us to locate structural breaks in the data, and to attribute these to either changes in the trend or the seasonal pattern. Estimating these components simultaneously did not achieve the same flexibility in the estimated components, nor in the location of the break points. The agreement between the estimated parametric trends from the iterated approach and the nonparametric STL trends is especially pleasing, as is the lack of residual structure around those parametric trends when compared to other trend estimates.

Acknowledgements Statistics New Zealand kindly supplied the data. We thank those who commented on presentations at Statistics New Zealand, the Reserve Bank of New Zealand, Victoria Management School, the ASC/NZSA 2006 Conference, and the TSEFAR 2006 Conference. We also thank Peter Thomson for some helpful suggestions that improved the paper.

References

Andrews, D. W. K. (1991). Heteroskedasticity and autocorrelation consistent covariance matrix estimation. *Econometrica, 59,* 817–858.

Andrews, D. W. K., & Monahan, J. C. (1992). An improved heteroskedasticity and autocorrelation consistent covariance matrix estimator. *Econometrica, 60,* 953–966.

Australian Bureau of Statistics. (2003). *Information paper: A guide to interpreting time series – Monitoring trends.* ABS Cat. No. 1349.0. Canberra: Australian Bureau of Statistics.

Bai, J., & Perron, P. (1998). Estimating and testing linear models with multiple structural changes. *Econometrica, 66,* 47–78.

Bai, J., & Perron, P. (2003). Computation and analysis of multiple structural change models. *Journal of Applied Econometrics, 18,* 1–22.

Box, G. E. P., & Jenkins, G. M. (1976). *Time series analysis, forecasting and control* (2nd ed.). Oakland: Holden-Day.

Box, G. E. P., & Tiao, G. C. (1975). Intervention analysis with applications to economic and environmental problems. *Journal of the American Statistical Association, 70,* 70–79.

Busetti, F., & Harvey, A. (2008). Testing for trend. *Econometric Theory, 24,* 72–87.

Cleveland, R. B., Cleveland, W. S., McRae, J. E., & Terpenning, I. (1990). STL: A seasonal-trend decomposition procedure based on loess. *Journal of Official Statistics, 6,* 3–73.

Dungey, M., Fry, R., & Martin, V. L. (2004). Currency market contagion in the Asia-Pacific region. *Australian Economic Papers, 43,* 379–395.

Findley, D. F., Monsell, B. C., Bell, W. R., Otto, M. C., & Chen, B. C. (1998). New capabilities and methods of the X-12-ARIMA seasonal-adjustment program. *Journal of Business and Economic Statistics, 16,* 127–177.

Franses, P. H. (1998). *Time series models for business and economic forecasting.* Cambridge: Cambridge University Press.

Hall, R., Feldstein, M., Bernanke, B., Frankel, J., Gordon, R., & Zarnowitz, V. (2001). *The business-cycle peak of March 2001.* Technical report, Business Cycle Dating Committee, National Bureau of Economic Research, USA. http://www.nber.org/cycles/november2001/.

Hamilton, J. D. (1994). *Time series analysis.* Princeton: Princeton University Press.

Harvey, A. C. (1989). *Forecasting, structural time series models and the Kalman filter.* Cambridge: Cambridge University Press.

Haywood, J., & Randal, J. (2004). *Stochastic seasonality, New Zealand visitor arrivals, and the effects of 11 September 2001.* Research Report 04-1, School of Mathematics, Statistics and Computer Science, Victoria University of Wellington, New Zealand.

Hoaglin, D. C., Mosteller, F., & Tukey, J. W. (Eds.) (1983). *Understanding robust and exploratory data analysis.* New York: Wiley.

Kaminsky, G. L., & Schmukler, S. L. (1999). What triggers market jitters? A chronicle of the Asian crisis. *Journal of International Money and Finance, 18,* 537–560.

Macaulay, F. R. (1931). *The smoothing of time series.* New York: National Bureau of Economic Research.

Makridakis, S., Wheelwright, S. C., & Hyndman, R. J. (1998). *Forecasting: Methods and applications* (3rd ed.). New York: Wiley.

NSW Department of Education (1985, April). 1987: *Perspectives: Looking at Education, 8*(4), pp. 3.

Pearce, D. (2001). Tourism. *Asia Pacific Viewpoint, 42,* 75–84.

R Development Core Team (2007). *R: A language and environment for statistical computing.* Vienna, Austria: R Foundation for Statistical Computing.

Schwarz, G. (1978). Estimating the dimension of a model. *The Annals of Statistics, 6,* 461–464.

Statistics New Zealand. (2005). *Tourism satellite account 2004.* Wellington: Statistics New Zealand.

US Department of State. (2004). *Three years after 9/11: Mixed reviews for war on terror.* http://www.globalsecurity.org/security/library/news/2004/09/wwwh40915.htm.

Zeileis, A. (2004). Econometric computing with HC and HAC covariance matrix estimators. *Journal of Statistical Software, 11*(10), 1–17.

Zeileis, A. (2006). Object-oriented computation of sandwich estimators. *Journal of Statistical Software, 16*(9), 1–16.

Zeileis, A., Kleiber, C., Krämer, W., & Hornik, K. (2003). Testing and dating of structural changes in practice. *Computational Statistics and Data Analysis, 44*, 109–123.

Zeileis, A., Leisch, F., Hornik, K., & Kleiber, C. (2002). Strucchange: An R package for testing for structural change in linear regression models. *Journal of Statistical Software, 7*(2), 1–38.

Forecasting the Risk of Insolvency Among Customers of an Automotive Financial Service

Rita Allais and Marco Bosco

Abstract The aim of our study is to present an application of Generalized Linear Models to the prevention of the risk of insolvency of an automotive financial service. In order to forecast the payments (by installment) of the customers, we use a logit multivariate regression model. Before fitting the model, we resort to sample logits, Generalized Additive Models and univariate logistic regression in order to identify the subset of best predictors and verify the assumptions underpinning the statistical model. For the estimated model, we use the Wald statistics to assess the significance of the coefficients, the Likelihood Ratio to test the goodness of fit of the model, and the Odds Ratio to interpret the meaning of the estimated coefficients. In order to verify the goodness of fit of the model, we utilize classifications tables and the Receiver Operating Characteristic curve. Finally, we externally validate the fitted model by means of a predictive-test on a training set.

Keywords Generalized additive model • Likelihood ratio • Logistic regression • Receiver operating characteristic curve • Wald statistics

1 Introduction

Our paper concerns the policies of control and prevention of the risks of insolvency of an automotive financial service. In order to forecast the performance of the customers' repayments (by instalment) we utilize a Generalized Linear Model. Typically, at the expiry of the contract, the finance company classifies a customer as being "good" or "bad" according to the correctness of his/her monthly re-payments.

R. Allais (✉)
Department of Social-Economic, Mathematical & Statistical Sciences, University of Turin, Corso Unione Sovietica, 218 bis, 10134 Turin, Italy
e-mail: allais@econ.unito.it

G. MacKenzie and D. Peng (eds.), *Statistical Modelling in Biostatistics and Bioinformatics*, Contributions to Statistics, DOI 10.1007/978-3-319-04579-5__7,
© Springer International Publishing Switzerland 2014

The company uses a performance indicator which is based on the regularity and type of the monthly re-payments.

Our goal is to establish the existence of a link between the performance indicator and some features of the customer and of his or her contract, so as to be able to forecast during the re-payment period, whether the customer will turn out to be a good one or a bad one.

Since the response is a binary random variable, we use a logit regression model to analyse our data. In order to identify, the subset of the best predictors for the response (i.e. those variables which are strongly correlated with the response) and to verify the assumptions of the statistical model (e.g., non-collinearity among the predictors, linearity between each predictor and the logit of the response) we adopt a step-by-step approach based on sample proportions and sample logits. For continuous predictors we need to resort to Generalized Additive Models (GAMs) in order to estimate the sample proportion. Furthermore, we check the results of univariate logistic regression.

After fitting the multivariate model, we verify the goodness of fit of the model by means of Odds Ratios, Wald statistics and the Likelihood Ratio (G-index). In order to verify the goodness of fit of the model, we analyse the behaviour of the Sensitivity and Specificity functions and construct the Receiver Operating Characteristic (ROC) curve. We also externally validate the fitted model by means of a predictive test on a training set.

2   The Response Variable and the Model

The financing house computes for each customer the value of the performance index I, defined on the real interval $[-1, 1]$, taking into account some feature of the customer related to the regularity of the re-payments, such as, the number of paid instalments, the number of unpaid instalments, and the number of instalments paid late. Furthermore, they classify a customer as bad if $I \leq 0.86$. Therefore we define the binary response random variable as

$$Y = \begin{cases} 0 & 1 - \theta, \\ 1 & \theta, \end{cases}$$

where $\theta = \mathbb{P}(I \leq 0.86)$.

For a binary response variable Y and a multiple explanatory variable $\mathbf{X} = (X_1, \ldots, X_p)$, let

$$\pi(\mathbf{x}) = \mathbb{E}[Y | \mathbf{X} = \mathbf{x}] = \mathbb{P}(Y = 1 | \mathbf{X} = \mathbf{x}).$$

To investigate the relationship between the response probability $\pi(\mathbf{x})$ and the covariate vector $\mathbf{x}$ it is convenient (see McCullagh and Nelder 1989) to construct a formal model thought capable of describing the effect on $\pi(\mathbf{x})$ of changes in $\mathbf{x}$. Furthermore we suppose that the dependence of a transformation $g(\pi)$ on $\mathbf{x}$ occurs through the linear combination

$$g(\pi) = \sum_{i=1}^{p} \beta_i x_i.$$

We select as link function the logit function

$$g(\mathbf{x}) = logit[\pi(\mathbf{x})] = \log \frac{\pi(\mathbf{x})}{1 - \pi(\mathbf{x})} = \beta_0 + \sum_{i=1}^{p} \beta_i x_i$$

and so we resort to the logistic regression model

$$\pi(\mathbf{x}) = \frac{\exp(\beta_0 + \sum_{i=1}^{p} \beta_i x_i)}{1 + \exp(\beta_0 + \sum_{i=1}^{p} \beta_i x_i)}.$$

If some of the independent variables are discrete, nominal scaled variables, then is inappropriate to include them in the model. This is because the numbers used to represent the various levels are merely identifiers, and have no numeric significance. In this situation the method of choice is to use a collection of dummy variables (Anderson 1984). Therefore, if X_j is a categorical predictor with M categories, defining, for each $h \in (1, \ldots, M)$, the dummy variable

$$X_h^j = \begin{cases} 0 & X_j \neq h, \\ 1 & X_j = h \end{cases}$$

and hence the logit function of the model becomes

$$g(\mathbf{x}) = \beta_0 + \sum_{i \neq j} \beta_i x_i + \sum_{h=1}^{M-1} \beta_h^j x_h^j. \tag{1}$$

We need a strategy to select the variables in order to identify the subset of best predictors for the logit regression model (Hosmer and Lemeshow 2013). The selection process should begin with a careful univariate analysis of each variable and subsequently, following the fit of the multivariate model, the importance of each variable included in the model should be verified. The univariate analysis involves fitting a univariate logistic regression model and studying the effect on Y of each predictor by itself and the interaction among variables using, for instance, plots of sample logits.

If X^j is a categorical predictor, with M categories, we define, $\forall h \in (1, \ldots, M)$ the sample logits

$$\tilde{g}(x^j) = \log \left[\frac{p_h}{1 - p_h} \right],$$

where (Agresti 2010) the sample proportion p_h is defined as

$$p_h = \frac{Nu\{y_i = 1 | x_i^j = h\}_{i=1,...,n}}{Nu\{x_i^j = h\}_{i=1,...,n}}.$$

For continuous covariates scatter diagrams are not very informative. Plotting a fitted smooth function for a continuous predictor may reveal a general trend without assuming a particular functional relationship. Hastie and Tibshirani (1990) introduced the use of a GAM for the analysis of binary data. GAM replaces the linear predictors of Generalized Linear Models by smooth function of the predictors:

$$g(\pi) = \sum_{j=1}^{p} s_j(x_j),$$

where $s_j(.)$ is an unspecified smooth function of predictor X^j.

3   The Database and the Variables

Our database consists of 151,443 customers, whose application has already been successfully scored, observed over a period of 4 years, and it includes 33 variables arising from merged different data sources. The percentage of bad customers in the database is 5.75 %. In order to construct the logit regression model, we consider 101,577 records letting the remainder (49,866) constitute the training-set, i.e. a randomly selected control group, hold out of sample, to test the final model.

Aiming to identify good predictors for the model, we decide not to resort to automatic methods, such as stepwise selection, which can lead to a biased set of predictors, but instead to use a step-by-step approach based on sample proportions and sample logits.

To this end, we shall distinguish among continuous (e.g., the price, the amount of the advance, the amount of the financing, the monthly income, the age, the annual interest rate, the net present value of the return on financing, etc.), ordinal (i.e., the number of monthly instalments, the number of incorrect payments during the first 3 months, the loyalty of the customer, classes of cubic capacity of the car, the family size of the customer, etc.) and dichotomous variables (i.e., the sex of the customer, real-estate ownership, the final destination of the car, method of payment, etc.). We shall furthermore choose those which are strongly correlated with the response but not correlated among themselves, showing no interaction in order to avoid problems of multicollinearity, and such that the assumption of linearity between each of them and the sample logit of the response holds.

We verify the assumption of linearity between each predictor and the logit function of the univariate form of model (1) by means of a plot of sample logit against each predictor. The assumption of no-interaction effects among the variables

Table 1 Correlation matrix for all the continuous predictors

	Price	Advance	Financing	Income	Age	Int.rate
Price	1.00	–	–	–	–	–
Advance	0.75	1.00	–	–	–	–
Financing	0.73	0.09	1.00	–	–	–
Income	0.15	0.13	0.09	1.00	–	–
Age	−0.11	−0.01	−0.14	0.12	1.00	–
Int.Rate	0.12	0.03	0.15	−0.09	−0.09	1.00

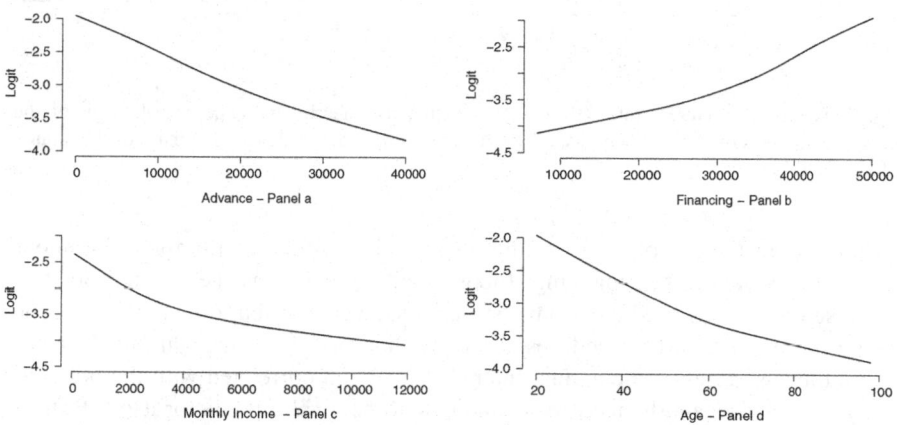

Fig. 1 Checking the linearity of the sample logit of the response versus the continuous predictors. The GAM approach

is checked by the plot of sample logit of one predictor conditioned by each level of another one.

Finally, we shall examine the results of the logit regression models obtained considering separately each of the selected predictors (Hosmer and Lemeshow 2013).

— *Continuous variables*

As continuous variables we consider the price of the car (PRICE), the amount of the advance (ADV), the amount of the financing (FIN), the monthly income of the customer (INC), the age of the customer (AGE), the annual interest rate (IRATE).

Table 1 shows the correlation matrix of these continuous variables. Since it is clear that ADV, FIN and PRICE are highly correlated among them, we decide to drop from our study the price of the car.

For these continuous variables, instead of reclassifying them into classes, we prefer to check their linearity with the sample logit of the response, simply inspecting a plot of the smoothed prediction of the mean provided by a GAM (Hastie and Tibshirani 1990). As displayed in Fig. 1, the assumption of

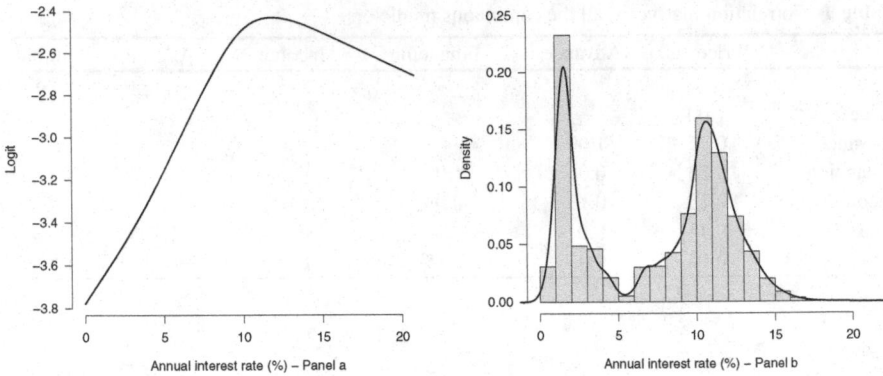

Fig. 2 The annual interest rate. (Panel **a**) Checking its linearity with the sample logit of the response via the GAM approach. (Panel **b**) Histogram and kernel density estimate of the annual interest rate

linearity in the sample logit of the response is verified for the four continuous predictors Advance, Financing, Income and Age. It must be pointed out that those continuous predictors have strongly skewed distributions; for this reason the results of GAM procedures are somewhat biased in the right tail. Our last continuous variable, the annual interest rate, is not correlated with the previous four predictors and hence it is a candidate to be a valid predictor itself. But we find that the relation between the sample logit of the response and the annual interest rate is not linear (see Fig. 2, panel a) and that its distribution is clearly bimodal (see Fig. 2, panel b), suggesting it comes from a mixture of two densities. Since we do not want to lose the prized information on customers' interest rate, we decide to transform this variable into a dichotomous one defined as

$$\text{IRATE} = \begin{cases} 0 & \text{if interest rate} \leq 0.05, \\ 1 & \text{otherwise.} \end{cases}$$

— *Discrete and ordinal variables*

As discrete and ordinal variables, we consider the number of monthly instalments (INST), the number of incorrect payments during the first 3 months (HIST), i.e., the history of the customer during his early 3 months and the loyalty of the customer (LOYAL). These variables are strongly correlated with the response and for them we have the following sample proportions of bad customers listed in Table 2.

These allow us to state that the assumption of linearity between the sample logit of the response and each variable is verified. We therefore consider all these three variables as good predictors.

— *Dichotomous variables*

As dichotomous variables, we consider the sex of the customer (SEX), the occupation state of the customer (OCCU), real-estate ownership (OWNER), the

Table 2 Sample proportions of bad customers—I

INST		HIST		LOYAL	
x_h	$p_h\%$	x_h	$p_h\%$	x_h	$p_h\%$
24	2.4	0	4.9	Low	8.1
36	4.7	1	4.0	Medium	3.8
48	8.8	2	5.5	High	3.4
60	13.8	3	7.6		

Table 3 Sample proportions of bad customers—II

SEX		OCCU		OWNER		DEST		SEGM	
x_h	$p_h\%$	x_h	$p_h\%$	x_h	$p_h\%$	x_h	$p_h\%$	x_h	$p_h\%$
Male	5.2	Empl.	3.1	No	8.4	Priv.	5.7	Low	5.3
Female	6.8	Self-empl.	7.1	Ye	4.8	Comm.	6.5	High	7.4
$(p_1 - p_0)\%$	+1.6		+4.0		−3.6		+0.8		+2.1

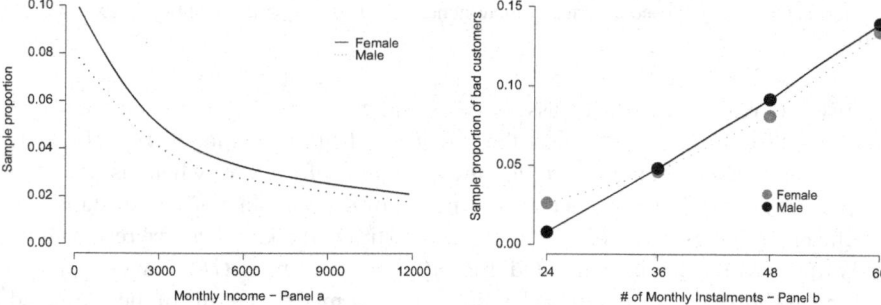

Fig. 3 (Panel **a**) Gam of sample proportion vs. INC by levels of SEX. (Panel **b**) Sample proportion vs. INST by levels of SEX

final destination of the car (DEST) and the segment of the car (SEGM). Among all the variables in the database, these are the most strongly correlated with the response and for them we have the following sample proportions of bad customers, see Table 3.

Since the increment of the DEST is negligible, we are likely to drop this variable as a predictor for the response. If we do so, we consider as predictors the dichotomous variables SEX, OCCU, OWNER, SEGM and IRATE.

In our study there is no evidence of interaction between predictors. The analysis is conducted, ignoring technicalities, simply by looking to see if the sample proportions of predictor X conditioned on each level of another predictor, say X^*, show the same behaviour. We do the same in the case of continuous predictors but we resort to GAMs in order to estimate the sample proportions. Figure 3 shows the approach we applied in the case of income (INC) versus sex and number of monthly instalments (INST) versus sex.

The next and last step consists in examining the results of univariate logit regression models, i.e., the models we obtain considering separately each predictor.

Table 4 Results of univariate logit model for the predictors

	Beta	OR	G-Index
ADV	−0.000167	0.9199*	1050.06
FIN	0.000130	1.0672*	1278.00
INC	−0.000274	0.8720*	305.33
AGE	−0.030860	0.9696	911.61
INST	0.051684	1.0530	2027.26
HIST	2.065065	7.8858	2757.48
LOYAL(Medium)	−0.793644	0.4522	854.85
LOYAL(High)	−0.899862	0.4070	854.84
SEX(Male)	0.122465	1.1303	180.84
OCCU(Self.)	0.895209	2.4478	786.78
OWNER(Yes)	−0.588468	0.5551	422.04
DEST(Comm.)	0.139410	1.1490	9.99
SEGM(High)	0.335890	1.3991	112.25
IRATE(High)	1.117891	3.0584	1234.84

The starred ORs are proposed in terms of increments of 500 euros; e.g. $OR(ADV) = exp(\beta_{ADV} \cdot 500)$

We use the Wald statistics to assess the significance of the coefficients and the Likelihood Ratio (G-index) to test the goodness of fit of the model (Harrell 2001; Balakrishnan 2013), being aware that these are not informative when, as here, the sample size is very large whence most if not all of the coefficients exhibit statistical significance. However, in order to interpret an estimated coefficient, we resort to the Odds Ratio, which can be computed, for any $i = 1, \ldots, p$, as $OR_i = exp(\beta_i)$.

Table 4 shows the results of each univariate logit model in terms of the estimated coefficients, the Odds-Ratios, eventually corrected by the unit of measure of the predictor, and the corresponding G-index for the model. The p-values associated to the Wald's test are all of order approximately $< 2e^{-16}$, except for the variable DEST for which is 0.013 %. This result together with the corresponding G-index (9.99) which is very low, justifies our previous idea that the contribution of the variable DEST to the response can be regarded as negligible and hence dropped from the final model.

This preliminary data analysis leads us finally to the identification of the best predictors to be considered in the logistic model.

4   The Estimated Logit Regression Model

At this point we consider 4 continuous, 2 discrete, 1 ordinal and 5 dichotomous predictors, so that the full 12 predictors logit regression model can be written as

$$g(x) = \beta_0 + \beta_1 \text{ ADV} + \beta_2 \text{ FIN} + \beta_3 \text{ INC} + \beta_4 \text{ AGE} + \beta_5 \text{ INST}+$$

$$\beta_6 \text{ HIST} + \beta_7 \text{ LOYAL(Medium)} + \beta_8 \text{ LOYAL(High)}+$$

Table 5 Estimates of the coefficients of the full model ordered by OR

	Beta	SE (beta)	OR
Const.	−3.3400	0.10500	
HIST	0.0194	0.04038	6.862
OCCU (self)	0.4289	0.04136	1.536
IRATE (high)	0.4224	0.04162	1.526
SEGM (high)	0.2033	0.04464	1.225
SEX (male)	0.1021	0.03181	1.108
FIN	0.0001	0.00001	1.036
INST	1.9260	0.00150	1.020
AGE	−0.0129	0.00131	0.987
ADV	−0.0002	0.00001	0.933
INC	−0.0002	0.00002	0.932
OWNER (yes)	−0.2606	0.03082	0.771
LOYAL (medium)	−0.4911	0.03152	0.612
LOYAL (high)	−0.6670	0.09473	0.513

$$\beta_9 \text{ SEX(Male)} + \beta_{10} \text{ OCCU(Self)} + \beta_{11} \text{ OWNER(Yes)} +$$

$$\beta_{12} \text{ SEGM(High)} + \beta_{13} \text{ IRATE(High)}.$$

Resorting to R software, defined the logit regression model via glm (Venables and Ripley 2002), we obtain estimates of the coefficients shown in Table 5 along with the correspondent standard errors.

We remark that all the p-values associated to the Wald's test applied to each coefficient are of order $< 2e^{-16}$, but for the predictor SEX for which it reduces to 0.133 %.

The G-index for the full model is 6,813.15 (on 13 d.f.) and due to the large sample size its p-value is clearly zero; so it does not tell us much about the goodness of fit of the model itself.

The elements of the matrix of the estimated covariances between the parameter estimates in the linear predictor of the model are all close to zero, suggesting non-collinearity among the predictors, as expected.

In order to have an idea about the contribution of each predictor to the response, we can consider (see Table 5) the Odds Ratios of each estimated coefficient ordered by their magnitude. Here, the ORs for ADV, FIN and INC are presented in terms of increments of 500 euros.

According to this classification, the best predictors are HIST, OCCU and IRATE. The very high value of the OR for HIST, and hence its heavy contribution to the predicted response, is clearly obvious if we recall the definition of HIST itself. Due to its low OR, we could drop LOYAL from the model. However, the society's staff argued that this predictor makes sense from the business point of view.

Table 6 Classification—I

	Observed Y	
Predicted $\hat{Y}$	0	1
0	$Nu(\hat{y}_i = 0 \mid y_i = 0)$	$Nu(\hat{y}_i = 0 \mid y_i = 1)$
1	$Nu(\hat{y}_i = 1 \mid y_i = 0)$	$Nu(\hat{y}_i = 1 \mid y_i = 1)$

Table 7 Classification—II

$\pi_0 = 0.50$	Observed Y			
Predicted $\hat{Y}$	Good	Bad	Good	Bad
Good	95,471	5,347	0.997	0.915
Bad	269	491	0.003	0.085

4.1 Classification Tables and the ROC Curve

Fixing a cut-off value π_0, we transform the n continuous fitted values $\hat{\pi}_i$ of the final model into n binary predicted $\hat{y}_i$ values according to

$$\hat{y}_i = \begin{cases} 0 & \hat{\pi}_i \leq \pi_0, \\ 1 & \hat{\pi}_i > \pi_0 \end{cases}$$

and in this way, we are able to construct the Classification Table, see Table 6.

If we now set the cut-off level $\pi_0 = 0.50$, we obtain the following Classification Table, see Table 7.

Hence, among the bad customers (5.75 % of the entire population), our model will correctly classify only 8.5 % of them as bad, while, among the good customers, it classifies 99.7 % of them correctly.

We can improve the predictive behaviour of the model looking for a different value for the cut-off. Varying $\pi \in [0, 1]$ and defining the functions

$$\text{Sensitivity}(\pi) = Nu(\hat{y}_i = 1 \mid y_i = 1)/Nu(y_i = 1),$$

$$\text{Specificity}(\pi) = Nu(\hat{y}_i = 0 \mid y_i = 0)/Nu(y_i = 0).$$

We can construct the ROC curve (Agresti 2010) plotting Sensitivity(π) as a function of $(1 - \text{Specificity}(\pi))$. The area under ROC curve is the Concordance-Index. The C-Index gives a measure of the concordance of predicted and observed values of the response and hence of the predictive power of the model. For our model we observe a value of the C-Index equal to 0.81 showing a quite good power of discrimination (see Fig. 4, panel b).

Analyzing the shape of the functions Sensitivity and Specificity, we can choose an optimal operating value for the cut-off. If we look at the plot of the two functions in Fig. 4, panel a, we may argue that a good cut-off point should lie approximately between 6 and 50 %. Thus we can re-define the optimal operating cut-off value as

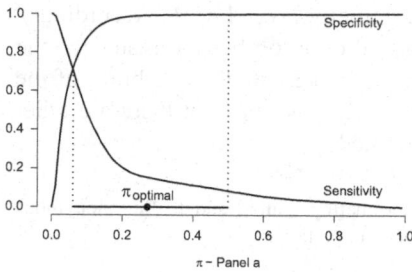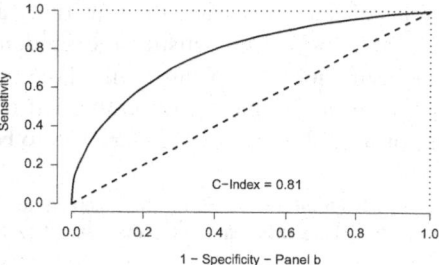

Fig. 4 Panel **a**: sensitivity and specificity functions and optimal cut-off point. Panel **b**: the Receiver Operating Characteristic curve and the C-Index

Table 8 Classification—III

$\pi_0 = 0.27$	Observed Y			
Predicted $\hat{Y}$	Good	Bad	Good	Bad
Good	94,857	4,952	0.991	0.848
Bad	882	886	0.009	0.152

Table 9 Classification—IV

$\pi_0 = 0.27$	Good	Bad	Good	Bad
Good	46,468	2,511	0.991	0.847
Bad	432	455	0.009	0.153

π_{optimal} such that Specificity$(\pi) = 0.99$. In our case, we obtain $\pi_{\text{optimal}} = 0.27$, corresponding to a value of Sensitivity$(\pi_{\text{optimal}}) = 0.15$. The new Classification Table with $\pi_0 = \pi_{\text{optimal}}$ is as Table 8.

Now, among the bad customers, our model will classify 15.2 % correctly as bad, while it correctly classifies 99.1 % of the good customers.

We remark that, comparing the two previous Classification Tables, the rate of bad customer classified as good decreases from 91.5 to 84.8 %.

Since our goal is to use the fitted logistic model to predict the behaviour of future customers, it seems natural to validate the fitted model on the training set. The percentage of bad customer in the training set is 5.95 % ($= 2966/49866$). The predictive power of the model on the training set is still good (C-index $= 0.80$) and for $\pi_0 = 0.27$ we have the following Classification Table, see Table 9.

We obtain (approximately) the same values for Sensitivity, Specificity and hence for C-Index: these results assess the goodness of fit of the proposed model.

5   Final Remarks

Despite a very detailed and thorough analysis of the available data, the identification of bad risk customers remains difficult. The current prediction model may be viewed in the same way as an Epidemiological screening test. In that context, such tests are acceptable only when the sensitivity and specificity exceed 85 %. Accordingly, the specificity result satisfies the Epidemiological criterion but the result for the sensitivity does not. Thus, while the current model forecasts the reliability of the customer during the repayment period in a fair way, it seems that there are other important risk factors which have yet to be identified.

Acknowledgements Authors are indebted to the coordinating editors and to the anonymous referees for carefully reading the manuscript and for their suggestions.

References

Agresti, A. (2010). *Analysis of ordinal categorical data* (2nd ed.). New York: Wiley.
Anderson, J. A. (1984). Regression and ordered categorical variables. *Journal for the Royal Statistical Society, B, 46*, 1–30.
Balakrishnan, N. (2013). *Handbook of the logistic distribution*. New York: CRC Press.
Harrell, F. E. (2001). *Regression modeling strategies*. New York: Springer.
Hastie, T., & Tibshirani, R. (1990). *Generalized additive models*. London: Chapman and Hall.
Hosmer, D. W., & Lemeshow, S. (2013). *Applied logistic regression* (3rd ed.). New York: Wiley.
McCullagh, P., & Nelder, J. A. (1989). *Generalized linear models*. London: Chapman and Hall.
Venables, W. N., & Ripley, B. D. (2002). *Modern applied statistics with S*. New York: Springer.

On Joint Modelling of Constrained Mean and Covariance Structures in Longitudinal Data

Jing Xu and Gilbert MacKenzie

Abstract A data-driven method for modelling the intra-subject covariance matrix is developed in the context of constrained marginal models arising in longitudinal data. A constrained iteratively re-weighted least squares estimation algorithm is applied. Some key asymptotic properties of the constrained ML estimates are given. We analyze a real data set in order to compare data-driven covariance modelling methods with classical menu-selection-based modelling techniques under a constrained mean model, extending the usual regression model for estimating generalized autoregressive parameters. Finally, we demonstrate, via a simulation study, that a correct choice of covariance matrix is required in order to minimise not only the bias, but also the variance, when estimating the constrained mean component.

Keywords Cholesky decomposition • Covariance modelling • Inequality constraints • Longitudinal data • Marginal models

1 Introduction

In longitudinal studies, constrained problems are often of interest in biomedicine and clinical trials. For example, in xenograft experiments, tumors in immunosuppressed mice usually continue to grow unchecked during the study period, leading to a larger mean size in the control group thereby generating a natural inequality constraint (Tan et al. 2005). Moreover, treatment effects arising in different groups in comparative clinical studies may form a natural ordering (Crowder and Hand 1990). Constrained problems of this type may be investigated using regression models with

J. Xu (✉)

Department of Mathematics, Statistics & Economics, Birkbeck College, London, UK

e-mail: j.xu@bbk.ac.uk

G. MacKenzie and D. Peng (eds.), *Statistical Modelling in Biostatistics and Bioinformatics*, Contributions to Statistics, DOI 10.1007/978-3-319-04579-5_8,
© Springer International Publishing Switzerland 2014

inequality constraints: see Xu and Wang (2008a,b), Fang et al. (2006), Tan et al. (2005), Shi et al. (2005) for constrained estimation and Pilla et al. (2006), Cysneiros and Paula (2004), Park et al. (1998), and Shin et al. (1996) for inequality-constrained hypothesis testing. The aim of this paper is to develop estimation methods for the parameters in constrained-mean covariance models.

Historically, intra-subject correlations have been modelled by menu selection techniques or by working correlation structures (Liang and Zeger 1986). The conventional approach is to select a particular covariance model from a menu of potential candidate structures, e.g., compound symmetry, AR(1), ARMA or unstructured covariance (Diggle et al. 2002). However, such procedures may not work well in practice. For example, misspecification of the working covariance structure may lead to a large loss of efficiency of the estimators of the mean parameters (Wang and Carey 2003). Although the unstructured covariance is assumed to approximate the true covariance structure, the number of nuisance parameters, say ρ_{jk}, in the resulting unstructured correlation matrix may be excessive and cause convergence problems in the iterative estimation process (Dobson 2002). We note, too, that when the true covariance structure is not contained in the menu set, this approach may fail to identify the optimum covariance structure suggested by the data (Pan and MacKenzie 2007). Therefore, in this paper, we adopted the data-driven method proposed by Pourahmadi (1999) to fit the covariance matrix in constrained models.

Accordingly, in Sect. 2 we formulate the constrained model and outline the data driven covariance modelling approach. In Sect. 3 we discuss constrained Maximum Likelihood Estimation, and outline some key elements of the relevant asymptotic theory for constrained estimators. In Sect. 4 we analyze data from a small diabetic study, consider two simulation studies in Sect. 5 and discuss the findings briefly in Sect. 6.

2 Model Formulation

2.1 Constrained Mean Covariance Model

Consider a balanced longitudinal study. Let m denote the common number of measurement times. The response vector for subject i is denoted by y_i. We assume that the y_i arise from the constrained marginal model

$$y_i = X_i\beta + \varepsilon_i \quad \text{for} \quad i = 1, \cdots, n \tag{1}$$

$$s.t. \quad A\beta \geqslant b,$$

where $s.t.$ means "subject to"; X_i is a known $m \times p$ design matrix for the ith individual; β is a $p \times 1$ vector of unknown coefficients to be estimated; A is a $k \times p$ matrix and $b = (b_1, \cdots, b_k)'$ is a $k \times 1$ vector; $\varepsilon_i = (\varepsilon_{i1}, \cdots, \varepsilon_{im})'$ are independently distributed as $N(0, \Sigma)$ for $i = 1, \cdots, n$. The inequality constraint set $\{\beta : A\beta \geq b\}$ is quite general, containing order restrictions as a special case.

2.2 Covariance Model

Since the subject-specific covariance matrix Σ is positive definite, there exists a unique lower triangular matrix, T, with 1's as main diagonal entries and a unique diagonal matrix, D, with positive diagonal entries such that $T\Sigma T' = D$. The below-diagonal entries of T are the negatives of the autoregressive coefficients, ϕ_{jk}, in $\hat{y}_{ij} = \mu_{ij} + \Sigma_{k=1}^{j-1}\phi_{jk}(y_{ik} - \mu_{ik})$, the linear least squares predictor of y_{ij} based on its predecessors $y_{i(j-1)}, \cdots, y_{i1}$. Here the μ_{ij}s are the expectations of the y_{ij}s. The diagonal entries of D are the innovation variances $\sigma_j^2 = var(y_{ij} - \hat{y}_{ij})$, where $1 \leq j \leq m$ and $1 \leq i \leq n$ (Pourahmadi 1999). The parameters ϕ_{jk} and $\varsigma_j \equiv \log \sigma_j^2$ are modelled as $\phi_{jk} = z'_{jk}\gamma$ and $\varsigma_j = h'_j\lambda$. Here γ and λ are vectors of order $q + 1$ and $d + 1$, respectively.

2.3 Joint Model

Thus, the constrained mean covariance model may be represented by an augmented regression model:

$$\mu_{ij} = x'_{ij}\beta \qquad \text{s.t.} \quad A\beta \geq b,$$
$$\phi_{jk} = z'_{jk}\gamma, \tag{2}$$
$$\varsigma_j = h'_j\lambda,$$

where β, γ and λ are the three regression parameters of scientific interest and only β is constrained. Typically, the design matrices are time- or lag-dependent i.e, $x'_{ij} = x(t)'_{ij}$, $z'_{jk} = z(lag)'_{jk}$ and $h'_j = h(t)'_j$. The latter two equations are said to define the class, C^*, of covariance structures when z'_{jk} is a polynomial in lag and h'_j is a polynomial in time, respectively (MacKenzie 2006). Now, our focus is on the effect of the constraints on simultaneous estimation of the parameters of interest.

The log-likelihood function for the parameters is given by

$$\ell(\beta, \gamma, \lambda) = -\frac{nm}{2}\log(2\pi) - \frac{n}{2}\log|T^{-1}DT'^{-1}| - \frac{1}{2}\sum_{i=1}^{n}r'_iT'D^{-1}Tr_i, \tag{3}$$

where $r_{ij} = y_{ij} - x'_{ij}\beta$ is the jth element of $r_i = y_i - X_i\beta$, the vector of residual, and the matrix X_i has row vectors $x'_{ij}(j = 1, 2, \cdots, m)$.

3   Constrained Maximum Likelihood Estimation

3.1   Estimation of Parameters

Denote the feasible solution set of the constrained model (2) by $S = \{\beta : A\beta \geqslant b\}$ and the function (3) by $\ell(\beta, \gamma, \lambda)$. Then the constrained ML estimation problem is

$$\max_{\beta \in S} \ell(\beta, \gamma, \lambda). \tag{4}$$

Based on the iteratively re-weighted least squares algorithm given by Pan and MacKenzie (2003), we present the following procedure for solving the constrained estimation problem (4).

Given γ and λ, the constrained regression parameters are determined by

$$\beta = \arg\min_{\beta \in S} \sum_{i=1}^{n} r_i' \Sigma^{-1} r_i. \tag{5}$$

Finding the optimal numerical solution for $\hat{\beta}$ in (5) is equivalent to solving a quadratic programming problem. Several methods are available in mathematical programming such as: the active set method, dual method and interior point method, (Fletcher 1971; Goldfarb and Ininani 1983). In practice, however, the *solve.QP* function in the *quadprog* package in the R language, can be used directly to obtain $\hat{\beta}$.

Secondly, given β and λ, the first order estimating equation for γ is

$$U_2(\gamma) = \sum_{i=1}^{n} Z_i^{*'} D^{-1} (r_i - Z_i^* \gamma) = 0, \tag{6}$$

where the matrix Z_i^*, of order $m \times (q + 1)$, has typical row $z_{ij}^{*'} = \sum_{k=1}^{j-1} r_{ik} z_{jk}'$. The estimates of γ can be obtained easily from Eq. (6). And finally, given β and γ, the estimating equation for λ is

$$U_3(\lambda) = \frac{1}{2} \sum_{i=1}^{n} H'(D^{-1} e_i - 1_m) = 0, \tag{7}$$

where $H = (h_1', h_2', \cdots, h_m')'$, $e_i = (e_{i1}, e_{i2}, \cdots, e_{im})'$ with $e_{ij} = (r_{ij} - \hat{r}_{ij})^2$ and $\hat{r}_{ij} = \sum_{k=1}^{j-1} \phi_{jk} r_{ik}$, are the $m \times (d + 1)$ matrix of covariates and the $m \times 1$ vector of squared fitted residuals, respectively, and 1_m is the $m \times 1$ vector of 1's. Equation (7) may be solved iteratively by the Newton–Raphson algorithm to obtain $\hat{\lambda}$.

By initializing at $\Sigma = I_m$, the iterative procedure proceeds within (5)–(7) until convergence. We refer to it as a constrained iteratively re-weighted least squares (CIRWLS) algorithm.

3.2 Asymptotic Properties

In this section some key asymptotic properties of the constrained estimates are only stated as they can be derived directly in the spirit of Xu and Wang (2008b). Those differences in computing certain moments, which are mostly due to the different but smoother reparameterisation of Σ, can also be found in Pourahmadi (2000).

All of the asymptotic results (as $n \to \infty$) take m, p, q and d to be fixed. Let parameter spaces $\mathcal{B}$, Γ and Λ, where $\beta \in \mathcal{B}$, $\gamma \in \Gamma$ and $\lambda \in \Lambda$, be compact subspaces of R^p, R^q and R^d. Let β_0 be the true parameter of β lying in $\mathcal{B}$ and $\alpha_0 = (\gamma_0', \lambda_0')'$ be the true parameter of $\alpha = (\gamma', \lambda')'$ lying in $\Gamma \times \Lambda$. Furthermore, we denote all of the unknown parameters by $\theta = (\beta', \gamma', \lambda')'$ and the unknown true values by $\theta_0 = (\beta_0', \gamma_0', \lambda_0')'$. Let a_j', $j = 1, \cdots, k$, be the rows of the matrix A. Define a $(p+q+d+3)$-dimensional vector $A_j = (a_j', 0, \cdots, 0)'$, for $j = 1, \cdots, k$. Then the constrained ML estimation problem (4) becomes

$$\max \ \ell(\theta): \qquad s.t. \quad A_j'\theta \geqslant b_j, j = 1, \cdots, k. \tag{8}$$

Here $A_j, j = 1, \cdots, k$ are assumed to be linearly independent. The optimization solution of the constrained estimators of problem (8) is denoted by $\hat{\theta}$. Moreover, for the remainder of the article, it is assumed that

Condition I. For all $\alpha \neq \alpha_0$ in $\Gamma \times \Lambda$,

$$\Sigma(\alpha) \neq \Sigma(\alpha_0),$$

where $\Sigma(\alpha) = T(\gamma)^{-1}D(\lambda)T'(\gamma)^{-1}$.

Condition I is needed to guarantee that the density function $f(y_i; \beta, \alpha)$ of Y_i is identifiable. Noting that the $(1, 1)$-th element in Σ is equal to the $(1, 1)$-th element in D, *Condition I* can be always satisfied given linear regression models of λ. The consistency of the maximum likelihood estimate is presented in Theorem 1.

Theorem 1. *Suppose that the design matrices X_i for $i = 1, 2, \cdots$, are bounded uniformly in the sense that there exists a real number c such that $|(X_i)_{ls}| \leq c$ where $(X_i)_{ls}$ is the (l, s)th element of X_i; the limit of $\frac{1}{n}\sum_{i=1}^{n} X_i' \Sigma^{-1}(\alpha) X_i$ exists for $\alpha \in \Gamma \times \Lambda$. Then the constrained ML estimators $\hat{\theta} = (\hat{\beta}', \hat{\gamma}', \hat{\lambda}')'$ are strongly consistent for the true value $\theta_0 = (\beta_0', \gamma_0', \lambda_0')'$; that is, $\hat{\theta} = (\hat{\beta}', \hat{\gamma}', \hat{\lambda}')' \to \theta_0 = (\beta_0', \gamma_0', \lambda_0')'$ almost surely as $n \to \infty$.*

Theorem 1 implies that $\hat{\theta}$ lies in a neighborhood of θ_0 when n is sufficiently large. Hence it is sufficient to discuss the properties of $\hat{\theta}$ in a small neighborhood of θ_0.

Next we give a brief description about the possible approximate representations of the constrained estimates $\hat{\theta}$ when n is sufficiently large. More details are available in Xu and Wang (2008b).

First denote the feasible solution set of the model (8) by $S = \{\theta : A'_j\theta \geqslant b_j, j = 1, \cdots, k\}$ which has the following subsets

$$S^\circ = \{\theta : A'_j\theta > b_j, j = 1, \cdots, k\};$$

$$S_j = \{\theta : A'_j\theta = b_j, A'_i\theta \geqslant b_i, i = 1, \cdots, k, i \neq j\};$$

$$S_{j_1, \cdots, j_t} = \cap^t_{l=1} S_{j_l}.$$

So the parameter θ_0 may be located in S°, or the relative interior parts of S_j or their intersections, $S_{j_1, \cdots, j_t}$.

Denoting the relative interior of a set, say K, by $ri(K)$ and recalling the consistency of $\hat\theta$, the following results obtain. If θ_0 is in S°, then $\hat\theta$ must be located in S° with a probability approaching to one for sufficiently large n. If θ_0 is in $ri(S_1) = \{\theta : A'_1\theta = b_1, A'_i\theta > b_i, i = 2, \cdots, k\}$, then $\hat\theta$ may be in S° or $ri(S_1)$ with a probability approaching to one for sufficiently large n. If θ_0 is in $ri(S_{12}) = (\theta : A'_1\theta = b_1, A'_2\theta = b_2, A'_j\theta > b_j, j = 3, \cdots, k)$, then most of $\hat\theta$ may be in S°, $ri(S_1)$, $ri(S_2)$ and $ri(S_{12})$. Other cases can be analyzed similarly. Then, if $\hat\theta$ is in, for instance, $ri(S_{12})$, the inequality-constrained problem (8) is reduced to an equality-constrained problem with a constraint set $\{A'_1\theta = b_1, A'_2\theta = b_2\}$. Thus, the approximate representation of $\hat\theta$ may be obtained by equality constrained optimization method.

In conclusion, for a given location of θ_0 except S°, the estimators $n^{\frac{1}{2}}(\hat\theta - \theta_0)$ will have different approximate representations, hence different asymptotic distributions (see Theorem 2), according to different locations of $\hat\theta$.

Theorem 2 explains that the constrained ML estimator $\hat\theta$ has a piecewise asymptotic normal distribution.

Theorem 2. *Suppose that*

$$V^{11}_n(\beta_0, \alpha_0) = \frac{1}{n} \sum_{i=1}^n E_0 \left[\frac{\partial \log f(Y_i; \beta, \alpha)}{\partial \beta} \frac{\partial \log f(Y_i; \beta, \alpha)'}{\partial \beta} \right] \Big|_{\substack{\beta = \beta_0 \\ \alpha = \alpha_0}} \to V_{11}(\beta_0, \alpha_0);$$

$$V^{22}_n(\beta_0, \alpha_0) = \frac{1}{n} \sum_{i=1}^n E_0 \left[\frac{\partial \log f(Y_i; \beta, \alpha)}{\partial \alpha} \frac{\partial \log f(Y_i; \beta, \alpha)'}{\partial \alpha} \right] \Big|_{\substack{\beta = \beta_0 \\ \alpha = \alpha_0}} \to V_{22}(\beta_0, \alpha_0),$$

where $f(y_i; \beta, \alpha)$ is the density function of Y_i; E_0 denotes the expectation operator with $\beta = \beta_0$ and $\alpha = \alpha_0$. All the matrices $V^{11}_n(\beta_0, \alpha_0)$, $V^{22}_n(\beta_0, \alpha_0)$ and $V_{11}(\beta_0, \alpha_0)$, $V_{22}(\beta_0, \alpha_0)$ are assumed to be positive definite. Further, let $V = \text{diag}(V_{11}(\beta_0, \alpha_0), V_{22}(\beta_0, \alpha_0))$ and $V_n = \text{diag}(V^{11}_n(\beta_0, \alpha_0), V^{22}_n(\beta_0, \alpha_0))$. The computation of V_n at the true value θ_0 is given in the appendix.

Then, under the same assumptions in Theorem 1, when $\hat\theta$ is in S°, the asymptotic distribution of $\hat\theta$ follows

$$n^{\frac{1}{2}}(\hat\theta - \theta_0) \xrightarrow{L} N(0, V^{-1})';$$

when $\hat{\theta}$ is not in $S°$, the asymptotic distribution of $\hat{\theta}$ follows

$$n^{\frac{1}{2}}(\hat{\theta} - \theta_0) \xrightarrow{L} N(0, CV^{-1}),$$

where $C = I - V^{-1}G(G'V^{-1}G)^{-1})G'$ with $G = (A_{j_1}, \cdots, A_{j_t})$ with $\{j_1, \cdots, j_t\} = \{i : A_i'\hat{\theta} = b_i, i = 1, \cdots, k\}$ and I being a $(p + q + d + 3)$-order identity matrix. Here "$\xrightarrow{L}$" stands for convergence in distribution.

4   Re-analysis of Diabetic Patient Data

4.1   The Data

We reanalyze data on a comparative study among diabetic groups given by Crowder and Hand (1990). These data have been analyzed by Shin et al. (1996) and Cysneiros and Paula (2004) in the context of inequality hypothesis testing. Originally, there were four patient groups, but following Shin et al. (1996) and Cysneiros and Paula (2004), we only consider three groups: the control group ($n_1 = 8$), the diabetic group without complications ($n_2 = 6$) and the diabetic group with hypertension ($n_3 = 7$). For each patient the response, a physical task, was measured at $1, 2, 3, 4, 5, 6, 8$ and 10 min. Additional responses were measured at 12 and 15 min, but these were dropped because a high proportion were missing. One additional missing response, at minute 8, was imputed by the mean response at that time. Accordingly, the data selected for analysis are balanced, but irregularly spaced. They comprise a challenging set because of the relatively small sample size. Data analysis and simulations in this paper were conducted in the R software package (Version 2.8.1). The function *solve.QP* adopted in programmes for constrained optimization is from the R package *quadprog* contributed by Berwin A. Turlach and Andreas Weingessel.

4.2   Joint Constrained Mean Covariance Regression Models

Scatterplots of the response against time suggest that three constant means may be appropriate for these data. Measurement times are rescaled to $j = 1, 2, \cdots, 8$. Let y_{ilj} be the observed physical task for the ith patient of the lth group at the time j. Here $l = 1, 2, 3$ is merely a group indicator. We assume model (2), namely: $y_{il} = \mu_l^* + \varepsilon_i$, where $\mu_l^* = \mu_l \times 1$ and μ_l is a scalar representing the common mean value in group l, where 1 is the $(m \times 1)$ unit vector. In particular, we have $\mu_1 \geq \mu_2 \geq \mu_3$. Moreover, we assume $\varepsilon_i \sim N(0, \Sigma)$ across subjects. Shin et al. (1996) and Cysneiros and Paula (2004) adopted similar conventions in their analysis.

Table 1 Diabetic patient data

j	1	2	3	4	5	6	7	8
1	*10.1*	0.973	0.969	0.978	0.932	0.931	0.887	0.879
2	0.970	*10.1*	0.966	0.954	0.895	0.901	0.812	0.808
3	0.533	0.404	*9.2*	0.975	0.925	0.930	0.851	0.844
4	0.633	−0.174	0.545	*9.9*	0.950	0.951	0.875	0.871
5	0.372	−0.346	0.106	0.904	*11.9*	0.966	0.915	0.905
6	−0.050	0.002	0.086	0.331	0.627	*11.3*	0.888	0.879
7	1.902	−1.157	0.187	−0.698	0.836	0.082	*18.5*	0.982
8	0.171	0.101	−0.139	0.282	−0.031	−0.021	0.997	*19.4*
$\hat{\sigma}^2$	10.1	0.5	0.5	0.3	1.1	0.6	2.0	0.7

Sample variances (along the main diagonal), correlations (above the main diagonal), generalized autoregressive parameters (below the main diagonal) and innovation variances (last row)

Table 1 shows the sample variances (main diagonal) and the sample correlation matrix (upper triangle) computed from the data. Inspection suggests that a model with a stationary covariance structure and strong correlation would be a reasonable model choice. Accordingly, classic covariance structures such as compound symmetry CS, $AR(1)$ and $ARMA(1, 1)$ are strong competitors for a *data-driven* covariance modelling approach.

We fitted model (2), using the group constraints described above and C^*, and estimated the generalized autoregressive parameters, ϕ_{jk}, $k < j$, $j = 2, \cdots, 8$, and innovation variances, σ_j^2, $j = 1 \cdots, 8$. The estimated generalized autoregressive parameters (Table 1, lower triangle) showed strong dependence on both indices j and k and we fitted the extended model

$$\phi_{jk} = \gamma_0 + \gamma_1 j + \cdots + \gamma_{q_1} j^{q_1} + \gamma_1^* k + \cdots + \gamma_{q_2}^* k^{q_2} + \gamma_1^{**}(j \times k) + \cdots + \gamma_{q_3}^{**}(j \times k)^{q_3},$$

in order to capture this structure. Here $j = 2, \cdots, 8$ and $k = 1, \cdots, 7$ and

$$\gamma = (\gamma_0, \gamma_1, \cdots, \gamma_{q_1}, \gamma_1^*, \cdots, \gamma_{q_2}^*, \gamma_1^{**}, \cdots, \gamma_{q_3}^{**})'$$

with $\dim(\gamma) = q = q_1 + q_2 + q_3$. This model extends the standard regression model in which γ^* and γ^{**} are absent. We call the class of covariance structures indexed by the extended model, C^{**}. In the context of these data, it is a rather ambitious model, but we sought a low order polynomial model in the indices and their interaction satisfying the usual marginality constraints.

4.3 Model Selection

In the sequel we label the standard covariance model $CM1$ and the extended model $CM2$. We fitted two versions of each: $CM1_a$ with $q = 3$ (generalized auto-regressive parameters) and $d = 3$ (innovation variances) and $CM1_b$ with $q = 5$

Table 2 Data-driven, regression-based, covariance modelling for Σ compared with several menu-selection methods

Structure of Σ	No. of parameters	$\hat{l}_{max}$	AIC	BIC
CS	2	−310.26	29.74	29.84
AR(1)	2	−269.46	25.85	25.95
ARMA(1,1)	3	−267.77	25.79	25.94
$CM1_a$	8	−262.28	25.74	26.14
$CM2_a$	11	−258.26	25.64	26.19
$CM1_b$	14	−250.11	25.15	25.85
$CM2_b$	15	−247.11	24.96	25.71

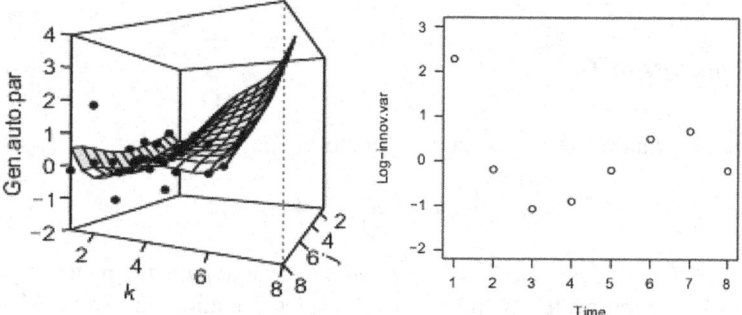

Fig. 1 Fitted regressograms for the diabetic patient data, model $CM2_b$. *Left*: fitted generalized autoregressive parameters and surface; *Right*: fitted log-innovation variances

and $d = 7$; $CM2_a$ with $q_1 = 2, q_2 = 2, q_3 = 2$ and $d = 3$ and $CM2_b$ with $q_1 = 5, q_2 = 4, q_3 = 1$ and $d = 3$. In addition, we fitted three stationary models: CS, $AR(1)$ and $ARMA(1, 1)$, making seven models in total.

We used the $BIC = -(2/n)\hat{\ell}_{max} + (q + d + 2)\log n/n$ as our model selection criterion and include the $AIC = -(2/n)\hat{\ell}_{max} + 2(q + d + 2)/n$ for comparison. The smaller the AIC or BIC value, the better the model. We systematically searched C^* for the optimum standard model (Pan and MacKenzie 2003) and found $CM1_b$ above. Then we searched the extended covariance class C^{**} and found $CM2_b$. The other two covariance models are included for the purposes of comparison. The stationary models were fitted directly using a specially written Fisher-scoring algorithm for constrained mean optimization.

The results are shown in Table 2. The model with the minimum BIC is $CM2_b$ and details of the fit are given in Fig. 1. However, the classical $AR(1)$ and $ARMA(1, 1)$ models are very close competitors. The extended covariance models, $CM2$, perform best in terms of BIC, but the AR(1) model, which fits two parameters, is preferred on the grounds of simplicity of interpretation. Overall, Table 2 allows us to exclude the CS model and adopt the $AR(1)$ model on the grounds that its BIC is close to that of the optimum model in C^{**} (MacKenzie 2006).

Finally, we remark that all of this model fitting is exploratory rather than confirmatory.

5 Simulation Studies

Two different simulation studies are conducted. The first study aims to investigate
how mis-specification of the covariance structure affects the estimates of the mean
($\pm s.e$) in the constrained model. We also present the results for unconstrained
models. The emphasis is on non-stationary covariance models. The objective of
the second study is to investigate the utility (if any) of the extended model $CM2$.
For simplicity, however, we only consider balanced and regular designs in these
simulation studies.

5.1 Simulation I

The simulated data were generated from the following model

$$y_{il}(t_j) = \mu_l + W_i(t_j) + \varepsilon_i(t_j)$$

for: $l = 1, 2, 3$; $i = 1, \cdots, n$; $j = 1, \cdots, m$; and where μ_l is the mean of group l.
The $W_i(t_j)$, generating the within subject serial correlation, are sampled from n
independent copies of a non-stationary Gaussian process. The $\varepsilon_i(t_j)$, measurement
error, are a set of $N = m \times n$ mutually independent Gaussian random variables and
$W_i(t_j)$ and $\varepsilon_i(t_j)$ are statistically independent.

We present representative results from our simulation study for the particular
case $n = 60$ ($n_l = 20$, $l = 1, 2, 3$), time points $t_j : j = 1, \cdots, m = 8$, with
a diabetic data-directed mean: $\mu_1 = 7.322$, $\mu_2 = 6.860$ and $\mu_3 = 4.191$. We
sampled the $W_i(t_j)$ from an $ARIMA(1, 1, 0)$ process. Denoting $W_i(t_j) - W_i(t_{(j-1)})$
by $\triangle W_i(t_j)$, the $\triangle W_i(t_j)$ can be represented as AR(1) model, i.e, $\triangle W_i(t_j) =
\rho \triangle W_i(t_{(j-1)}) + Z_i(t_j)$. We set $\rho = \exp(-0.5)$. The $Z_i(t_j)$ white noise random
variables were generated with $E(Z_i(t_j)) = 0$ and $Var(Z_i(t_j)) = \sigma^2(1-\rho^2)$, to give
$Var(\triangle W_i(t_j)) = \sigma^2$ and we set $\sigma = 3$. The random variables $\varepsilon_i(t_j)$ are mutually
independent with $E(\varepsilon_i(t_j)) = 0$ and $Var(\varepsilon_i(t_j)) = 1$.

In contrast to the stationary covariance structure in the diabetic patient data, our
simulated data have a non-stationary covariance structure as the variance of $y_i(t_j)$
increases with time t_j and correlations between $y_i(t_j)$ and $y_i(t_{j+k})$ also increases
with time t_j for a given lag k. For the constrained case we have $\mu_1 \geqslant \mu_2 \geqslant \mu_3$. The
number of replications was 500.

The following models were fitted: $CM1$ with $q = 3$ and $d = 3$, CS, $AR(1)$ and
$ARMA(1, 1)$. The results are shown in Table 3. The data-driven covariance model,
$CM1$, performs much better than the other three models in the constrained and
unconstrained cases. In particular, the smaller biases and reduced standard errors
should be noted, particularly in the constrained case. In the unconstrained case, the
bias is negligible for all models, but the standard errors in $CM1$ are 33–40% of
those produced by the other models.

Table 3 Simulation I. Average maximum likelihood estimates and standard errors: for the true model and four completing models in constrained and unconstrained cases

| Est. | True | Constrained | | | |
		CM1	CS	AR1	ARMA
$\hat{\mu}_1$	7.322	7.433(0.732)	7.843(1.853)	7.827(1.820)	7.830(1.826)
$\hat{\mu}_2$	6.860	6.731(0.723)	6.505(1.619)	6.512(1.603)	6.513(1.613)
$\hat{\mu}_3$	4.191	4.150(0.843)	3.928(2.011)	3.938(1.996)	3.934(2.006)
$\hat{l}$	−1,120.048	−1,134.989	−1,686.788	−1,332.732	−1,280.458
AIC	37.435	38.100	56.293	44.491	42.782
BIC	37.540	38.379	56.363	44.561	42.887
Est.	True	Unconstrained			
		CM1	CS	AR1	ARMA
$\hat{\mu}_1$	7.322	7.306(0.832)	7.312(2.268)	7.318(2.215)	7.324(2.219)
$\hat{\mu}_2$	6.860	6.855(0.824)	6.861(2.034)	6.851(2.008)	6.847(2.019)
$\hat{\mu}_3$	4.191	4.153(0.848)	4.102(2.222)	4.107(2.191)	4.106(2.201)
$\hat{l}$	−1,120.048	−1,134.784	−1,686.543	−1,332.593	−1,280.318
AIC	37.435	38.100	56.285	44.486	42.777
BIC	37.540	38.379	56.355	44.556	42.882

It is generally well known that constrained models produce a smaller mean square error for the estimates of mean, but that this may conceal a larger bias (Liew 1976; Xu and Wang 2008a). So the bias here must arise in part from the constraints imposed. However, it is interesting to note that the data-driven model produces much smaller biases compared with the menu-selection models in the constrained case. Accordingly, we may conclude that covariance mis-specification exacerbates the bias in the mean caused by the imposed constraints.

5.2 Simulation II

We simulated the data for the three groups data from the model

$$y_{il}(t_j) = \mu_l + u_i + \varepsilon_i(t_j)$$

for: $l = 1, 2, 3$; $i = 1, \cdots, n$; $j = 1, \cdots, m$. The random variables u_i are mutually independent with $E(u_i) = 0$ and $Var(u_i) = v^2$. The random variables $\varepsilon_i(t_j)$ are mutually independent with $E(\varepsilon_i(t_j)) = 0$ and $Var(\varepsilon_i(t_j)) = \tau^2$. These two types of random variables are independent. The remaining assumptions are the same as in *Simulation I*. Denote by I and J the $m \times m$ identity matrix and the $m \times m$ unit matrix. Let $\rho = v^2/(v^2 + \tau^2)$ and $\sigma^2 = v^2 + \tau^2$. Then, $\Sigma = \sigma^2\{(1-\rho)I + \rho J\}$ has a Compound Symmetric structure. The modified Cholesky decomposition of this matrix Σ is $T \Sigma T' = D$ where

Table 4 Simulation II. Maximised log-likelihood estimates and *AIC* and *BIC*: comparison of *CM2* and *CM1* under a Compound Symmetry model

Est.	$var(u_i) = 2^2, var(\varepsilon_i) = 1$			$var(u_i) = 3^2, var(\varepsilon_i) = 1$		
	True	CM2	CM1	True	CM2	CM1
$\hat{l}$	−785.809	−786.336	−804.336	−809.615	−819.084	−843.160
AIC	26.260	26.478	27.082	27.054	27.569	28.372
BIC	26.330	26.757	27.361	27.124	27.849	28.651

$$T = \begin{pmatrix} 1 & 0 & 0 & \dots 0 \\ -\frac{\rho}{1+\rho} & 1 & 0 & \dots 0 \\ -\frac{\rho}{1+2\rho} & -\frac{\rho}{1+2\rho} & 1 & \dots 0 \\ \vdots & \vdots & \vdots & \vdots \\ -\frac{\rho}{1+(m-2)\rho} & -\frac{\rho}{1+(m-2)\rho} & -\frac{\rho}{1+(m-2)\rho} & \dots 1 \end{pmatrix}$$

and

$$D = \mathrm{diag}\{\sigma^2, \sigma^2(1 - \frac{\rho^2}{1+\rho}), \sigma^2(1 - \frac{\rho^2}{1+2\rho}), \cdots, \sigma^2(1 - \frac{(m-1)\rho^2}{1+(m-1)\rho})\}.$$

Notice that in T the values in every sub-diagonal decrease when the indices j and k increase. Accordingly, this suggests modelling both indices simultaneously using *CM2*, rather than *CM1* which uses just one value to fit every sub-diagonal. Imposing the inequality restriction on the model, we set $q1 = 1$, $q2 = 1$ and $q3 = 1$ and $d = 3$ for *CM2* and $q = 3$ and $d = 3$ for *CM1*. Furthermore, we consider two different cases: $var(u_i) = 2^2$ and $var(u_i) = 3^2$.

The results are in Table 4 and show, as expected, that model *CM2* is closer to the true model than model *CM1* in sense of the likelihood and the AIC and BIC criteria, although its superiority is not particularly compelling in the scenarios studied.

6 Discussion

This is our first foray into joint mean-covariance modelling, where the mean is subject to inequality constraints. The asymptotic theory for constrained estimators is much more complicated than the standard theory. Accordingly, we generalized the work of Xu and Wang (2008a,b) on fixed effect estimation with inequality constraints by adding a data-driven marginal covariance model via the modified Cholesky decomposition and applied many of the covariance modelling techniques developed in Pan and MacKenzie (2003) to analyse the diabetic data. For some covariance structures, the generalized autoregressive coefficients, ϕ_{jk}, vary with j and k simultaneously and we extended the usual model to capture this variation, with some limited success. In all of the analyses undertaken, the covariance models performed well and the technique is clearly feasible even when dealing with small sample sizes. Its real strength lies, perhaps, in modelling non-stationary features where variances increase over time, and measurements equidistant in time are not equi-correlated, as has been demonstrated in the analysis of Kenward (1987)'s cattle data (Pourahmadi 2000; Pan and MacKenzie 2006). In the constrained mean context we point to the smaller standard errors obtained and to the reduction in bias as obvious advantages of the method. We have clearly demonstrated that misspecification of the covariance structure can impact adversely on the estimation of the mean component (MacKenzie 2006).

This first paper has only addressed the constrained mean marginal model and naturally it has not been possible to tackle other covariance modelling issues which will form the subject of future work.

Acknowledgements This paper is one of several emanating from the BIO-SI project (07/MI/012) supported by Science Foundation Ireland (SFI), see www3.ul.ie/bio-si. Dr. Xu is a SFI postdoctoral research fellow and Professor MacKenzie is the principal investigator. The authors gratefully acknowledge Professor Jianxin Pan, Manchester University, UK, for helpful discussions and thank Professor Martin Crowder, Imperial College, London,UK, for supplying the interesting data set.

Appendix

Computation of V_n

Since the log-likelihood function $L(Y_1, \cdots, Y_n; \theta)$ is regular with respect to its first and second derivatives, i.e.,

$$E \partial L / \partial \theta = 0 \quad \text{and} \quad -E \partial^2 L / \partial \theta \partial \theta' = E \partial L / \partial \theta \partial L / \partial \theta',$$

the covariance matrix V_n can be obtained by computing the expectation of the second order derivatives of $L(Y_1, \cdots, Y_n; \theta)$ at the true value $\theta = \theta_0$.

It is easy to verify that

$$v_n^{11} = -n^{-1} E_0 \partial^2 L / \partial \beta \beta' \Big|_{\theta = \theta_0} = n^{-1} \sum_{i=1}^{n} X_i' \Sigma_i^{-1} (\gamma_0, \lambda_0) X_i,$$

where E_0 denotes the expectation operator at the point $\theta = \theta_0$.

Setting $r_{i[j-1]} = (r_{i1}, \cdots, r_{i(j-1)})'$ and $Z_{i[j-1]}^* = (z_{ij1}, \cdots, z_{ij(j-1)})'$ for $j = 1, \cdots, m_i$, then we have

$$v_n^{22} = -n^{-1} E_0 \partial^2 L / \partial \gamma \gamma' \Big|_{\theta=\theta_0}$$

$$= n^{-1} E_0 \sum_{i=1}^{n} Z_i^{*'} D_i^{-1} Z_i^* \Big|_{\theta=\theta_0}$$

$$= n^{-1} E_0 \sum_{i=1}^{n} \sum_{j=2}^{m_i} \sigma_{ij}^{-2} z_{ij}^* z_{ij}^{*'} \Big|_{\theta=\theta_0}$$

$$= n^{-1} E_0 \sum_{i=1}^{n} \sum_{j=2}^{m_i} \sigma_{ij}^{-2} Z_{i[j-1]}^{*'} r_{i[j-1]}' r_{i[j-1]} Z_{i[j-1]}^* \Big|_{\theta=\theta_0}$$

$$= n^{-1} \sum_{i=1}^{n} \sum_{j=2}^{m_i} \exp(-h_{ij}' \lambda_0) Z_{i[j-1]}^{*'} \Sigma_{i[j-1]}(\gamma_0, \lambda_0) Z_{i[j-1]}^*,$$

where $\Sigma_{i[j-1]} = E_0(\varepsilon_{i[j-1]}' \varepsilon_{i[j-1]})$ with $\varepsilon_{i[j-1]} = (\varepsilon_{i1}, \cdots, \varepsilon_{i(j-1)})'$.

Noticing that $e_{ij} = (r_{ij} - \hat{r}_{ij})^2 = T_{ij}' r_i r_i' T_{ij}$ with T_{ij}' is the j-th row of T_i and defining R_i by $R_i = diag\{e_{i1}, \cdots, e_{im_i}\}$, then we get

$$v_n^{33} = -n^{-1} E_0 \partial^2 L / \partial \lambda \lambda' \Big|_{\theta=\theta_0}$$

$$= (2n)^{-1} E_0 \sum_{i=1}^{n} H_i' D_i^{-1} R_i H_i \Big|_{\theta=\theta_0}$$

$$= (2n)^{-1} \sum_{i=1}^{n} H_i' D_i^{-1}(\lambda_0) diag\{T_{i1}' \Sigma_i(\gamma_0, \lambda_0) T_{i1}, \cdots, T_{im_i}' \Sigma_i(\gamma_0, \lambda_0) T_{im_i}\} H_i.$$

After some matrix algebra, we can see that the factors containing random error in the elements of the matrices $\partial^2 L / \partial \beta \partial \gamma'$, $\partial^2 L / \partial \beta \partial \lambda'$ and $\partial^2 L / \partial \gamma \partial \lambda'$ are the residual vectors $r_i, i = 1, \cdots, n$, the expectations of which are zero at the true value $\theta = \theta_0$. Thus

$$v_n^{kl} = 0 \quad \text{for} \quad k \neq l \quad \text{with} \quad k, l = 1, 2, 3.$$

References

Crowder, M. J., & Hand, D. J. (1990). *Analysis of repeated measures*. London: Chapman and Hall.
Cysneiros, F. J. A., & Paula, G. A. (2004). One sided tests in linear models with multivariate t-distribution. *Communications in Statistics: Simulation and Computation, 33*, 747–771.
Diggle, P. J., Heagerty, P., Liang, K. Y., & Zeger, S. L. (2002). *Analysis of longitudinal data* (2nd ed.). London: Oxford.

Dobson, A. J. (2002). *An introduction to generalized linear models* (2nd ed.). London: Chapman and Hall.

Fang, H., Tian, G., Xiong, X., & Tan, M. (2006). A multivariate random-effects model with restricted parameters: Application to assessing radiation therapy for brain tumours. *Statistics in Medicine, 25*, 1948–1959.

Fletcher, R. (1971). A general quadratic programming algorithm. *Journal of the Institute of Mathematics and its Applications, 7*, 76–91.

Goldfarb, D., & Ininani, A. (1983). A numerical stable dual method for solving strictly convex quadratic programs. *Mathematical Programming, 27*, 1–33.

Kenward, M. G. (1987) A method for comparing profiles of repeated measurements. *Applied Statistics, 36*, 296–308.

Liang, K. Y., & Zeger, G. (1986). Longitudinal data analysis using generalized linear models. *Biometrika, 73*, 13–22.

Liew, C. K. (1976). Inequality constrained least squares estimations. *Journal of the American Statistical Association, 71*, 13–22.

MacKenzie, G. (2006). In discussion of double hierarchical generalized linear models. *Journal of the Royal Statistical Society. Series: C, 55*, 139–185.

Pan, J., & MacKenzie, G. (2003). On modelling mean-covariance structure in longitudinal studies. *Biometrika, 90*, 239–244.

Pan, J., & MacKenzie, G. (2006). Regression models for covariance structures in longitudinal studies. *Statistical Modelling, 7*, 49–71.

Pan, J., & MacKenzie, G. (2007). Modelling conditional covariance in the linear mixed model. *Statistical Modelling, 7*, 49–71.

Park, T., Shin, D. W., & Park, C. G. (1998). A generalized estimating equations approach for testing ordered group effects with repeated measurements. *Biometrics, 54*, 1645–1653.

Pilla, R. S., Qu, A., & Loader, C. (2006). Testing for order-restricted hypotheses in longitudinal data. *Journal of the Royal Statistical Society. Series: B, 68*, 437–455.

Pourahmadi, M. (1999). Joint mean-covariance models with applications to longitudinal data: Unconstrained parameterisation. *Biometrika, 86*, 677–690.

Pourahmadi, M. (2000). Maximum likelihood estimation of generalised linear models for multivariate normal covariance matrix. *Biometrika, 87*, 425–435.

Shi, N. Z., Zheng, S. R., & Guo, J. (2005). The restricted em algorithm under inequality restrictions on the parameters. *Journal of Multivariate Analysis, 92*, 53–76.

Shin, D. W., Park, C. G., & Park, T. (1996). Testing for ordered group effects with repeated measurements. *Biometrika, 83*, 688–694.

Tan, M., Fang, H., Tian, G., & Houghton, P. J. (2005). Repeated-measures models with constrained parameters for incomplete data in tumour xenograft experients. *Statistics in Medicine, 24*, 109–119.

Wang, Y. G., & Carey, V. (2003). Working correlation structure misspecification, estimation and covariate design: Implications for generalized estimating equations performance. *Biometrika, 90*, 29–41.

Xu, J., & Wang, J. (2008b). Maximum likelihood estimation of linear models for longitudinal data with inequality constraints. *Communication in Statistics-Theory and Methods, 37*, 931–946.

Xu, J., & Wang, J. (2008a). Two-stage estimation of inequality-constrained marginal linear models with longitudinal data. *Journal of Statistical Planning and Inference, 138*, 1905–1918.

Part III
Statistical Model Development

Hierarchical Generalized Nonlinear Models

Roger W. Payne

Abstract Hierarchical generalized linear models allow non-Normal data to be modelled in situations when there are several sources of error variation. They extend the familiar generalized linear models to include additional random terms in the linear predictor. However, they do not constrain these terms to follow a Normal distribution nor to have an identity link, as is the case in the more usual generalized linear mixed model. They thus provide a much richer set of models, that may seem more intuitively appealing. Another extension to generalized linear models allows nonlinear parameters to be included in the linear predictor. The fitting algorithm for these generalized nonlinear models operates by performing a nested optimization, in which a generalized linear model is fitted for each evaluation in an optimization over the nonlinear parameters. The optimization search thus operates only over the (usually relatively few) nonlinear parameters, and this should be much more efficient than a global optimization over the whole parameter space. This paper reviews the generalized nonlinear model algorithm, and explains how similar principles can be used to include nonlinear fixed parameters in the mean model of a hierarchical generalized linear model, thus defining a *hierarchical generalized nonlinear model*.

Keywords Hierarchical generalized linear models • Hierarchical generalized nonlinear models

R.W. Payne (✉)
Department of Computational and Systems Biology, Rothamsted Research, Harpenden, Herts AL5 2JQ, UK

VSN International, 5 The Waterhouse, Waterhouse Street, Hemel Hempstead, Herts HP1 1ES, UK
e-mail: Roger.Payne@vsni.co.uk

G. MacKenzie and D. Peng (eds.), *Statistical Modelling in Biostatistics and Bioinformatics*, Contributions to Statistics, DOI 10.1007/978-3-319-04579-5_9,
© Springer International Publishing Switzerland 2014

1 Introduction

The methodology of hierarchical generalized linear models (HGLMs) was devised by Lee and Nelder (1996) to provide a flexible and efficient framework for modelling non-Normal data in situations when there are several sources of error variation. They extend the familiar generalized linear models (GLMs) to include additional random terms in the linear predictor.

In an ordinary regression the model to be fitted is

$$y = \mu + \varepsilon,$$

where μ is the mean predicted by a model

$$\mu = X\beta,$$

(e.g. $a+b\times x$), and ε is the residual with Normal distribution $N(0, \sigma^2)$. Equivalently, we can write that y has Normal distribution $N(\mu, \sigma^2)$.

In a GLM the expected value of y is still

$$E(y) = \mu,$$

but model now defines the *linear predictor*

$$\eta = X\beta$$

with μ and η related by the *link function g*

$$\eta = g(\mu)$$

and y has a distribution with mean μ from the exponential family; see McCullagh and Nelder (1989).

In a HGLM, the expected value $E(y)$ is still μ, and this is still related to the linear predictor by a link function $g()$. The vector y still has a distribution from the exponential family, but this is currently limited to binomial, gamma, Normal or Poisson. The linear predictor now contains additional random terms

$$\eta = X\beta + \sum_i Z_i v_i$$

which have their own link functions

$$v_i = v(u_i)$$

and the vectors of random effects u_i have beta, Normal, gamma or inverse gamma distributions (these being the distributions that are conjugate to the distributions available for y). For details see Lee et al. (2006).

The analysis involves fitting an augmented GLM, known as the *augmented mean model*, to describe the mean vector μ. This has units corresponding to the original data units, together with an additional unit for each effect of a random term. The augmented mean model is fitted as a GLM, but there may be different link functions and distributions operating on the additional units from those on the original units. The link function is the function $v()$, while the distribution is the one to which the distribution of u_i is conjugate; see Chap. 6 of Lee et al. (2006) for details. The data values for the extra units contain the inverse-link transformations of the expected values of the random distributions. The HGLM algorithm also involves further GLMs, with gamma distributions and usually with logarithmic links, to model the dispersion for each random term (including the residual dispersion parameter ϕ). The models are connected, in that the y-variates for the dispersion models are deviance contributions from the augmented mean model divided by one minus their leverages, while the reciprocals of the fitted values from the dispersion models act as weights for the augmented mean model. So the models are fitted alternately until convergence, as shown in Table 7.3 of Lee et al. (2006).

The methodology has been implemented in GenStat, as a suite of procedures (i.e. sub-programs written in the GenStat language); see Payne et al. (2006b). From its 9th Edition GenStat also includes data files and programs to run many of the worked examples from Lee et al. (2006).

1.1 Generalized Nonlinear Models

Another extension to GLMs allows for the inclusion of nonlinear parameters in the linear predictor; see Lane (1996), or Sect. 3.5.8 of Payne et al. (2006a). The linear predictor is still

$$\eta = X\beta = \sum x_i \beta_i,$$

but some of the x_i's may now be nonlinear functions of other explanatory variables and parameters that must be estimated separately. For example, an exponential curve can be written as

$$a + b \times x,$$

where $x = \theta^r$ for parameter θ and explanatory vector r. The methodology also allows for nonlinear parameters in the link function (for example to model natural mortality or immunity in probit analysis) or in the offset variate (for example for survival models).

The nonlinear parameters are fitted by standard optimization methods such as Gauss–Newton or Newton–Raphson. So, deviances are calculated on grids of trial values of nonlinear parameters, as the algorithm finds its way to the optimum. Each point on the grid involves fitting a GLM, but this is a relatively quick and straightforward operation. So the process is much more efficient than a global optimization over the whole parameter space of both nonlinear and linear parameters. Furthermore, because the model essentially remains a GLM, all the familiar inference techniques can be used, for example to assess the fit, or to determine which parameters are needed in the model.

1.2   Hierarchical Generalized Nonlinear Models

The same idea can be used to define a hierarchical generalized nonlinear model (HGNLM). The linear predictor is

$$\eta = X\beta + \sum_i Z_i v_i$$

as before, but some columns of X may be derived as nonlinear functions of other explanatory variables and parameters. Again the nonlinear parameters are fitted by standard optimization methods, but now it is the augmented mean model that is fitted at each point of the grids of trial nonlinear parameter values.

2   Example

As an example we use the Cake data from Cochran and Cox (1957), also analysed in Lee et al. (2006). The data concern an experiment carried out at Iowa State College in which three recipes were used to prepare the cake mixtures. Fifteen replicates were performed. In each of these a batch of mixture was produced using each recipe, and then subdivided into enough for six different cakes which were each baked at a different temperature: 175, 185, 190, 205, 215 or 225 °C. The analysis variate is the angle at which the cakes break. The experiment thus has the structure of a split-plot design with batch as the whole-plot factor, corresponding to recipe as the whole-plot treatment factor, and temperature as the sub-plot treatment factor. Cochran and Cox (1957) analyse the data in this way, using a standard linear mixed model, but Lee et al. (2006) suggest that the breaking angles are non-Normal and fit a gamma generalized linear mixed model. Currently HGNLMs can be fitted only with conjugate HGLMs, i.e., those in which the distribution of the random effects is the conjugate of the distribution of y. So instead, below, we fit a gamma/inverse-gamma HGLM (which may, in any case, be an intuitively more appealing model).

The first command, SPLOAD in line 2, loads the data from a GenStat spread-sheet. HGRANDOMMODEL defines the random terms using the model formula Replicate/Batch, giving random terms Replicate (replicates) and Replicate.

Batch (batches within replicates). HGFIXEDMODEL defines the fixed terms using the model formula Recipe*Temperature, giving terms Recipe and Temperature representing the main effects of recipe and temperature, and Recipe. Temperature representing their interaction (this is an interaction as both main effects occur earlier in the model). HGANALYSE then fits the model.

Output from GenStat

```
1   " Cake data (see Lee, Nelder & Pawitan (2006) Sections 5.5 and 6.4.1) "
2   SPLOAD       'Cake.gsh'
```

Loading Spreadsheet File

Catalogue of file Cake.gsh

Data imported from GenStat Server on: 21-Jun-2005 12:27:25
Sheet Type: vector

Index	Type	Nval	Name
1	factor	270	Replicate
2	factor	270	Batch
3	factor	270	Recipe
5	factor	270	Temperature
6	variate	270	Angle

Note: Missing indices are used by unnamed or system structures. These store ancillary information, for example factor labels.

```
3   " fit a gamma inverse-gamma HGLM "
4   HGRANDOMMODEL  [DISTRIBUTION=inversegamma; LINK=log] Replicate/Batch
5   HGFIXEDMODEL   [DISTRIBUTION=gamma; LINK=log] Recipe*Temperature
6   HGANALYSE      [PRINT=model,fixed,dispersion,likelihood] Angle
```

Hierarchical Generalized Linear Model

Response variate: Angle

Mean Model

Fixed terms: Recipe*Temperature
Distribution: gamma

Link: logarithm
Random terms: Replicate/Batch
Distribution: inversegamma
Link: logarithm
Dispersion: free

Dispersion Model

Distribution: gamma
Link: logarithm

Estimates from the Mean Model

Covariate	estimate	s.e.	t(252)
constant	3.3737	0.05884	57.341
Recipe 2	−0.0783	0.05617	−1.395
Recipe 3	−0.0541	0.05617	−0.963
Temperature 185	0.0933	0.05053	1.846
Temperature 195	0.0614	0.05053	1.216
Temperature 205	0.1491	0.05053	2.951
Temperature 215	0.2874	0.05053	5.688
Temperature 225	0.1928	0.05053	3.816
Recipe 2 .Temperature 185	−0.0094	0.07146	−0.131
Recipe 2 .Temperature 195	0.0978	0.07146	1.368
Recipe 2 .Temperature 205	0.0286	0.07146	0.400
Recipe 2 .Temperature 215	−0.0495	0.07146	−0.693
Recipe 2 .Temperature 225	0.0818	0.07146	1.145
Recipe 3 .Temperature 185	−0.0512	0.07146	−0.716
Recipe 3 .Temperature 195	0.0745	0.07146	1.043
Recipe 3 .Temperature 205	−0.0388	0.07146	−0.543
Recipe 3 .Temperature 215	−0.0648	0.07146	−0.907
Recipe 3 .Temperature 225	0.0576	0.07146	0.806

Estimates from the Dispersion Model

Estimates of Parameters

Parameter	estimate	s.e.	t(*)	antilog of estimate
phi	−3.9584	0.0947	−41.79	0.01909
lambda Replicate	−3.541	0.394	−8.99	0.02900
lambda Replicate.Batch	−5.401	0.342	−15.80	0.004514

Message: s.e.s are based on dispersion parameter with value 1.

Likelihood Statistics

$-2 \times h(y\|v)$	1,507.637
$-2 \times h$	1,351.700
$-2 \times P_v(h)$	1,614.954
$-2 \times P_{\beta,v}(h)$	1,696.710
$-2 \times EQD(y\|v)$	1,506.777
$-2 \times EQD$	1,350.735
$-2 \times P_v(EQD)$	1,613.989
$-2 \times P_{\beta,v}(EQD)$	1,695.744

Initially temperature has been fitted as a factor, with no account taken of the actual values represented by its levels. If we form predictions for the temperatures and plot these against the temperature values, the relationship appears to be fairly linear, as can be seen in Fig. 1. So the next analysis instead fits regression coefficients of temperature (including interactions with recipe, i.e., to investigate whether the regression coefficient differs according to the recipe).

Output from GenStat

```
7   " form and plot predictions at the various temperatures "
8   HGPREDICT    [PRINT=prediction,se; PREDICTION=Mean] Temperature
```

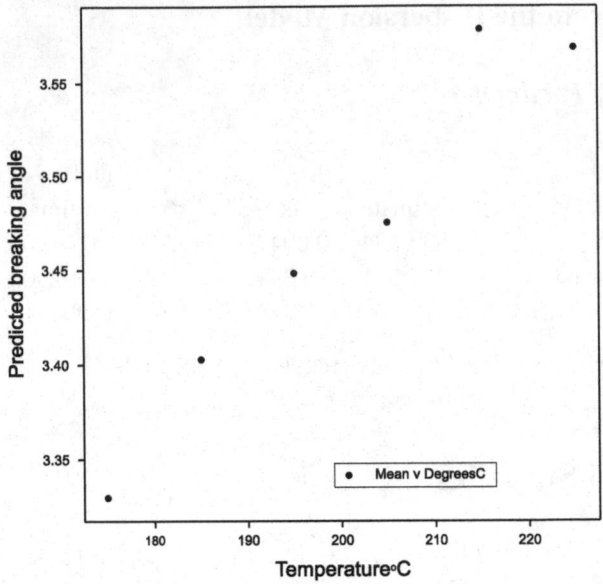

Fig. 1 Predicted breaking angle by temperature °C

Predictions from Regression Model

The standard errors are appropriate for interpretation of the predictions as summaries of the data rather than as forecasts of new observations.

Response variate: Angle

	Mean	se
Temperature		
175	3.330	0.04909
185	3.403	0.04909
195	3.448	0.04909
205	3.475	0.04909
215	3.579	0.04909
225	3.569	0.04909

Message: s.e's, variances and lsd's are approximate, since the model is not linear.
Message: s.e's are based on the residual deviance.

```
 9  PEN           1; SYMBOL=2; CSYMBOL=1; CFILL=1
10  FRAME         1,2; BOX=include; BOXKEY=bounded;\
11                XLOWER=0,0.5; XUPPER=1,0.95; YLOWER=0,0.1; YUPPER=1,0.2
12  XAXIS         1; TITLE='Temperature~^{o}C'
13  YAXIS         1; TITLE='Predicted breaking angle'
14  GETATTRIBUTE  [ATTRIBUTE=levels] Temperature; SAVE=TempAtt
15  VARIATE       DegreesC; VALUES=TempAtt['levels']
16  DGRAPH        Mean; DegreesC
```

```
17   " fit a linear relationship with temperature "
18   CALCULATE     TempC = Temperature
19   HGRANDOMMODEL [DISTRIBUTION=inversegamma; LINK=log] Replicate/Batch
20   HGFIXEDMODEL  [DISTRIBUTION=gamma; LINK=log] Recipe*TempC
21   HGANALYSE     [PRINT=model,fixed,dispersion,likelihood] Angle
```

Hierarchical Generalized Linear Model

Response variate: Angle

Mean Model

Fixed terms: Recipe∗TempC
Distribution: gamma
Link: logarithm
Random terms:
Replicate/Batch
Distribution: inversegamma
Link: logarithm
Dispersion: free

Dispersion Model

Distribution: gamma
Link: logarithm

Estimates from the Mean Model

	estimate	s.e.	t(264)
constant	2.5621	0.1788	14.329
Recipe 2	−0.1697	0.2453	−0.692
Recipe 3	−0.1263	0.2453	−0.515
TempC	0.0047	0.0009	5.486
TempC.Recipe 2	0.0006	0.0012	0.474
TempC.Recipe 3	0.0003	0.0012	0.278

Estimates from the Dispersion Model

Estimates of Parameters

Parameter	estimate	s.e.	t(∗)	antilog of estimate
phi	−3.9451	0.0922	−42.78	0.01935
lambda Replicate	−3.540	0.394	−8.99	0.02902
lambda Replicate.Batch	−5.410	0.344	−15.75	0.004473

Message: s.e.s are based on dispersion parameter with value 1.

Likelihood Statistics

$-2 \times h(y\|v)$	1,523.414
$-2 \times h$	1,366.924
$-2 \times P_v(h)$	1,629.995
$-2 \times P_{\beta,v}(h)$	1,681.544
$-2 \times EQD(y\|v)$	1,522.544
$-2 \times EQD$	1,365.947
$-2 \times P_v(EQD)$	1,629.019
$-2 \times P_{\beta,v}(EQD)$	1,680.567

```
 22  HGPREDICT      [PRINT=*; PREDICTION=LinMean] TempC; LEVELS=DegreesC
```

The nonlinearity with temperature can be assessed using the change in the likelihood statistic $-2 \times P_v(h)$; see Sect. 6.5 of Lee et al. (2006). The difference in the statistic between the two models is $1629.995 - 1614.954 = 15.041$ corresponding to a change of 12 in the number of fixed parameters. So there is scant evidence of nonlinearity. However, it may still be worth trying a nonlinear relationship, for interest and to illustrate the HGNLM methodology. So in the next section of the example, we use the HGNONLINEAR procedure (added in the 10th Edition of GenStat *for Windows*) to define a Box-Cox transformation of temperature: BoxCoxTemp is the derived column to include in the design matrix X, and BoxCox is the nonlinear parameter. Notice that, to avoid potential overflows in the calculation, the temperatures are first divided by 100. We then refit the model with BoxCoxTemp fixed (taking the estimated value of BoxCox) so that we can form predictions to compare in a plot with the predictions made originally for each individual temperature and those made assuming a linear model. (GenStat does not currently allow predictions to be formed from nonlinear GLMs.)

Output from GenStat

```
 23  " try a Box-Cox transformation of temperature
-24    (scaled to avoid overflow) "
 25  CALCULATE     xtemp = TempC / 100
 26  EXPRESSION    [VALUE=BoxCoxTemp = (BoxCox==0) * LOG(xtemp) +\
 27                (BoxCox/=0) * (xtemp**BoxCox-1)/(BoxCox+(BoxCox==0))]\
 28                BoxCoxCalc
 29  SCALAR        BoxCox; VALUE=-1
 30  CALCULATE     #BoxCoxCalc
 31  HGFIXEDMODEL  [DISTRIBUTION=gamma; LINK=log] Recipe*BoxCoxTemp
 32  HGNONLINEAR   [CALCULATION=BoxCoxCalc; VECTORS=BoxCoxTemp,xtemp]\
 33                BoxCox; INITIAL=-1; STEP=0.01
 34  HGANALYSE     [PRINT=model,fixed,dispersion,likelihood] Angle
```

Hierarchical Generalized Linear Model

Response variate: Angle

Mean Model

Fixed terms: Recipe*BoxCoxTemp
Distribution: gamma
Link: logarithm
Random terms:
Replicate/Batch
Distribution: inversegamma
Link: logarithm
Dispersion: free

Dispersion Model

Distribution: gamma
Link: logarithm

Estimates from the Mean Model

	estimate	s.e.	t(263)
BoxCox	−1.523	2.699	−0.5643
constant	2.373	1.208	1.9641
Recipe 2	−0.198	0.330	−0.6013
Recipe 3	−0.128	0.301	−0.4248
BoxCoxTemp	2.665	4.884	0.5457
BoxCoxTemp.Recipe 2	0.338	0.924	0.3664
BoxCoxTemp.Recipe 3	0.163	0.746	0.2185

Estimates from the Dispersion Model

Estimates of Parameters

Parameter	estimate	s.e.	t(∗)	antilog of estimate
phi	−3.9446	0.0924	−42.68	0.01936
lambda Replicate	−3.540	0.394	−8.99	0.02902
lambda Replicate.Batch	−5.412	0.344	−15.75	0.004462

Message: s.e.s are based on dispersion parameter with value 1.

Likelihood Statistics

$-2 \times h(y\|v)$	1,522.585
$-2 \times h$	1,365.968
$-2 \times P_v(h)$	1,629.083
$-2 \times P_{\beta,v}(h)$	1,642.647
$-2 \times EQD(y\|v)$	1,521.714
$-2 \times EQD$	1,364.991
$-2 \times P_v(EQD)$	1,628.106
$-2 \times P_{\beta,v}(EQD)$	1,641.670

```
 35   " reanalyse using the Box-Cox transformed temperatures
-36     (i.e. taking the Box-Cox parameter as fixed) to allow
-37      so that predictions can be calculated "
 38   CALCULATE    #BoxCoxCalc
 39   HGRANDOMMODEL [DISTRIBUTION=inversegamma; LINK=log] Replicate/Batch
 40   HGFIXEDMODEL  [DISTRIBUTION=gamma; LINK=log] Recipe*BoxCoxTemp
```

Fig. 2 Predicted breaking
angle by temperature °C

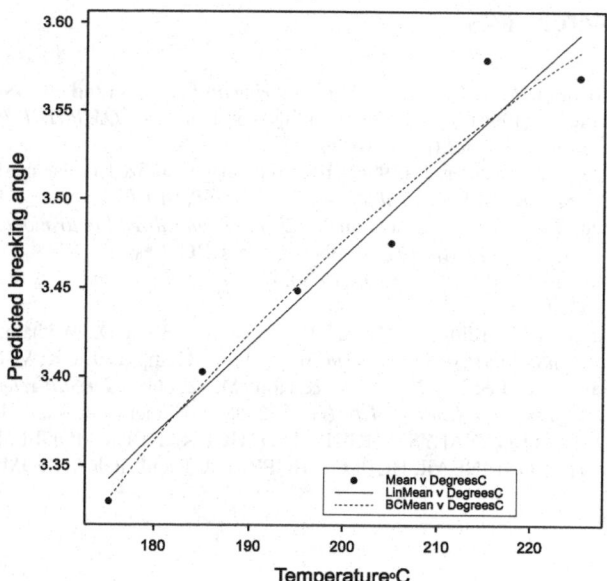

```
41  HGANALYSE      [PRINT=*] Angle
42  " make predictions "
43  CALCULATE      BoxCoxLevs = LOG(DegreesC/100)*(BoxCox==0) \
44                 + ((DegreesC/100)**BoxCox-1)/(BoxCox+(BoxCox==0))*(BoxCox/=0)
45  HGPREDICT      [PRINT=*; PREDICTION=BCMean] BoxCoxTemp; LEVELS=BoxCoxLevs
46  " plot predictions "
47  PEN            2,3; SYMBOL=0; CLINE=1; METHOD=monotonic; LINESTYLE=1,2
48  XAXIS          1; TITLE='Temperature~^{o}C'
49  DGRAPH         Mean,LinMean,BCMean; DegreesC; PEN=1,2,3
```

The plot in Fig. 2 shows some nonlinearity in the Box-Cox model, but this is only slight, and that is borne out by the fact that the likelihood statistic $-2 \times P_v(h)$ is virtually unchanged, at 1,629.083. Nevertheless, the example does illustrate the potential usefulness of being able to assess nonlinearity of fixed terms in an HGLM.

3 Conclusion

HGNLMs provide a further enhancement to the HGLM methodology in the 10th Edition of GenStat *for Windows*. Additional information can be found at http://genstat.co.uk/.

References

Cochran, W., & Cox, G. (1957). *Experimental designs* (2nd ed.). New York: Wiley.

Lane, P. (1996). Generalized nonlinear models. In *COMPSTAT 1996 Proceedings in Computational Statistics* (pp. 331–336).

Lee, Y., & Nelder, J. (1996). Hierarchical generalized linear models (with discussion). *Journal of the Royal Statistical Society Series B, 58,* 619–678.

Lee, Y., Nelder, J., & Pawitan, Y. (2006). *Generalized linear models with random effects: Unified analysis via H-likelihood.* Boca Raton: CRC Press.

McCullagh, P., & Nelder, J. (1989). *Generalized linear models* (2nd ed.). London: Chapman and Hall.

Payne, R., Harding, S., Murray, D., Soutar, D., Baird, D., Welham, S., et al. (2006a) *The guide to GenStat release 9, part 2 statistics.* Hemel Hempstead, UK: VSN International.

Payne, R., Lee, Y., Nelder, J., & Noh, M. (2006b). *GenStat release 10 reference manual, part 3, procedure library PL18* (pp. 372–389). Hemel Hempstead, UK: VSN International [procedures HGANALYSE, HGDISPLAY, HGDRANDOMMODEL, HGFIXEDMODEL, HGKEEP, HGNONLINEAR, HGPLOT, HGPREDICT and HGRANDOMMODEL].

Comparing Robust Regression Estimators to Detect Data Clusters: A Case Study

Alessandra Durio and Ennio Isaia

Abstract It is well known that in all situations involving the study of large data sets where a substantial number of outliers or clustered data are present, regression models based on M-estimators are likely to be unstable. Resorting to the inherent properties of robustness of the estimates based on the Integrated Square Error criterion we compare the results arising from L_2 estimates with those obtained from some common M-estimators. The discrepancy between the estimated regression models is measured by means of a new concept of similarity between functions and a system of statistical hypothesis. A Monte Carlo Significance test, is introduced to test the similarity of the estimates. Whenever the hypothesis of similarity between models is rejected, a careful investigation of the data structure is necessary to check for the presence of clusters, which can lead to the consideration of a mixture of regression models. Concerning this, we shall see how L_2 criterion can be applied in fitting a finite mixture of regression models. The requisite theory is outlined and the whole procedure is applied to a case study concerning the evaluation of the risk of fire and the risk of electric shocks of electronic transformers.

Keywords Minimum integrated square error • Mixture of regression models • Robust regression • Similarity between functions

1 Introduction

Regression is one of the widespread tools used to establish the relationship between a set of predictor variables and a response variable. However, in many circumstances, careful data preparation may not be possible and hence data may

A. Durio (✉)
Department of Economics & Statistics "S. Cognetti de Martiis", University of Turin, Lungo Dora Siena 100/A, 10124 Turin, Italy
e-mail: alessandra.durio@unito.it

G. MacKenzie and D. Peng (eds.), *Statistical Modelling in Biostatistics and Bioinformatics*, Contributions to Statistics, DOI 10.1007/978-3-319-04579-5__10,
© Springer International Publishing Switzerland 2014

be heavily contaminated by a substantial number of outliers. In these situations, the estimates of the parameters of the regression model obtained by the Maximum Likelihood criterion are fairly unstable.

The development of robust methods is underlined by the appearance of a wide number of papers and books on the topic including: Huber (1981), Rousseeuw and Leroy (1987), Staudte and Sheather (1990), Davies (1993), Dodge and Jurečkova (2000), Seber and Lee (2003), Rousseeuw et al. (2004), Jurečkova and Picek (2006), Maronna et al. (2006) and Fujisawa and Eguchi (2006).

The approach based on minimizing the Integrated Square Error is particularly helpful in those situations where, due to large sample size, careful data preparation is not feasible and hence data may contain a substantial number of outliers (Scott 2001). In this sense the L_2E criterion can be viewed as an efficient diagnostic tool in building useful models.

In this paper we suggest a procedure of regression analysis whose first step consists in comparing the results arising from L_2 estimates with those obtained from some common M-estimators. Afterwards, if a particular test of hypothesis leads us to reject the conjecture of similarity between the estimated regression models, we investigate the data for the presence of clusters by analyzing the L_2 minimizing function. The third step of the procedure consists in fitting a mixture of regression models via the L_2 criterion.

Below, we introduce the Integrated Square Error minimizing criterion for regression models, define a new concept of similarity between functions and introduce a Monte Carlo Significance (M.C.S.) test. We also illustrate the whole procedure by means of some simulated examples involving simple linear regression models. Finally, we present an analysis of a case study concerning the evaluation of the risk of fire and the risk of electric shocks in electronic transformers.

2 Parametric Linear Regression Models and Robust Estimators

Let $\{(x_{i1}, \ldots, x_{ip}, y_i)\}_{i=1,\ldots,n}$ be the observed data set, where each observation stems from a random sample drawn from the $p + 1$ random variable $(X_1, \ldots, X_p, Y)$. The regression model for the observed data set being studied is $y_i = m_{\boldsymbol{\beta}}(\mathbf{x}_i) + \varepsilon_i$, with $i = 1, \ldots, n$, where the object of our interest is the regression mean

$$m_{\boldsymbol{\beta}}(\mathbf{x}_i) = \mathbb{E}[Y | \mathbf{x}_i] = \beta_0 + \sum_{j=1}^{p} \beta_j \mathbf{x}_{ij} \tag{1}$$

and the errors $\{\varepsilon_i\}_{i=1,\ldots,n}$ are assumed to be independent random variables with zero mean and unknown finite variances.

2.1 Huber M-Estimator

The presence of outliers is a problem for regression techniques; these may occur for many reasons. An extreme situation arises when the outliers are numerous and they arise as a consequence of clustered data. For example, a large proportion of outliers may be found, if there is an omitted unknown categorical variable (e.g. gender, species, geographical location, etc.) where the data behave differently in each category. In parametric estimation, the estimators with good robustness proprieties relative to maximum likelihood are the M-estimators. The class of M-estimators of the vector $\boldsymbol{\beta}$ is defined as (e.g., Hampel et al. 2005)

$$\hat{\boldsymbol{\beta}}_M = \arg\min_{\boldsymbol{\beta}} \sum_{i=1}^{n} \rho\left(y_i - m_{\boldsymbol{\beta}}(\mathbf{x}_i)\right), \qquad (2)$$

where $\rho : \mathbb{R} \to \mathbb{R}$ is absolutely continuous convex function with derivative ψ.

If we assume that the r.v.s ε_i are independent and identically distributed as the r.v. $\varepsilon \sim \mathcal{N}(0, \sigma)$, the least-squares estimator gives the Maximum Likelihood Estimate (*MLE*) of the vector $\boldsymbol{\beta}$, i.e.:

$$\hat{\boldsymbol{\beta}}_{MLE} = \arg\min_{\boldsymbol{\beta}} \sum_{i=1}^{n} \left[y_i - m_{\boldsymbol{\beta}}(\mathbf{x}_i)\right]^2.$$

Since in the presence of outliers MLEs are quite unstable, i.e., inefficient and biased, for our purpose in the class of M-estimators we shall resort to the robust Huber M-estimator (*HME*) for which

$$\rho(y_i - m_{\boldsymbol{\beta}}(\mathbf{x}_i)) = \begin{cases} \dfrac{1}{2}(y_i - m_{\boldsymbol{\beta}}(\mathbf{x}_i))^2 & \text{if } |y_i - m_{\boldsymbol{\beta}}(\mathbf{x}_i)| \le k, \\ k\,|y_i - m_{\boldsymbol{\beta}}(\mathbf{x}_i)|\,(1 - \dfrac{k}{2}) & \text{if } |y_i - m_{\boldsymbol{\beta}}(\mathbf{x}_i)| > k, \end{cases}$$

where the tuning constant k is generally set to $1.345\,\sigma$.

2.2 L_2-Based Estimator

We investigate estimation methods in parametric linear regression models based on the minimum Integrated Square Error and the minimum L_2 metric. In the α-family of estimators proposed by Basu et al. (1998), L_2 estimator, briefly L_2E, is the more robust to outliers, even if it is less efficient than *MLE*.

Given the r.v. X, with unknown density $f(x|\boldsymbol{\theta}_0)$, for which we introduce the model $f(x|\boldsymbol{\theta})$, the estimate for $\boldsymbol{\theta}_0$ minimizing the L_2 metric will be:

$$\hat{\boldsymbol{\theta}}_{L_2E} = \arg\min_{\boldsymbol{\theta}} \int_{\mathbb{R}} [f(x|\boldsymbol{\theta}) - f(x|\boldsymbol{\theta}_0)]^2 \, dx =$$

$$= \arg\min_{\boldsymbol{\theta}} \left[\int_{\mathbb{R}} f^2(x|\boldsymbol{\theta}) \, dx - 2\,\mathbb{E}\left[f(x|\boldsymbol{\theta}_0)\right] \right] = \qquad (3)$$

$$= \arg\min_{\boldsymbol{\theta}} \left[\int_{\mathbb{R}} f^2(x|\boldsymbol{\theta}) \, dx - \frac{2}{n} \sum_{i=1}^{n} f(x_i|\boldsymbol{\theta}) \right],$$

where, the so-called expected height of the density, $\mathbb{E}\left[f(x|\boldsymbol{\theta}_0)\right]$ is replaced with its estimate $\hat{\mathbb{E}}\left[f(x|\boldsymbol{\theta}_0)\right] = n^{-1}\sum_{i=1}^{n} f(x_i|\boldsymbol{\theta})$ and where (Basu et al. 1998),

$$\int_{\mathbb{R}} f^2(x|\boldsymbol{\theta}) \, dx = \frac{1}{n} \sum_{i=1}^{n} \int_{\mathbb{R}} f^2(x_i|\boldsymbol{\theta}) \, dx_i . \qquad (4)$$

We turn now our attention to illustrate how the estimates based on L_2 criterion can be applied to parametric regression models. Assuming that the random variables $Y|\mathbf{x}$ are distributed as a $\mathcal{N}(m_{\boldsymbol{\beta}_0}(\mathbf{x}), \sigma_0)$, i.e. $f_{Y|\mathbf{x}}(y|\boldsymbol{\beta}_0, \sigma_0) = \phi(y|m_{\boldsymbol{\beta}_0}(\mathbf{x}), \sigma_0)$, the L_2 estimates of the parameters in $\boldsymbol{\beta}_0$ and σ_0 are given by Eq. (3), which in this case becomes

$$(\hat{\boldsymbol{\beta}}, \hat{\sigma})_{L_2E} = \arg\min_{\boldsymbol{\beta},\sigma} \left[\int_{\mathbb{R}} \phi^2(y|m_{\boldsymbol{\beta}}(\mathbf{x}), \sigma) \, dy - \frac{2}{n} \sum_{i=1}^{n} \phi(y_i|m_{\boldsymbol{\beta}}(\mathbf{x}_i), \sigma) \right]$$

$$= \arg\min_{\boldsymbol{\beta},\sigma} \left[\frac{1}{2\sigma\sqrt{\pi}} - \frac{2}{n} \sum_{i=1}^{n} \phi(y_i|m_{\boldsymbol{\beta}}(\mathbf{x}_i), \sigma) \right], \qquad (5)$$

since from Eq. (4)

$$\int_{\mathbb{R}} \phi^2(y|m_{\boldsymbol{\beta}}(\mathbf{x}), \sigma) \, dy = \frac{1}{n} \sum_{i=1}^{n} \int_{\mathbb{R}} \phi^2(y_i|m_{\boldsymbol{\beta}}(\mathbf{x}_i), \sigma) \, dy_i = \frac{1}{2\sigma\sqrt{\pi}} .$$

Clearly Eq. (5) is a feasible computationally closed-form expression so that L_2 criteria can be performed by any standard non-linear optimization procedure, for example, the nlm routine in the R library. However, it is important to recall that, whatever the algorithm, convergence to the global optimum can depend strongly on the starting values.

3   The Similarity Index and the M.C.S Test

To compare the L_2E performance with respect to some other common estimators we resort to an index of similarity between regression models introduced in Durio and Isaia (2010). In order to measure the discrepancy between the two estimated regression models, the index of similarity takes into account the *space region*

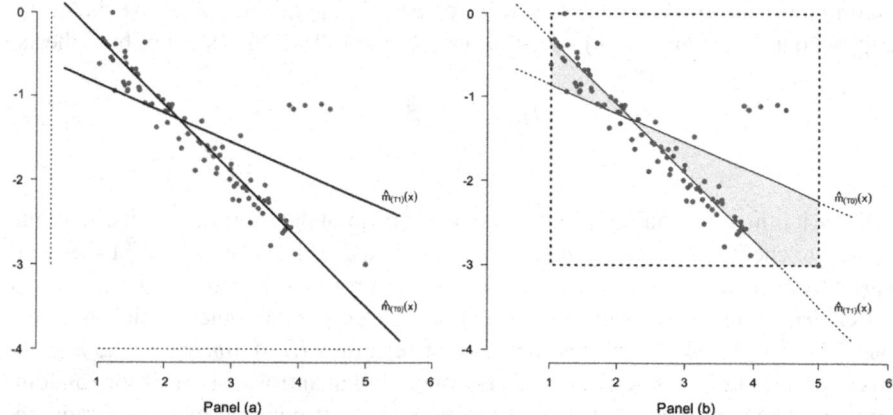

Fig. 1 Data points and two estimated regression models $\hat{m}_{T0}(x)$ and $\hat{m}_{T1}(x)$. In panel (**b**) the domains $\boldsymbol{D}^{p+1}$ and $\boldsymbol{C}^{p+1}$ upon which the $sim(T_0, T_1)$ statistic is computed

between $\hat{m}_{T_0}(\mathbf{x})$ and $\hat{m}_{T_1}(\mathbf{x})$ with respect to the space region where the whole of the data points lie. Let T_0 and T_1 be two regression estimators and $\hat{\boldsymbol{\beta}}_{T_0}, \hat{\boldsymbol{\beta}}_{T_1}$ the corresponding vectors of the estimated parameters. Introducing the sets:

$$I^p = \left[\min(x_{i1}); \max(x_{i1}) \right] \times \ldots \times \left[\min(x_{ip}); \max(x_{ip}) \right],$$

$$I = [\min(y_i); \max(y_i)] = [a; b],$$

we define the *similarity index* as

$$sim(T_0, T_1) \stackrel{def}{=} \frac{\int_{\boldsymbol{D}^{p+1}} d\mathbf{t}}{\int_{\boldsymbol{C}^{p+1}} d\mathbf{t}}$$

$$\boldsymbol{C}^{p+1} = I^p \times I \tag{6}$$

$$\boldsymbol{D}^{p+1} = \left\{ (\mathbf{x}, y) \in \mathbb{R}^{p+1} : \zeta(\mathbf{x}) \le y \le \xi(\mathbf{x}), \mathbf{x} \in I^p \right\} \cap \boldsymbol{C}^{p+1}$$

with $\zeta(\mathbf{x}) = min\left(\hat{m}_{T_0}(\mathbf{x}), \hat{m}_{T_1}(\mathbf{x}) \right)$ and $\xi(\mathbf{x}) = max\left(\hat{m}_{T_0}(\mathbf{x}), \hat{m}_{T_1}(\mathbf{x}) \right)$.

Figure 1 shows how the similarity index given by Eq. (6) can be computed in the simple case where $p = 1$. In panel (a) we have the cloud of data points and the two estimated models $\hat{\boldsymbol{\beta}}_{T_0}$ and $\hat{\boldsymbol{\beta}}_{T_1}$. The shaded area of panel (b) corresponds to $\int_{\boldsymbol{D}^{p+1}} d\mathbf{t}$, while the integral $\int_{\boldsymbol{C}^{p+1}} d\mathbf{t}$ is given by the area of the dotted rectangle, in which data points lay.

In order to compute the integrals of Eq. (6), we employ the fast and accurate algorithm proposed by Durio and Isaia (2010).

If the vectors $\hat{\boldsymbol{\beta}}_{T_0}$ and $\hat{\boldsymbol{\beta}}_{T_1}$ are close to each other, then $sim(T_0, T_1)$ will be close to zero. On the other hand, if the estimated regression models $\hat{m}_{T_0}(\mathbf{x})$ and $\hat{m}_{T_1}(\mathbf{x})$ are dissimilar we are likely to observe a value of $sim(T_0, T_1)$ far from zero. We therefore propose to use the $sim(T_0, T_1)$ statistic to verify the following system of hypothesis

$$\begin{cases} H_0 : \boldsymbol{\beta}_0 = \hat{\boldsymbol{\beta}}_{T_0} \\ H_1 : \boldsymbol{\beta}_0 \neq \hat{\boldsymbol{\beta}}_{T_0} \end{cases} \tag{7}$$

Since it is not reasonable to look for an exact form of the $sim(T_0, T_1)$ distribution, in order to check the above system of hypothesis we utilise a simplified M.C.S. test originally suggested by Barnard (1963) and later proposed by Hope (1968).

Let $sim_{T_0 T_1}$ denote the value of the $sim(T_0, T_1)$ statistic computed on the observed data. The simplified M.C.S. test consists of rejecting H_0 if $sim_{T_0 T_1}$ is the $m\alpha$-th most extreme statistic relative to the corresponding quantities based on the random samples of the reference set, where the reference set consists of $m - 1$ random samples, of size n each, generated under the null hypothesis, i.e., drawn at random from the model $\hat{m}_{T_0}(\mathbf{x})$ with $\sigma = \hat{\sigma}_{T_0}$. In other words we generate $m - 1$ random samples under H_0 and for each of them we compute $sim^*_{T_0 T_1}$ and we shall reject the null hypothesis, at the α significance level, if and only if the value of the test statistic $sim_{T_0 T_1}$ is greater than all the $m - 1$ values of $sim^*_{T_0 T_1}$. We remark that if we set $m\alpha = 1$ and fix $\alpha = 0.01$, we have $m - 1 = 99$ (while fixing $\alpha = 0.05$ would yield $m - 1 = 19$).

4 Simple Linear Regression and Examples

Since for our case study we shall consider the simple linear regression model $y_i = \beta_0 + \beta_1 x_i + \varepsilon_i$, the L_2 criterion according to Eq. (5) reduces to the following computationally closed-form expression

$$(\hat{\boldsymbol{\beta}}, \hat{\sigma})_{L_2 E} = \underset{\beta, \sigma}{\arg\min} \left[\frac{1}{2\sigma\sqrt{\pi}} - \frac{2}{n} \sum_{i=1}^{n} \phi(y_i | \beta_0 + \beta_1 x_i, \sigma) \right]. \tag{8}$$

In the following we introduce two simulated examples in order to demonstrate the behaviour of the L_2 criterion in the presence of outliers and in the presence of clustered data. To evaluate its performance, we shall use the Maximum Likelihood estimator and the robust Huber M estimator. Given $T_1 = L_2 E$, we shall perform the M.C.S. test two times: the first one, fixing $T_0 = MLE$, for $sim(MLE, L_2 E)$, the second one fixing $T_0 = HME$, for $sim(HME, L_2 E)$. We remark that, as $p = 1$, in both situations we have $I^p = [\min(x_i); \max(x_i)]$ and that clearly the integrals of Eq. (6) are defined on bi-dimensional domains.

Example I. Let us consider a simulated dataset of $n = 200$ points generated according to the model $Y = X + \varepsilon$, where $X \sim \mathcal{U}(0, 10)$ and $\varepsilon \sim \mathcal{N}(0, 0.8)$. We then introduce $m = 10(30)$ points according to the model $Y = -3 + X + \varepsilon$,

Table 1 Results of simulated Example I

	$m = 10$			$m = 30$		
	MLE	*HME*	L_2E	*MLE*	*HME*	L_2E
$\hat{\beta}_0$	0.3078	0.1616	0.0353	0.2884	0.2081	0.0139
$\hat{\beta}_1$	0.9054	0.9509	0.9886	0.8635	0.8944	0.9975
$\hat{\sigma}$	0.9889	0.9972	0.7926	1.2352	1.2389	0.9712

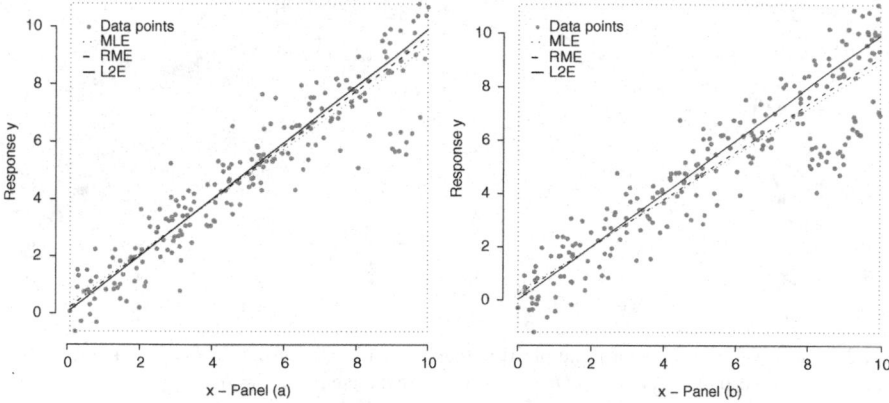

Fig. 2 Data points of Example I and estimated models $\hat{m}_{ML}(x)$, $\hat{m}_{HM}(x)$ and $\hat{m}_{L2}(x)$. In panel (**a**) we set $m = 10$ outliers while in panel (**b**) $m = 30$

where $X \sim \mathcal{U}(8, 10)$ and $\varepsilon \sim \mathcal{N}(0, 0.4)$, so that *they can be considered as outliers.* Resorting to the estimators *ML*, *HM* and L_2 we obtain the following estimates of the parameters β_0, β_1 and σ listed in Table 1 (also see Fig. 2).

Applying the M.C.S. test, with $\alpha = 0.01$, to the estimated models $\hat{m}_{ML}(x)$ and $\hat{m}_{L2}(x)$, we reject the null hypothesis of system (7) as we have $sim_{ML,L2} = 0.0203 > \max(sim^*_{ML,L2}) = 0.0128$. Turning our attention to models $\hat{m}_{HM}(x)$ and $\hat{m}_{L2}(x)$, the M.C.S. test leads us to accept the null hypothesis since $sim_{HM,L2} = 0.0091 < \max(sim^*_{HM,L2}) = 0.0123$.

In the case we add $m = 30$ outliers to the sample data, the results of the M.C.S. tests lead us to different conclusions. In both situations we reject the null hypothesis of system (7) as we have

$$sim_{ML,L2} = 0.0364 > \max(sim^*_{ML,L2}) = 0.0159$$

$$sim_{HM,L2} = 0.0289 > \max(sim^*_{HM,L2}) = 0.0103$$

When the outliers are few, the estimated regression model $\hat{m}_{HM}(x)$ and $\hat{m}_{L2}(x)$ do not differ significantly. This is not the case when the number of outliers increases; in this sense it seems that L_2 estimator can be helpful in cluster detection.

Table 2 Results of simulated
Example II

	MLE	*HME*	$L_2 E$
$\hat{\beta}_0$	2.6755	2.4956	1.7340
$\hat{\beta}_1$	0.4607	0.5086	0.6856
$\hat{\sigma}$	1.4021	1.4074	1.1633

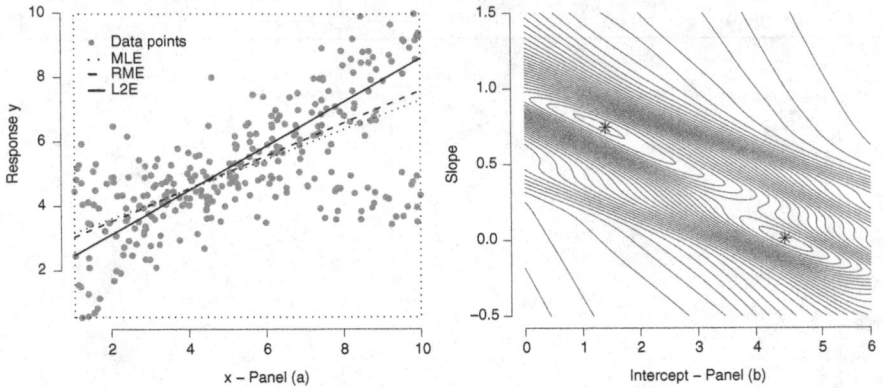

Fig. 3 (**Panel a**) Data points of Example II and estimated models $\hat{m}_{ML}(x)$, $\hat{m}_{HM}(x)$ and $\hat{m}_{L2}(x)$. (**Panel b**) Contour plot of function $g(\boldsymbol{\beta}|\sigma^*)$ of Eq. (9) evaluated at $\sigma^* = 0.5\,\hat{\sigma}_{L_2E}$

Example II. Let us consider a dataset of $n = 300$ points, 200 of which arise from model $Y = 1 + 0.8\,X + \varepsilon_1$ while the remaining from model $Y = 5 - 0.2\,X + \varepsilon_2$, where $\varepsilon_1 \sim \mathcal{N}(0, 1)$, $\varepsilon_2 \sim \mathcal{N}(0, 0.5)$ and $X \sim \mathcal{U}(1, 10)$. Again, resorting to the estimators *ML*, *HM* and L_2 we obtain the following estimates of the parameters β_0, β_1 and σ listed in Table 2 (also see Fig. 3, panel a). Considering the models $\hat{m}_{ML}(x)$ and $\hat{m}_{L2}(x)$ the M.C.S. test, with $\alpha = 0.01$, indicates that they can be considered dissimilar, as we observe $sim_{ML,L2} = 0.0582 > \max(sim^*_{ML,L2}) = 0.0210$. This is still true if we consider the estimated models $\hat{m}_{HM}(x)$ and $\hat{m}_{L2}(x)$, in fact from the M.C.S. test we have $sim_{HM,L2} = 0.0451 > \max(sim^*_{MH,L2}) = 0.0156$. Also in this situation the L_2 estimator seems to be helpful in detecting clusters of data when compared with the Maximum Likelihood and the Huber M estimators.

5 Mixture of Regression Models via L_2

It seems to the authors that the properties of robustness of L_2 estimates, as outlined above, can be helpful in pointing out the presence of clusters in the data, e.g. Durio and Isaia (2007).

This in the sense that whenever sample data belong to two (or more) clusters, $\hat{m}_{L2}(\mathbf{x})$ will always tend to fit the cluster with the heaviest number of data points and hence big discrepancies between $\hat{m}_{ML}(\mathbf{x})$ and $\hat{m}_{L2}(\mathbf{x})$ will be likely to be observed, as illustrated by the previous examples. Investigating more accurately function (5) for a fixed value of σ it can be seen that in all situations where sample data are clustered it can show more than one local minimum. A simple way forward is to investigate the behaviour of the function

$$g(\boldsymbol{\beta}|\sigma^*) = \frac{1}{2\sigma\sqrt{\pi}} - \frac{2}{n}\sum_{i=1}^{n}\phi(y_i|m_{\boldsymbol{\beta}}(\mathbf{x}_i),\sigma^*) \tag{9}$$

for different values of σ^* on its parameter space, for instance, the interval $]0, 2 \cdot \hat{\sigma}_{L_2E}]$. In fact, whenever sample data are clustered, function $g(\boldsymbol{\beta}|\sigma^*)$ given by Eq. (9) shows one absolute and one or more local points of minimum.

Whenever the presence of clusters of data is detected by L_2 criterion, we can use L_2 estimator assuming that the model that best fits the data is a mixture of $K \geq 2$ regression models. Assuming that each data point $(\mathbf{x}_i, y_i)$ comes from the k-th regression model $y_i = m_{\boldsymbol{\beta}_k}(\mathbf{x}_i) + \varepsilon_{ik}$ with probability p_k, we suppose that the random variables $Y|\mathbf{x}$ are distributed as a mixture of K Gaussian random variables, i.e.,

$$f_{Y|\mathbf{x}}(y|\boldsymbol{\theta}_0) = \sum_{k=1}^{K} p_k^0\,\phi(y|m_{\boldsymbol{\beta}_k^0}(\mathbf{x}),\sigma_k^0). \tag{10}$$

We are now able to derive the following closed-form expression for the estimates of $\boldsymbol{\theta}_0 = [\boldsymbol{p}^0, \boldsymbol{\beta}^0, \boldsymbol{\sigma}^0]$; in fact, according to Eq. (9) and recalling Eq. (4), we have

$$\hat{\boldsymbol{\theta}}_{L_2E} = \underset{p,\beta,\sigma}{\arg\min} \left[\frac{1}{n}\sum_{i=1}^{n}\sum_{j=1}^{K}\sum_{h=1}^{K} p_j\,p_h\,\phi(0|m_{\boldsymbol{\beta}_j}(\mathbf{x}_i) - m_{\boldsymbol{\beta}_h}(\mathbf{x}_i),\sigma_j^2 + \sigma_h^2) - \right.$$

$$\left. - \frac{2}{n}\sum_{i=1}^{n}\sum_{k=1}^{K} p_k\,\phi(y_i|m_{\boldsymbol{\beta}_k}(\mathbf{x}_i),\sigma_k^2) \right]. \tag{11}$$

Solving Eq. (11) we obtain the estimates of the vector of the weights, i.e. $\hat{\boldsymbol{p}} = [p_1,\dots,p_K]^T$, the vector of the parameters, i.e. $\hat{\boldsymbol{\beta}} = [\beta_{0_1},\dots,\beta_{d_1},\dots,\beta_{0_K},\dots, \beta_{d_K}]^T$ and the vector of the standard deviations of the error of each component of the mixture, i.e. $\hat{\boldsymbol{\sigma}} = [\sigma_1,\dots,\sigma_K]^T$.

Example II (continued). Referring to the situation of Example II, for which $\hat{\sigma}_{L_2} = 1.1633$, the contour plot of function $g(\boldsymbol{\beta}|\sigma^*)$ of Eq. (9) and displayed in Fig. 3, panel b, evaluated at $\sigma^* = 0.5\,\hat{\sigma}_{L_2E}$, shows the existence of one absolute minimum corresponding to the estimates of the parameters of the model $Y = 1 + 0.8\,X + \varepsilon_1$ and one local minimum close to the values of the parameters of the model $Y = 5 - 0.2\,X + \varepsilon_2$. We therefore consider a mixture of $K = 2$ simple linear regression models. Since in this situation Eq. (10) becomes

$$f_{Y|\mathbf{x}}(y|\boldsymbol{\theta}_0) = p_1^0\,\phi(y|\beta_{0_1}^0 + \beta_{1_1}^0\,x,\sigma_1^0) + p_2^0\,\phi(y|\beta_{0_2}^0 + \beta_{1_2}^0\,x,\sigma_2^0),$$

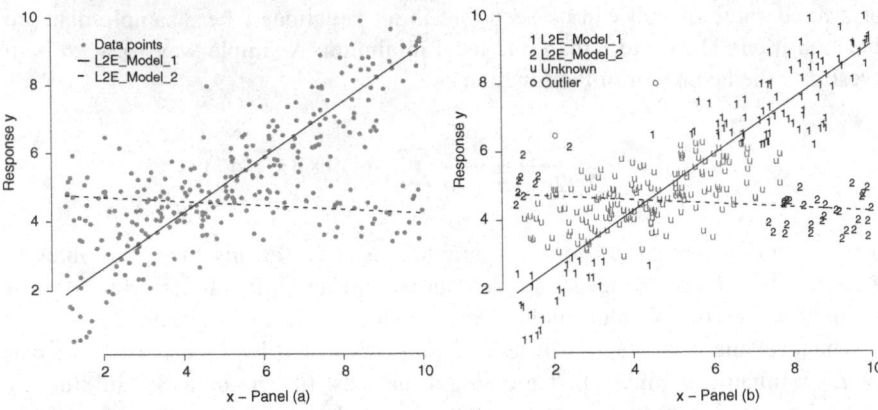

Fig. 4 (Panel **a**) Data points and estimated components of the mixture of two simple regression models via L_2. (Panel **b**) Data points assignment according to the "quick classification rule" with $\gamma = 3$

the L_2 estimates of the vector $\boldsymbol{\theta}_0$, according to Eq. (11), will be given by solving

$$\hat{\boldsymbol{\theta}}_{L_2E} = \arg\min_{p,\beta,\sigma} \left[\frac{p_1^2\sigma_2 + p_2^2\sigma_1}{2\sigma_1\sigma_2\sqrt{\pi}} + \frac{2}{n}\sum_{i=1}^{n} p_1 p_2 \phi(0|\beta_{0_1} + \beta_{1_1}x_i - \beta_{0_2} - \beta_{1_2}x_i, \sigma_1^2 + \sigma_2^2) - \right.$$

$$\left. - \frac{2}{n}\sum_{i=1}^{n} \left(p_1\,\phi(y_i|\beta_{0_1} + \beta_{1_1}\,x_i, \sigma_1^2) + p_2\,\phi(y_i|\beta_{0_2} + \beta_{1_2}\,x_i, \sigma_2^2) \right) \right]. \tag{12}$$

From numerical minimization of Eq. (12), we obtain (see Fig. 4, panel a) the following estimates of the eight parameters of the mixture

L_2E Model_1: $\quad \hat{p}_1 = 0.646 \quad \hat{\beta}_{0_1} = 1.0281 \quad \hat{\beta}_{1_1} = 0.8109 \quad \hat{\sigma}_1 = 0.8411$
L_2E Model_2: $\quad \hat{p}_2 = 0.354 \quad \hat{\beta}_{0_2} = 4.8267 \quad \hat{\beta}_{1_2} = -0.0576 \quad \hat{\sigma}_2 = 0.5854$

which are quite close to the true values of the parameters.

From a practical point of view, it would be interesting to be able to highlight which data points belong to each component of the mixture; to this end we resort to a *quick classification rule* based on the assumption that the density of the errors follows a Normal distribution, i.e. $\forall\, i = 1, \ldots, n$

$$\text{if } |\hat{\varepsilon}_{i_1}| \leqq \gamma\,\hat{\sigma}_1 \wedge |\hat{\varepsilon}_{i_2}| > \gamma\,\hat{\sigma}_2 \quad \rightarrow (x_i, y_i) \in \text{Model } L_2E - I$$

$$\text{if } |\hat{\varepsilon}_{i_1}| > \gamma\,\hat{\sigma}_1 \wedge |\hat{\varepsilon}_{i_2}| \leqq \gamma\,\hat{\sigma}_2 \quad \rightarrow (x_i, y_i) \in \text{Model } L_2E - II$$

$$\text{if } |\hat{\varepsilon}_{i_1}| \leqq \gamma\,\hat{\sigma}_1 \wedge |\hat{\varepsilon}_{i_2}| \leqq \gamma\,\hat{\sigma}_2 \quad \rightarrow (x_i, y_i) \in \text{Unknown model}$$

$$\text{if } |\hat{\varepsilon}_{i_1}| > \gamma\,\hat{\sigma}_1 \wedge |\hat{\varepsilon}_{i_2}| > \gamma\,\hat{\sigma}_2 \quad \rightarrow (x_i, y_i) \in \text{Outlier}, \tag{13}$$

where γ is an appropriate quantile of a $\mathcal{N}(0, 1)$.

Table 3 Classification I

	L_2 estimates of $\hat{p}$	Quick rule	
L_2E Model_1	64.6 %	34.6 %	(103)
L_2E Model_2	35.4 %	12.7 %	(38)
Unknown model	–	52.7 %	(157)

Fixing $\gamma = 3$, if we apply the *quick rule* and drop two points that are classified as outliers we obtain (see Fig. 4, panel b) the following classification table, see Table 3. Clearly, the high percentage of not assigned points (52.7%) is due to the specific structure of the two clusters which are quite confused.

6   The Case Study

A firm operating in the field of diagnosis and decontamination of *electronic transformers fluids* assesses the risks of fluid degradation, electric shocks, fire or explosion, PCB contamination, decomposition of cellulosic insulation, etc. With the aid of well-known models and relying on the results of chemical analysis, the firm's staff estimate the value of the risk on continuous scales.

In order to determine if their methods of assigning risk values are independent of specific characteristics of the transformers (age, voltage, fluid mass, etc.) we conducted an analysis based on a database of 1,215 records of diagnosis containing oil chemical analysis, technical characteristics and risk values.

Taking into account the *risk of fire (Y)* and the *risk of electric shocks (X)*, it was natural to suppose a linear dependence between the two variables, i.e., we considered the simple regression model with $m_\beta(x_i) = \beta_0 + \beta_1 x_i$.

Resorting to the estimators *ML, HM* and L_2 we obtained the following estimates of the parameters β_0, β_1 and σ listed in Table 4.

Although the estimates of the vector of the parameters β are quite close, the corresponding three estimated models differ in some way, e.g., Fig. 5, panel a.

Computing the values of the *sim*() statistics, the M.C.S. test led us to the conclusion that the L_2 estimated model can be considered dissimilar from both $\hat{m}_{ML}(x)$ and $\hat{m}_{HM}(x)$ models, as

$$sim_{ML,L2} = 0.0220 > \max(sim^*_{ML,L2}) = 0.0051$$

$$sim_{HM,L2} = 0.0203 > \max(sim^*_{HM,L2}) = 0.0031$$

Probing more deeply, we found that function $g(\beta|\sigma^*)$ of Eq. (9) presents two points of minimum for $\sigma^* = 0.5\,\hat{\sigma}_{L_2E} = 0.0755$, as shown in Fig. 5, panel b.

Therefore we decided to model our data by means of a mixture of two simple regression models. Considering the L_2 criterion and solving Eq. (12), we found that about 57 %($= \hat{p}_1$ %) of the data points follow the model

$$\hat{m}_{\beta_1}(x) = -0.4042 + 1.7705\,x \qquad \rightarrow \qquad L_2E \ \text{Model\_1}$$

Table 4 Estimates of the parameters after resorting

	MLE	HME	L_2E
$\hat{\beta}_0$	−0.4321	−0.4423	−0.5330
$\hat{\beta}_1$	1.7110	1.7199	1.8115
$\hat{\sigma}$	0.1472	0.1471	0.1509

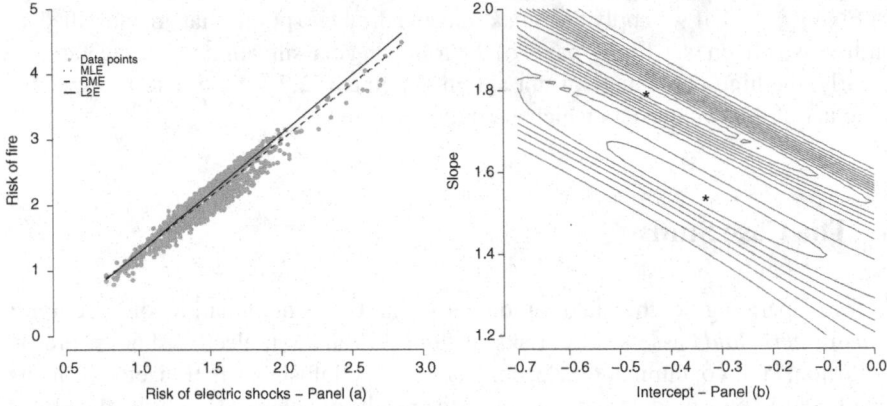

Fig. 5 Case study. (Panel **a**) Data points and estimated models $\hat{m}_{ML}(x)$, $\hat{m}_{HM}(x)$ and $\hat{m}_{L2}(x)$. (Panel **b**) Contour plot of function $g(\beta|\sigma^*)$ of Eq. (9) evaluated at $\sigma^* = 0.5\,\hat{\sigma}_{L_2E}$, with $\hat{\sigma}_{L_2E} = 0.151$

for which $\hat{\sigma}_1 = 0.0547$, while the remaining 43 %($= \hat{p}_2$ %) of the data points follow the model

$$\hat{m}_{\beta_2}(x) = -0.3955 + 1.5847\,x \qquad \rightarrow \qquad L_2E \text{ Model\_2}$$

for which $\hat{\sigma}_2 = 0.0775$. Panel a of Fig. 6 shows the two estimates models.

Applying the *quick rule* we were able to classify the data according to whether they followed the first or the second regression model. From the L_2 estimates of $\hat{p}$ and the *quick rule* (dropping two points that were classified as outliers) we obtained the following classification table, see Table 5.

In order to classify the 266 (= 22.0 %) points belonging, according to the *quick rule*, to the *Unknown Model*, we had to investigate more deeply the specific characteristics of the transformers themselves.

Examining our database, we found that 40 % of the transformers has a fluid mass ≤500 kg and the L_2 criterion gave us an estimate of 43 % for the weight of points belonging to L_2E Model_1 while our *quick rule* assigned the 36.9 % of data points to L_2E Model_2.

Furthermore, our *quick classification rule* assigns 419 out of the 448 points (93.5 %) to L_2E Model_2 and these have a fluid mass less (or equal) than 500 kg, while all the 499 transformers imputed to L_2E Model_1 have a fluid mass greater than 500 kg, see Table 6.

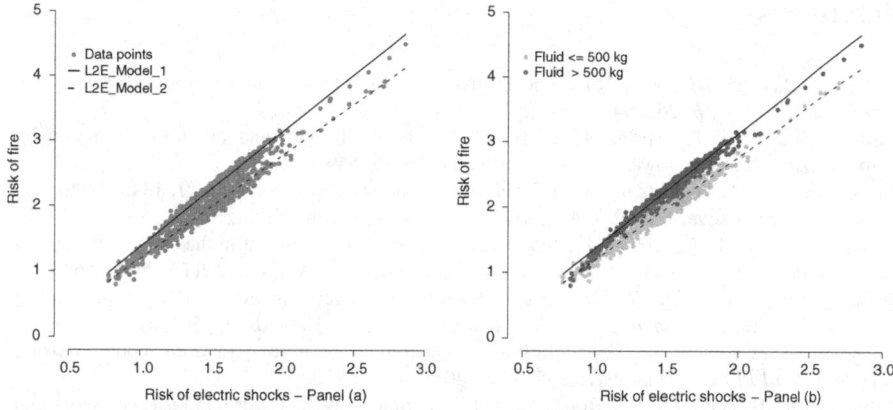

Fig. 6 Case study. (Panel **a**) Data points and estimated models $\hat{m}_{\beta_1}(x)$ and $\hat{m}_{\beta_2}(x)$. (Panel **b**) Final data points assignment according to the fluid mass of the electrical transformers

Table 5 Classification II

	L_2 estimates of $\hat{p}$	Quick rule	
L_2E Model_1	57.0 %	41.1 %	(499)
L_2E Model_2	43.0 %	36.9 %	(448)
Unknown model	–	22.0 %	(266)

Table 6 Fluid mass of the model

	Fluid mass $\leqq$ 500 kg	Fluid mass > 500 kg
L_2E Model_1	0 (0.0 %)	499 (100 %)
L_2E Model_2	419 (93.5 %)	29 (6.5 %)
Unknown model	65 (24.4 %)	201 (75.6 %)

From the above, we decided to use the *fluid mass as clustering variable* and so we assigned the transformers with a fluid mass equal or less than 500 kg to Model L_2E Model_2 while the transformers with a fluid mass greater than 500 kg were assigned to the L_2E Model_1 regression line. The final assignment is shown in Fig. 6, panel b.

These results allowed us to state that, at fixed level of risk of electric shocks, the risk of fire was evaluated in a different way for the two groups of transformers, i.e., the relationship between the two variables depended on the fluid mass of the transformers.

However, the chemical staff of the firm could not find any scientific reason to explain the different risks of fire in the two types of transformers, so they decided to change the model used by assigning different weights to the hydrocarbon variable in order to better reflect the differential risks of fire.

Acknowledgements The authors are indebted to the coordinating editors and to the anonymous referees for carefully reading the manuscript and for their many important remarks and suggestions.

References

Barnard, G. A. (1963). Contribution to the discussion of paper by m.s. bartlett. *Journal of the Royal Statistical Society, B, 25*, 294.

Basu, A., Harris, I. R., Hjort, N., & Jones, M. (1998). Robust and efficient estimation by minimizing a density power divergence. *Biometrika, 85*, 549–559.

Davies, P. L. (1993). Aspects of robust linear regression. *Annals of Statistics, 21*, 1843–1899.

Dodge, Y., & Jurečkova, J. (2000). *Adaptive regression*. New York: Springer.

Durio, A., & Isaia, E. D. (2007). A quick procedure for model selection in the case of mixture of normal densities. *Journal of Computational Statistics & Data Analysis, 51*(12), 5635–5643.

Durio, A., & Isaia, E. D. (2010). Clusters detection in regression problems: A similarity test between estimate. *Communications in Statistics Theory and Methods, 39*, 508–516.

Fujisawa, H., & Eguchi, F. (2006). Robust estimation in the normal mixture model. *Journal of Statistical Planning Inference, 136*, 3989–4011.

Hampel, F. R., Ronchetti, E. M., Rousseeuw, R.,J., & Stahel, W. A. (2005). *Robust regression and outlier detection*. New York: Wiley.

Hope, A. C. (1968). A simplified monte carlo significance test procedure. *Journal of the Royal Statistical Society, B, 30*, 582–598.

Huber, P. J. (1981). *Robust statistics*. New York: Wiley.

Jurečkova, J., & Picek, J. (2006). *Robust statistical methods with R*. Boca Raton: Chapman & Hall.

Maronna, R., Martin, D., & Yohai, V. (2006). *Robust statistics: Theory and methods*. New York: Wiley.

Rousseeuw, P. J., & Leroy, A. M. (1987). *Robust regression and outlier detection*. New York: Wiley.

Rousseeuw, P. J., Van Alest, S., Van Driessen, K., & Agulló, J. (2004). Robust multivariate regression. *Technometric, 46*, 293–305.

Scott, D. W. (2001). Parametric statistical modeling by minimum integrated square error. *Technometrics, 43*, 274–285.

Seber, G. A. F., & Lee, A. J. (2003). *Linear regression analysis* (2nd ed.). New York: Wiley.

Staudte, R. G., & Sheather, S. J. (1990). *Robust estimation and testing*. New York: Wiley.

Finite Mixture Model Clustering of SNP Data

Norma Bargary, J. Hinde, and A. Augusto F. Garcia

Abstract Finite mixture models have been used extensively in clustering applications, where each component of the mixture distribution is assumed to represent an individual cluster. The simplest example describes each cluster in terms of a multivariate Gaussian density with various covariance structures. However, using finite mixture models as a clustering tool is highly flexible and allows for the specification of a wide range of statistical models to describe the data within each cluster. These include modelling each cluster using linear regression models, mixed effects models, generalized linear models, etc. This paper investigates using mixtures of orthogonal regression models to cluster biological data arising from a study of the sugarcane plant.

Keywords Clustering • Finite-mixtures models • Orthogonal regression • SNP data

1 Introduction

Sugarcane is the highest tonnage crop among cultivated plants. Almost 70 % of the world's sugar supply is derived from sugarcane while the remaining 30 % comes from sugar beet. Sugarcane is cultivated in approximately 110 different countries and is an important industrial crop in many regions such as Brazil and South Asia, where approximately 50 % of all sugarcane production occurs. According to Palhares et al. (2012), sugarcane is a cost-effective renewable resource produced for use as sugar, in animal feeds, alcohols and fertilizers. In addition, there is an increased emphasis in its use as a bio-fuel which requires a crop with high yield

N. Bargary (✉)
Department of Mathematic & Statistics, University of Limerick, Limerick, Ireland
e-mail: norma.bargary@ul.ie

G. MacKenzie and D. Peng (eds.), *Statistical Modelling in Biostatistics and Bioinformatics*, Contributions to Statistics, DOI 10.1007/978-3-319-04579-5__11,
© Springer International Publishing Switzerland 2014

and fibre content. Thus there is an interest in developing breeds with high sugar yield, increased resistance to drought, high fibre content, etc. Such work requires identifying gene(s) that contribute to these complex traits that could possibly provide DNA markers for use in marker-assisted breeding. One of the primary issues in examining the genetic make-up of the sugarcane genome is its polyploid structure. Polyploidy implies that the sugarcane plant has multiple sets of chromosomes rather than two as for diploid organisms (such as humans). For example, the *S. spontaneous* breed has between 5 and 16 sets of chromosomes, while the species *S. officinarum* has 8 sets of chromosomes. Each chromosome carries a particular form of each gene, i.e., an allele for that gene. For example, the gene for eye colour has a number of alleles; blue, brown, green, grey. The particular combination of these alleles results in different genotypes, and consequently phenotypes in each individual. Since sugarcane is polyploid, individual alleles can appear in varying numbers and combinations, resulting in much genetic variation in sugarcane. It is therefore difficult to obtain information about its complex genetic makeup. A primary aim is to identify the many different alleles and associated genotypes and phenotypes for the various sugarcane crossbreeds. One way of doing this is through the analysis of single nucleotide polymorphisms (SNPs).

SNPs occur during cell division, when an existing cell divides in two by first copying its DNA so the new cells will each have a complete set of genetic instructions. Cells sometimes make mistakes (called SNPs) during the copying process and these lead to variations in the DNA sequence at particular locations. An SNP is a single base pair mutation at a specific locus and typically consists of two alleles. Much research has centered on the identification of new SNPs since they act as markers to identify genomic regions controlling traits of interest and can be used for genotyping (Olivier 2005). Figure 1 gives an example for a sample of diploid individuals. Here the intensities for two alleles (C and G for example) of a particular SNP are measured for a number of individuals and plotted on the x and y-axes respectively. These observations can be clustered into three clear groups; one group along the y-axis, one along the x-axis and one along the line corresponding to $\pi/4$. Since diploid individuals have two sets of chromosomes and each chromosome has one of the two alleles (either C or G), there are three possible genotypes for this SNP. If the alleles on both chromosomes are the same, the individual is said to be homozygous with possible genotypes G/G or C/C. If an individual has different alleles on each chromosome they are said to be heterozygous with genotype G/C. The group along the y-axis consists of individuals with genotype G/G (since the contribution from the C allele is essentially 0), the group along the x-axis consists of individuals with genotype C/C, and the group along the line $\pi/4$ consists of individuals with genotype G/C. Therefore the clusters produced contain information about the genotype of each individual. In addition, the proportion of individuals within each cluster are related to expected segregation ratios and to the ploidy level (the number of chromosomes) of the individuals measured, while the angles between the clusters are also informative for this reason. In this simple example, the expected segregation ratio is 1:2:1 for the G/G:G/C:C/C genotypes and the angle between the clusters is $\pi/4$ (since the intensity of the G allele and C allele

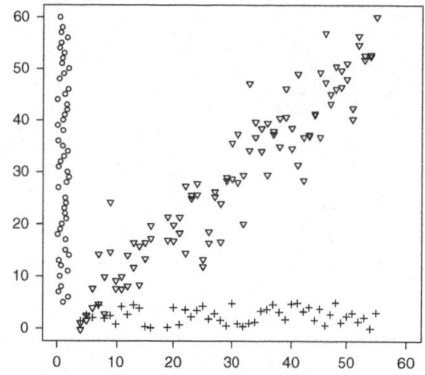

in this group will be equal). Thus, by comparing the proportions of individuals in each cluster with the expected segregation ratio and examining the angles between the clusters, it would be possible to infer that these individuals are diploid if that information was not already available.

Such an approach would also prove useful in the analysis of sugarcane since SNPs occur frequently in the sugarcane genome, approximately 1 in every 50 bases. However, its polyploid structure results in a much more complex problem. The ploidy level, on which segregation ratios etc. are based, is generally unknown and thus it is difficult to determine the number of unique genotypes that exist among individuals. This information could have implications for sugarcane breeding since high yield potential may be due to the presence of a specific allele, or a particular number of copies of a specific allele(s) present at a gene locus, or possibly a combination of both. Cordeiro et al. (2006) state that the frequency of a SNP base (A, T, C, G) at a locus is determined by

- the number of chromosomes carrying the gene;
- the number of different alleles for a gene;
- the frequency of each allele possessing each SNP base.

In sugarcane, the proportional frequency of each SNP base varies depending on the number of alleles containing the SNP locus. The frequency of a SNP base at a gene locus will be determined by both the number of chromosomes carrying the gene, the number of different alleles and the frequency of each allele possessing each SNP base. This in turn provides information about the ploidy level and genetic make-up of the sugarcane plant.

Figure 2 displays the data collected for two of the SNPs analyzed in this paper. Each point represents the intensity of two SNP bases, h.L is the intensity of the C allele and h.H is the intensity of the G allele. The data on the LHS in Fig. 2 can clearly be clustered into two groups—the group along the *y*-axis and the group along the line with a particular (unknown) angle. These groups correspond to two genotypes and thus clustering is essential for genotyping. In the example shown on

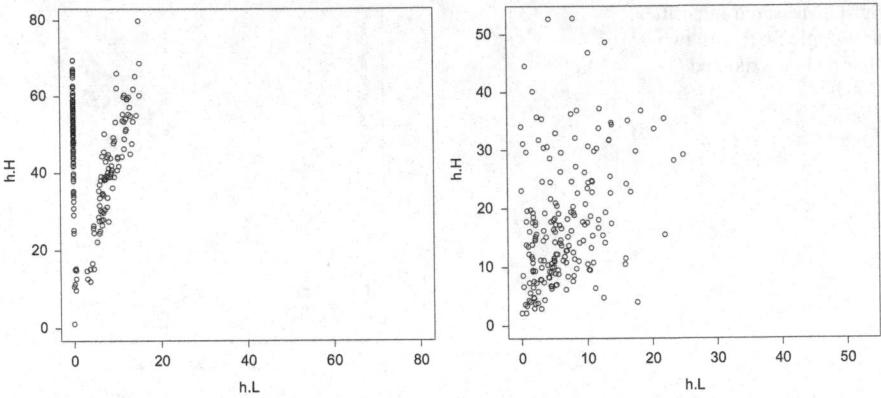

Fig. 2 *LHS*: Raw data for SNP Contig89b17; *RHS*: Raw data for SNP Contig2312b2

the RHS in Fig. 2, it is not clear how many clusters (i.e. genotypes) are present and therefore the aim of this research is to develop a technique that can:

(1) provide a probabilistic clustering to identify individuals that have high probability of belonging to a particular cluster (i.e. individuals that have a particular genotype) and those that are regarded as an unclear genotype;
(2) determine the number of clusters present;
(3) calculate the proportion of individuals in each cluster;
(4) determine the angles between clusters.

The above criteria suggest that using an appropriate clustering algorithm may prove useful for these data. Clustering methods such as k-means clustering (Hartigan and Wong 1978), hierarchical clustering (Eisen et al. 1998; Spellman et al. 1998), clustering on self-organizing maps (Kohonen 1997; Tamayo et al. 1999), model-based clustering (Fraley and Raftery 2002; McLachlan et al. 2002, 2003, 2006), fuzzy c-means clustering (Futschik and Carlisle 2005) and tight clustering (Tseng and Wong 2005), have been used extensively in many applications to group observations such that individuals within a cluster are more alike than individuals in different clusters. Here we use model-based clustering, a parametric clustering technique that assumes a particular statistical model for the data within each cluster. In the simplest case, the data in each cluster are assumed to have a normal distribution, however, more elaborate models can also be used. These include mixtures of linear regression models, mixtures of mixed effects models (Celeux et al. 2005; Ng et al. 2006), mixtures of generalized linear models (Leisch 2004; Grün and Leisch 2008), etc. In contrast, this paper uses finite mixtures of orthogonal regression lines to cluster SNP data arising from the analysis of the genetic traits of sugarcane.

The remainder of the paper is outlined as follows. Section 2 describes finite mixture models and discusses the use of orthogonal regression lines to describe the data within each cluster. Section 3 presents the results of applying the proposed method to SNP data arising from sugarcane. Section 4 provides a brief discussion.

2   Methodology

2.1   Finite Mixture Models

Model-based clustering assumes that the data $\mathbf{y} = (\mathbf{y}_1, \ldots, \mathbf{y}_n)$ arise from a mixture of G components

$$f(\mathbf{y}_i; \mathbf{\Theta}) = \sum_{g=1}^{G} \pi_g f_g(\mathbf{y}_i; \boldsymbol{\theta}_g),$$

where $f(\mathbf{y}_i; \mathbf{\Theta})$ is the density of the data, $f_g(\mathbf{y}_i; \boldsymbol{\theta}_g)$ is the density of the data in the gth component, which if assumed to be a normal distribution has parameters $\boldsymbol{\theta}_g = (\boldsymbol{\mu}_g, \boldsymbol{\Sigma}_g)$, and π_g are mixing proportions such that

$$\sum_g \pi_g = 1.$$

To fit the latter model, it is necessary to obtain estimates of $(\boldsymbol{\theta}_1, \ldots, \boldsymbol{\theta}_G, \pi_1, \ldots, \pi_G)$, which is typically achieved using the Expectation–Maximization (EM) algorithm of Dempster et al. (1977).

The EM algorithm determines maximum likelihood estimates of the parameters in a statistical model by maximizing the log-likelihood in the presence of "missing" data. The missing data in a clustering context are the vectors of cluster membership probabilities $\mathbf{z}_i = (z_{i1}, \ldots, z_{iG})$ such that

$$z_{ig} = \begin{cases} 1 \text{ if gene } i \text{ belongs to cluster } g, \\ 0 \text{ otherwise.} \end{cases}$$

The EM algorithm maximizes the "complete data" log-likelihood

$$\ell_C(\boldsymbol{\theta}_g, \pi_g, z_{ig} | \mathbf{y}) = \sum_{i=1}^{n} \sum_{g=1}^{G} z_{ig} [\log \pi_g f_g(\mathbf{y}_i | \boldsymbol{\theta}_g)],$$

by iterating between the E-step, where the z_{ig} values are replaced with their expected values conditional on the current model parameter estimates $\hat{z}_{ig} = E[z_{ig} | \mathbf{y}_i, \boldsymbol{\theta}_1, \ldots, \boldsymbol{\theta}_G]$, and the M-step, where the model parameters $(\boldsymbol{\theta}_1, \ldots, \boldsymbol{\theta}_G, \pi_1, \ldots, \pi_G)$ are updated given the current $\hat{z}_{ig}$ values.

2.2 Finite Mixtures of Least Squares Regression Lines

For these data, fitting a regression line to the data in each cluster would facilitate determining the number of clusters and the angles between clusters (as the angles between the regression lines describing the data in each cluster), which contains information about the number of different alleles, the corresponding genotypes and phenotypes and the ploidy level as required. Here, the data for each individual consists of a p-length vector $\mathbf{y}_i = (\text{h.H}, \text{h.L})$, where $p = 2$. To cluster the data using a mixture of regression lines, it was initially assumed that one of the measured variables, h.L or h.H, was the response variable y and the other was the explanatory variable x. Information from the geneticists indicated that the regression lines should pass through the origin and thus it was assumed that a linear regression line through the origin

$$y_i = \beta_1 x_i + \varepsilon_i$$

could be fitted to the data in each cluster. The cluster densities were then univariate normal such that

$$f_g(y_i | \beta_{1g} x_i, \sigma_g^2) = N(\beta_{1g} x_i, \sigma_g^2),$$

where β_{1g} is the slope in the gth component and σ_g^2 is the variance. The process was repeated by reversing the roles of h.H and h.L, i.e., if h.H was the assumed response variable in the first analysis, it was treated as the explanatory variable in the second analysis. The results of both analyses were then compared.

Using h.L as the response variable y and h.H as the explanatory variable x yielded more interpretable results than using $y = $ h.H and $x = $ h.L. This was primarily due to the presence of many h.L values that had the same corresponding h.H value, resulting in a regression line parallel to the y-axis when $y = $ h.H was used. Such lines have infinite slope and thus cannot be estimated by standard least squares. In addition, for these data it is not clear which variable is the true response variable and which is the true explanatory variable and both values contain some measurement error/noise. As a result an alternative approach using finite mixtures of *orthogonal* regression lines is proposed.

2.3 Finite Mixtures of Orthogonal Regression Lines

Total Least Squares (also known as errors in variables or rigorous least squares) is a regression method where observational errors on both the dependent variable and p independent variables are taken into account during model fitting. Computation of the total least squares regression line is achieved using the singular value decomposition (SVD) as described in the general case as follows. Let

$$y = X\beta$$

be a system of equations that we wish to solve for β, where X is $n \times p$ and y is $n \times 1$. Therefore, we wish to find β that minimizes the matrix of errors E for X and vector of errors r for y. That is,

$$\text{argmin}_{E,r} \|[E \ r]\|_F, \quad (X + E)\beta = y + r,$$

where $[E \ r]$ is the augmented matrix and $\| \cdot \|_F$ is the Frobenius norm.

Golub and Van Loan (1980) show that this can be achieved using a SVD of $[X \ y]$ such that

$$[X \ y] = \begin{bmatrix} U_X \ U_y \end{bmatrix} \begin{bmatrix} D_X & 0 \\ 0 & D_y \end{bmatrix} \begin{bmatrix} V_{XX} & V_{Xy} \\ V_{yX} & V_{yy} \end{bmatrix}^T$$

and setting some of the singular values to zero;

$$[(X + E) \ (y + r)] = \begin{bmatrix} U_X \ U_y \end{bmatrix} \begin{bmatrix} D_X & 0 \\ 0 & 0_{1\times1} \end{bmatrix} \begin{bmatrix} V_{XX} & V_{Xy} \\ V_{yX} & V_{yy} \end{bmatrix}^T.$$

This implies

$$[E \ r] = - \begin{bmatrix} U_X \ U_y \end{bmatrix} \begin{bmatrix} 0_{1\times1} & 0 \\ 0 & D_X \end{bmatrix} \begin{bmatrix} V_{XX} & V_{Xy} \\ V_{yX} & V_{yy} \end{bmatrix}^T$$

$$= - \begin{bmatrix} X \ y \end{bmatrix} \begin{bmatrix} V_{Xy} \\ V_{yy} \end{bmatrix} \begin{bmatrix} V_{Xy} \\ V_{yy} \end{bmatrix}^T$$

and

$$[(X + E) \ (y + r)] \begin{bmatrix} V_{Xy} \\ V_{yy} \end{bmatrix} = 0.$$

If V_{yy} is nonsingular, right multiply both sides by $-V_{yy}^{-1}$ to get:

$$[(X + E) \ (y + r)] \begin{bmatrix} -V_{Xy}V_{yy}^{-1} \\ -V_{yy}V_{yy}^{-1} \end{bmatrix} = [(X + E) \ (y + r)] \begin{bmatrix} \beta \\ -I_{1\times1} \end{bmatrix} = 0$$

and thus

$$\hat{\beta} = -V_{Xy}V_{yy}^{-1}.$$

Since the sugarcane data is two-dimensional, Deming regression (a special case of total least squares where there is one dependent variable y and one independent variable x), is appropriate. Then both x and y are assumed to be measured with error such that

$$x_i = x_i^* + \epsilon_i,$$
$$y_i = y_i^* + \eta_i,$$

where ϵ_i and η_i are independent and the ratio of their variances

$$\delta = \frac{\sigma_\epsilon^2}{\sigma_\eta^2}$$

is assumed to be known. For our purposes we use orthogonal regression (through the origin), which assumes $\delta = 1$. Applying the estimation approach outlined above implies that $\hat{\beta}_1 = -V_{Xy}/V_{yy}$ and V_{Xy}/V_{yy} are scalars rather than matrices.

Once the slope of the orthogonal regression line is determined using the above method, it is necessary to determine the fitted values. This requires finding the equation of the line that passes through the original data point (x_i, y_i) but orthogonal to the fitted regression line with slope given by $\hat{\beta}_1$. The point at which both lines intersect gives the fitted point. Let $\hat{y}_i = \hat{x}_i \hat{\beta}_1$ denote the line with slope $\hat{\beta}_1$ that passes through the origin (i.e. the fitted orthogonal regression line). Then the equation of the line orthogonal to this will have slope $-1/\hat{\beta}_1$ and corresponding equation

$$\hat{y}_i = -\frac{\hat{x}_i}{\hat{\beta}_1} + b.$$

This line passes through our original data point (x_i, y_i) implying that

$$b = y_i + \frac{x_i}{\hat{\beta}_1}$$

and

$$\hat{y}_i = -\frac{\hat{x}_i}{\hat{\beta}_1} + y_i + \frac{x_i}{\hat{\beta}_1}.$$

The point at which the two lines intersect is given by:

$$\hat{x}_i \hat{\beta}_1 = -\frac{\hat{x}_i}{\hat{\beta}_1} + y_i + \frac{x_i}{\hat{\beta}_1},$$
$$\hat{x}_i \hat{\beta}_1^2 = -x_i + y_i \hat{\beta}_1 + x_i,$$

$$\hat{x}_i = \frac{y_i \hat{\beta}_1 + x_i}{1 + \hat{\beta}_1^2},$$

$$\hat{y}_i = \hat{x}_i \hat{\beta}_1.$$

Therefore the fitted point is

$$\left(\hat{x}_i = \frac{y_i \hat{\beta}_1 + x_i}{1 + \hat{\beta}_1^2}, \quad \hat{y}_i = \hat{x}_i \hat{\beta}_1 \right).$$

The corresponding residuals are

$$r_{ix} = x_i - \hat{x}_i,$$

$$r_{iy} = y_i - \hat{y}_i,$$

and since orthogonal regression assumes the variances σ_η^2 and σ_ϵ^2 are equal (but independent), an overall estimate of σ^2 is given by,

$$\hat{\sigma}^2 = \frac{\sum\limits_{i=1}^{n}(x_i - \hat{x}_i)^2 + \sum\limits_{i=1}^{n}(y_i - \hat{y}_i)^2}{2(n-1)}.$$

Implementing this in a clustering context requires maximizing the "complete-data" log-likelihood

$$\ell_C(\boldsymbol{\theta}_g, \pi_g, z_{ig}|x_i, y_i) = \sum_{i=1}^{n}\sum_{g=1}^{G} z_{ig}[\log \pi_g f_g(x_i, y_i|\boldsymbol{\theta}_g)], \qquad (1)$$

where $f_g(x_i, y_i|\boldsymbol{\theta}_g)$ is now a bivariate normal distribution such that

$$f_g(x_i, y_i|\boldsymbol{\theta}_g) = N(\boldsymbol{\mu}_g, \boldsymbol{\Sigma}_g),$$

and

$$\boldsymbol{\mu}_g = \begin{pmatrix} \mu_{Xg} \\ \mu_{Yg} \end{pmatrix}, \quad \boldsymbol{\Sigma}_g = \begin{pmatrix} \sigma_{\eta g}^2 & 0 \\ 0 & \sigma_{\epsilon g}^2 \end{pmatrix} = \begin{pmatrix} \sigma_g^2 & 0 \\ 0 & \sigma_g^2 \end{pmatrix},$$

since $\sigma_{\epsilon g}^2 = \sigma_{\eta g}^2$. Estimates of $\mu_{Xg} = \hat{x}_{ig}$ and $\mu_{Yg} = \hat{y}_{ig}$ are given by

$$\hat{x}_{ig} = \frac{y_i \hat{\beta}_{1g} + x_i}{1 + \hat{\beta}_{1g}^2}, \qquad (2)$$

$$\hat{y}_{ig} = \hat{x}_{ig} \hat{\beta}_{1g}. \qquad (3)$$

The estimated regression coefficients $\hat{\beta}_{1g}$, $g = 1, \ldots, G$ are found for each component via SVD where the data values (x_i, y_i) are multiplied by their estimated weights in component g, $\sqrt{\hat{z}_{ig}}$, such that

$$[\mathbf{X}_{wgt} \ \mathbf{y}_{wgt}] = [\mathbf{U}_X \ \mathbf{U}_y] \begin{bmatrix} \mathbf{D}_X & \mathbf{0} \\ \mathbf{0} & \mathbf{D}_y \end{bmatrix} \begin{bmatrix} \mathbf{V}_{XX} & \mathbf{V}_{Xy} \\ \mathbf{V}_{yX} & \mathbf{V}_{yy} \end{bmatrix}^T, \tag{4}$$

where $\mathbf{X}_{wgt} = (\sqrt{\hat{z}_{ig}}x_1, \sqrt{\hat{z}_{ig}}x_2, \ldots, \sqrt{\hat{z}_{ig}}x_n)^T$, $\mathbf{y}_{wgt} = (\sqrt{\hat{z}_{ig}}y_1, \sqrt{\hat{z}_{ig}}y_2, \ldots, \sqrt{\hat{z}_{ig}}y_n)^T$.

Then

$$\hat{\beta}_{1g} = -V_{Xy}/V_{yy}$$

and σ_g^2 is estimated using

$$\hat{\sigma}_g^2 = \frac{\sum\limits_{i=1}^{n} \hat{z}_{ig}(x_i - \hat{x}_{ig})^2 + \sum\limits_{i=1}^{n} \hat{z}_{ig}(y_i - \hat{y}_{ig})^2}{2\sum\limits_{i=1}^{n} \hat{z}_{ig}}. \tag{5}$$

The following outlines the EM algorithm for the orthogonal regression problem.
Steps in EM algorithm for orthogonal regression:

(1) Initialize $\hat{z}_{ig}$, e.g. by randomly allocating each individual to a particular cluster.
(2) **M-step:**

- For each cluster g, calculate $\hat{\beta}_{1g}$ using (4), $\hat{\sigma}_g^2$ using (5) and

$$\hat{\pi}_g = \frac{\sum\limits_{i=1}^{n} \hat{z}_{ig}}{n}.$$

- Calculate the fitted values for the ith individual in each component using (2) and (3).

(3) **E-step:**

- For each component, calculate $f_g(x_i, y_i | \hat{\boldsymbol{\mu}}_g, \hat{\boldsymbol{\Sigma}}_g)$ (a bivariate normal distribution). Since $\sigma_{\epsilon g}^2$ and $\sigma_{\eta g}^2$ are assumed to be independent and equal, this implies that

$$f_g(x_i, y_i | \hat{\boldsymbol{\mu}}_g, \hat{\boldsymbol{\Sigma}}_g) = f_g(x_i | \hat{x}_{ig}, \hat{\sigma}_g^2) \ f_g(y_i | \hat{y}_{ig}, \hat{\sigma}_g^2),$$

i.e., the product of two univariate normal distributions.
- Update the individual weights using

$$\hat{z}_{ig*} = \frac{\hat{\pi}_g f_g(x_i, y_i | \hat{\mu}_g, \hat{\Sigma}_g)}{\sum\limits_{h=1}^{G} \hat{\pi}_h f_h(x_i, y_i | \hat{\mu}_g, \hat{\Sigma}_g)}.$$

(4) Iterate between Steps 2 and 3 until convergence.

2.4 Choosing the Number of Clusters

Cluster analysis requires choosing the number of clusters G and model-based clustering facilitates using model-selection criteria such as the Akaike Information Criterion (AIC) or Bayesian Information Criterion (BIC) to determine an optimal value for G. Typically in cluster analysis the BIC is used and is written as

$$\text{BIC} = -2\log L + d \log n;$$

where $\log L$ is given in (1), d = number of parameters to be estimated in the model and n is the sample size. Here d consists of G slope parameters $\hat{\beta}_{1g}$, $g = 1, \ldots, G$, G variance parameters $\hat{\sigma}_g^2$, $g = 1, \ldots, G$ and $G - 1$ mixing proportions $\pi_1, \ldots, \pi_{G-1}$, implying that $d = 3G - 1$. The model fitting process is repeated for varying values of G and the value for G corresponding to the solution with minimum BIC is typically chosen. However, in many instances in this work, a drop in BIC could be attributed to a solution having many empty clusters. As a result, the statistical "elbow" in the BIC plot was identified and the value for G at which this "elbow" occurred was then chosen as the number of clusters.

3 Results

The proposed method was applied to five different SNPs: Contig89b17, Contig168b1, Contig628b21, Contig875b2 and Contig2312b2. The aim was to determine the number of clusters, the estimated orthogonal regression lines modelling the data in each cluster and the angle between the resulting clusters. In each case the algorithm was run using either h.H or h.L as the response variable, to determine if the clustering results were consistent when the roles of the variables were reversed. The results presented in this section are for $y = h.H$ and $x = h.L$; however, it should be noted that the results obtained from reversing the roles of h.H and h.L were identical (as expected). The number of clusters was determined using the BIC and outright assignment of data points into clusters was achieved using the map function in the mclust package. This function assigns point i to cluster g such that

$$\hat{z}_{ig} = \begin{cases} 1 & \text{if } g = \arg\max_h \hat{z}_{ih}, \\ 0 & \text{otherwise.} \end{cases}$$

To ensure the EM algorithm did not converge to a local optimum, the algorithm was run from five initial starting points obtained by randomly allocating individuals to clusters. The solution with maximum log-likelihood from these five starting positions was retained. The angles between adjacent clusters were calculated using

$$\phi = \arctan\left(\frac{m_2 - m_1}{1 + m_1 m_2}\right) \times \frac{180}{\pi},$$

where m_1 and m_2 are the slopes of the orthogonal regression lines describing the data in these two clusters.

3.1 Contig89b17

The top of Fig. 3 displays the raw data and BIC plot for Contig89b17. The BIC plot indicated that there were three clusters in these data (the reduction in BIC at later stages is due to a number of empty clusters for each solution). The corresponding cluster assignments and estimated orthogonal regression lines for each cluster are given in the bottom of Fig. 3. It is clear that the proposed method can fit a regression line to the group parallel to the y-axis, which was not possible using mixtures of least squares regression lines. The estimated slopes of the orthogonal regression lines (from right to left) were $\hat{\beta}_{11} = 4.294$, $\hat{\beta}_{12} = 5.496$ and $\hat{\beta}_{13} = 6,377.499$, and thus the angle between Cluster 1 and Cluster 2 ($\phi_{C1,C2}$) was calculated using

$$\phi_{C1,C2} = \arctan\left(\frac{\hat{\beta}_{12} - \hat{\beta}_{11}}{1 + \hat{\beta}_{11}\hat{\beta}_{12}}\right)$$

$$= \arctan\left(\frac{5.496 - 4.294}{1 + 4.294\,5.496}\right) \times \frac{180}{\pi}$$

$$= 2°80'.$$

The angle between Cluster 2 and Cluster 3 was

$$\phi_{C2,C3} = \arctan\left(\frac{6377.499 - 5.496}{1 + (5.496)(6377.499)}\right) \times \frac{180}{\pi} = 10°30'.$$

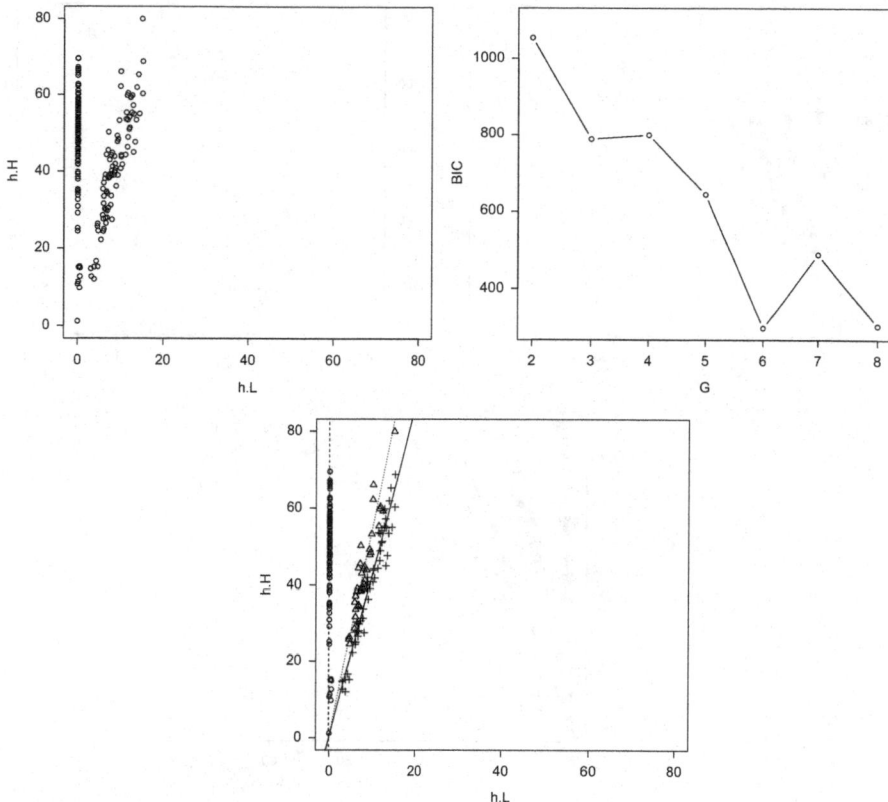

Fig. 3 *Top LHS*: Raw data for SNP Contig89b17. *Top RHS*: BIC plot for SNP Contig89b17. *Bottom*: Cluster allocations and fitted orthogonal regression line for SNP Contig89b17

3.2 *Contig168b1*

The analysis was repeated for SNP Contig168b1. In this case, the BIC plot indicated that there were five clusters (top of Fig. 4) in this dataset. The corresponding cluster assignments and estimated orthogonal regression lines for each cluster are shown in the bottom of Fig. 4. The estimated slopes of the orthogonal regression lines (from right to left) were $\hat{\beta}_{11} = 2.050$, $\hat{\beta}_{12} = 2.840$, $\hat{\beta}_{13} = 3.813$, $\hat{\beta}_{14} = 5.654$ and $\hat{\beta}_{15} = 33.992$. The corresponding angles between adjacent clusters (from right to left) were

$$\phi_{C1,C2} = 6°61' \quad \phi_{C3,C4} = 4°67'$$
$$\phi_{C2,C3} = 4°70' \quad \phi_{C4,C5} = 8°34'$$

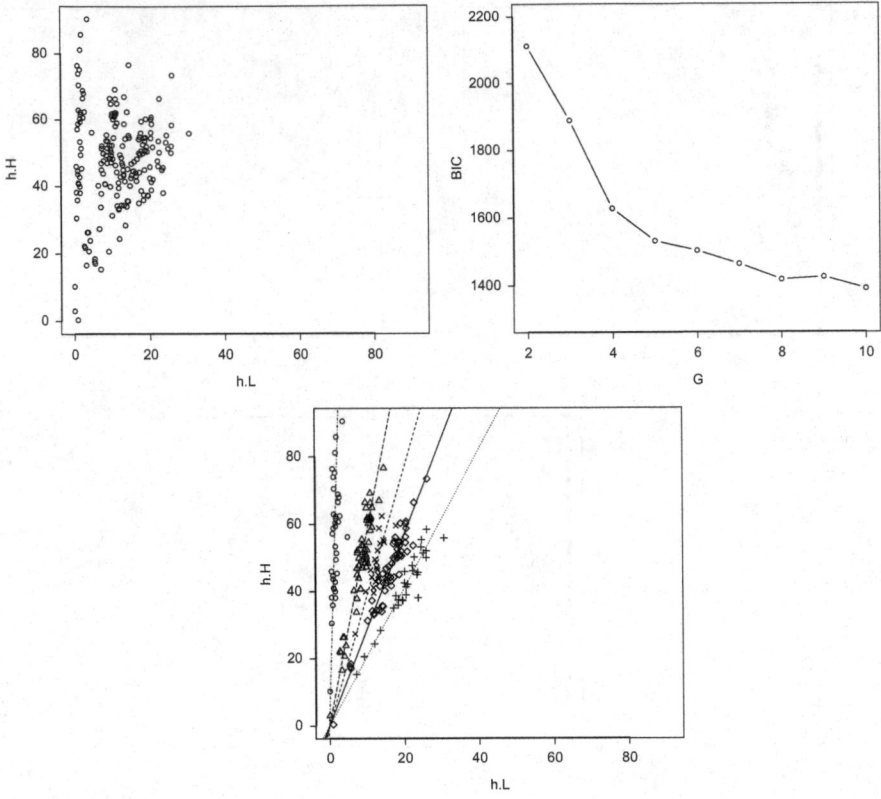

Fig. 4 *Top LHS*: Raw data for SNP Contig168b1. *Top RHS*: BIC plot for SNP Contig168b1. *Bottom*: Cluster allocations and fitted orthogonal regression line for SNP Contig168b1

3.3 Contig628b21

For this SNP, there was an obvious group of individuals parallel to the y-axis. Again it can be seen that the proposed methodology could cluster the data in this group without difficulty. The BIC plot in Fig. 5 indicated that there were three clusters in this dataset, with the cluster assignments and estimated orthogonal regression lines for each cluster displayed in the bottom of Fig. 5. From right to left, the estimated slopes of the orthogonal regression lines were $\hat{\beta}_{11} = 4.075$, $\hat{\beta}_{12} = 8.491$ and $\hat{\beta}_{13} = 1,087.018$. The angles between adjacent clusters (from right to left) were

$$\phi_{C1,C2} = 7°7'$$

$$\phi_{C2,C3} = 6°66'$$

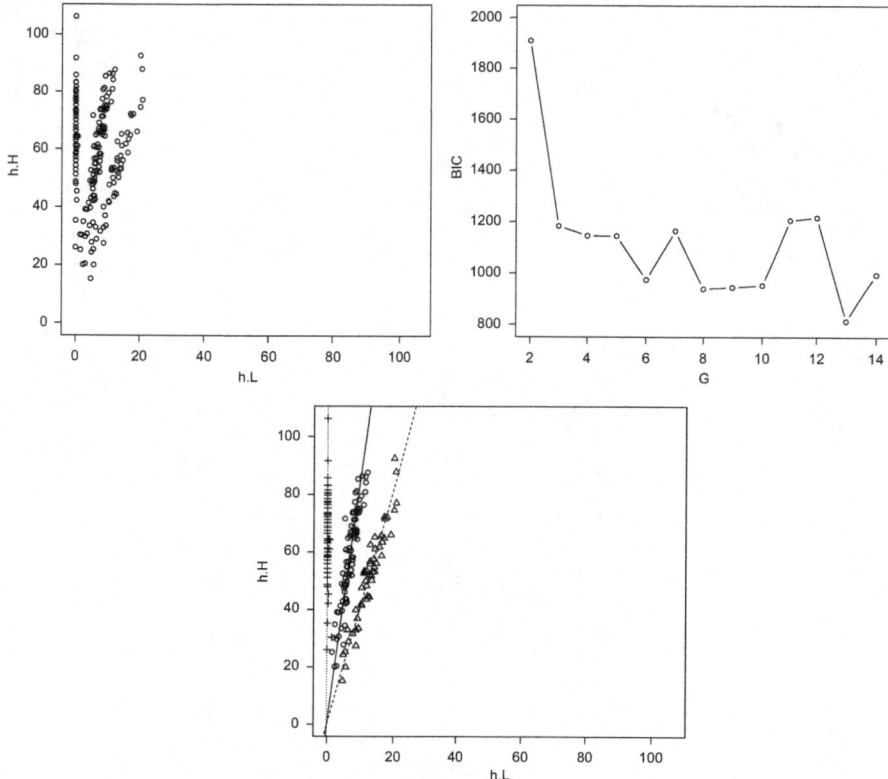

Fig. 5 *Top LHS*: Raw data for SNP Contig628b21. *Top RHS*: BIC plot for SNP Contig628b21. *Bottom*: Cluster allocations and fitted orthogonal regression line for SNP Contig628b21

3.4 Contig875b2

The data for this SNP did not exhibit a particularly obvious grouping structure; however, there were a number of points close to the y-axis which were quite different from the remaining data. The proposed method clustered all of these observations into the same cluster, described by an orthogonal regression line that was virtually parallel to the y-axis. The BIC plot for these data indicated that choosing $G = 6$ clusters was appropriate, with estimated slopes (from right to left) given by $\hat{\beta}_{11} = 1.532$, $\hat{\beta}_{12} = 1.874$, $\hat{\beta}_{13} = 2.394$, $\hat{\beta}_{14} = 2.858$, $\hat{\beta}_{15} = 4.906$ and $\hat{\beta}_{16} = 114.623$. The drop in BIC from $G = 10$ onwards was attributable to a number of empty clusters arising in the clustering solution (Fig. 6). The angles between adjacent clusters were calculated as

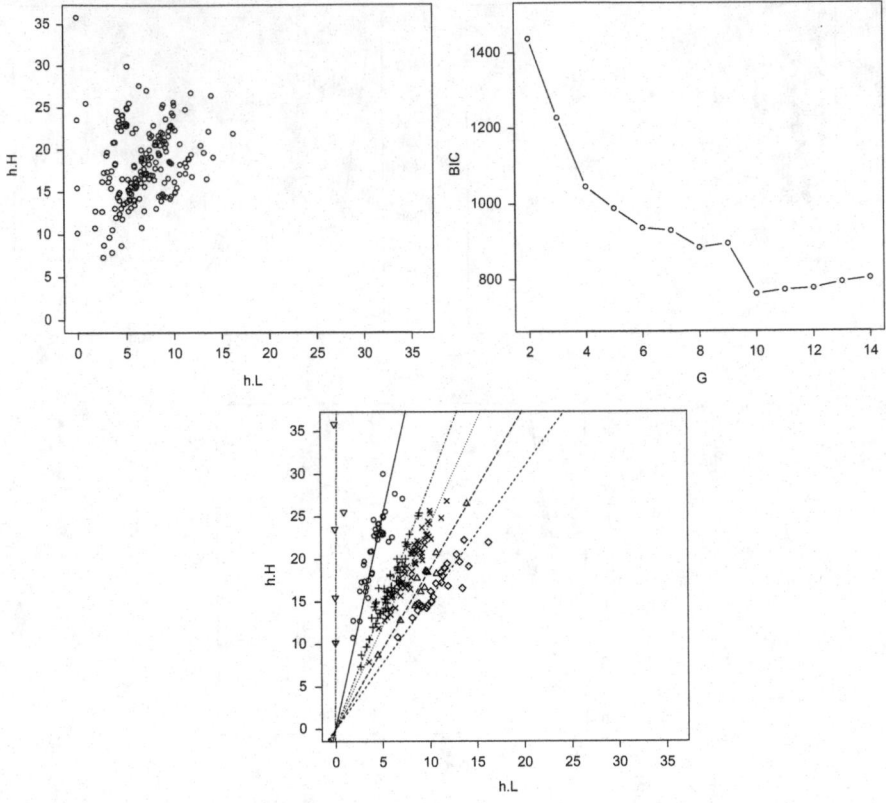

Fig. 6 *Top LHS*: Raw data for SNP Contig875b2. *Top RHS*: BIC plot for SNP Contig875b2.
Bottom: Cluster allocations and fitted orthogonal regression line for SNP Contig875b2

$$\phi_{C1,C2} = 5°05' \quad \phi_{C4,C5} = 7°77'$$
$$\phi_{C2,C3} = 5°42' \quad \phi_{C5,C6} = 11°02'$$
$$\phi_{C3,C4} = 3°38'$$

3.5 Contig2312b2

Finally, the algorithm was applied to SNP Contig2312b2. This was the most
complex dataset, since there was no clear grouping structure evident a priori.
Examining the BIC plot, $G = 8$ clusters were chosen with estimated regression lines
and cluster memberships displayed in the bottom of Fig. 7. The slope coefficients
(from right to left) for the eight clusters were $\hat{\beta}_{11} = 0.582$, $\hat{\beta}_{12} = 1.186$,

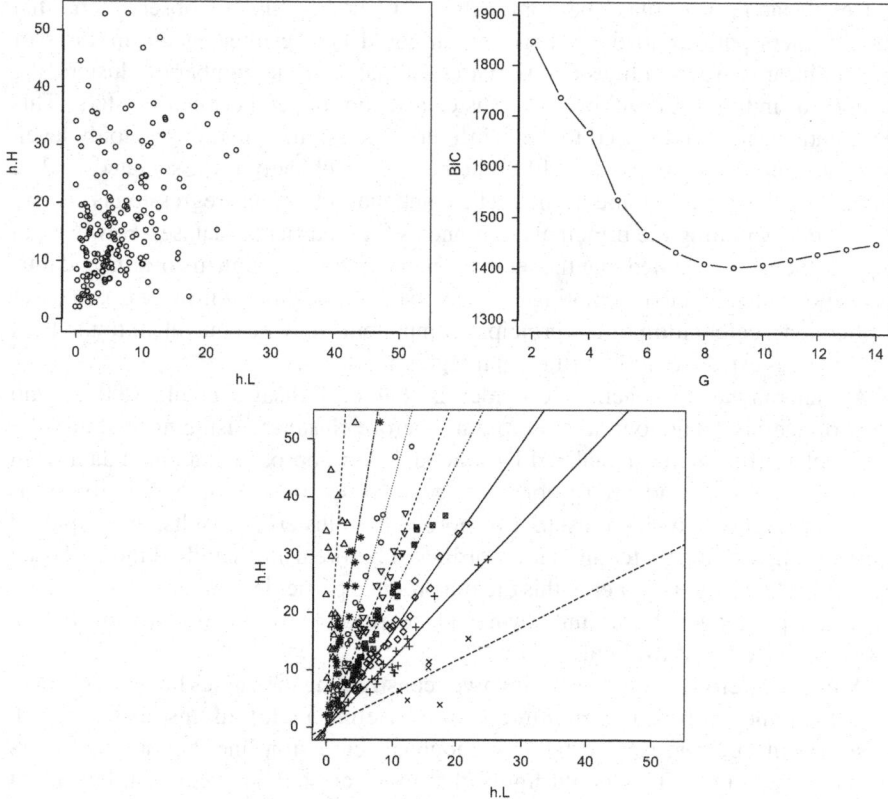

Fig. 7 *Top LHS*: Raw data for SNP Contig2312b2. *Top RHS*: BIC plot for SNP Contig2312b2. *Bottom*: Cluster allocations and fitted orthogonal regression line for SNP Contig2312b2

$\hat{\beta}_{13} = 1.645$, $\hat{\beta}_{14} = 2.283$, $\hat{\beta}_{15} = 2.890$, $\hat{\beta}_{16} = 4.214$, $\hat{\beta}_{17} = 7.116$ and $\hat{\beta}_{18} = 19.111$, with corresponding angles between adjacent clusters given by

$$\phi_{C1,C2} = 19°66' \quad \phi_{C4,C5} = 4°57' \quad \phi_{C7,C8} = 5°00'$$
$$\phi_{C2,C3} = 8°86' \quad \phi_{C5,C6} = 5°74'$$
$$\phi_{C3,C4} = 7°63' \quad \phi_{C6,C7} = 5°35'$$

4   Discussion

This paper has presented a simple but effective way of clustering bivariate SNP data using mixtures of orthogonal regression lines, where both variables are assumed to be measured with error and there is no natural distinction between the response and explanatory variable. The approach can handle groups of observations that form clusters parallel to the y-axis, which could not be fitted using mixtures of simple linear regression lines and provides estimates of the number of clusters, the number of individuals within each cluster and the angles between clusters. This information can then be used to make inferences about the (unknown) ploidy level, the segregation ratios and the different genotypes/phenotypes associated with a particular sugarcane genome. It should be noted that orthogonal regression is closely related to calculating the principal components for a particular dataset. However, in this instance it is assumed that the regression line passes through the origin, and thus this is not equivalent to calculating the principal components (Joliffe 2002). In other applications, calculation of the principal components may be equivalent to the total least squares estimate of the orthogonal regression lines.

An alternative approach to consider is that of Fujisawa et al. (2004), who transformed SNP data to polar co-ordinates before clustering using normal mixture model clustering with a penalized likelihood. Their approach examined data from a diploid organism and used prior knowledge (based on the known ploidy level) about the angles between clusters to improve the clustering results. We explored transforming these data to angular co-ordinates before using standard model-based clustering; however, in our case this did not produce particularly interpretable results since the ploidy level was unknown and no prior knowledge about the angles between clusters was available.

A future extension of this work involves constraining the angles between clusters to be the same (or based on multiple(s) of a baseline angle). In this instance, each cluster would be represented by an orthogonal regression line, but some clusters may now be empty. This could imply that more clusters are required, but might more accurately reflect the polyploid structure and perhaps explain the behavior of the BIC encountered in the analysis presented.

Acknowledgements Norma Bargary (nee Coffey) carried out this work at the National University of Ireland, Galway while supported by Science Foundation Ireland under Grant No. 07/MI/012 (BIO-SI project). The authors would also like to thank Dr. Anete P. Souza who carried out the laboratory work and is the co-ordinator of the project that produced the data analyzed.

References

Celeux, G., Martin, O., & Lavergne, C. (2005). Mixture of linear mixed models for clustering gene expression profiles from repeated microarray experiments. *Statistical Modelling, 5*, 243–267.

Cordeiro, G., Eliott, F., McIntyre, C., Casu, R. E., & Henry, R. J. (2006). Characterization of single nucleotide polymorphisms in sugarcane ESTs. *Theoretical and Applied Genetics, 113*, 331–343.

Dempster, A., Laird, N., & Rubin, D. (1977). Maximum likelihood from incomplete data via the EM algorithm. *Journal of the Royal Statistical Society, Series B, 39*, 1–38.

Eisen, M., Spellman, P., Brown, P., & Botstein, D. (1998) Cluster analysis and display of genome-wide expression patterns. *Proceeding of the National Academy of Sciences of the USA, 95*, 14863–14868.

Fraley, C., & Raftery, A. (2002). Model-based clustering, discriminant analysis, and density estimation. *Journal of the American Statistical Association, 97*, 611–631.

Fujisawa, H., Eguchi, S., Ushijima, M., Miyata, S., Miki, Y., Muto, T., et al. (2004). Genotyping of single nucleotide polymorphism using model-based clustering. *Bioinformatics, 20*, 718–726.

Futschik, M., & Carlisle, B. (2005). Noise-robust soft clustering of gene expression time-course data. *Journal of Bioinformatics and Computational Biology, 3*, 965–988.

Golub, G., & Van Loan, C. (1980). An analysis of the total least squares problem. *SIAM Journal of Numerical Analysis, 17*, 883–893.

Grün, B., & Leisch, F. (2008). FlexMix Version 2: Finite mixtures with concomitant variables and varying and constant parameters. *Journal of Statistical Software, 28*, 1–35.

Hartigan, J., & Wong, M. (1978). A k-means clustering algorithm. *Applied Statistics, 28*, 100–108.

Joliffe, I. (2002). *Principal component analysis*. New York: Springer.

Kohonen, T. (1997). *Self-organizing maps*. New York: Springer.

Leisch, F. (2004). FlexMix: A general framework for finite mixture models and latent class regression in R. *Journal of Statistical Software, 11*, 1–18.

McLachlan, G., Bean, R., & Peel, D. (2002). A mixture model-based approach to the clustering of microarray expression data. *Bioinformatics, 18*, 413–422.

McLachlan, G., Ng, S., & Bean, R. (2006). Robust cluster analysis via mixture models. *Austrian Journal of Statistics, 35*, 157–174.

McLachlan, G., Peel, D., & Bean, R. (2003). Modelling high-dimensional data by mixtures of factor analyzers. *Computational Statistics and Data Analysis, 41*, 379–388.

Ng, S., McLachlan, G., Wang, K., Ben-Tovim Jones, L., & Ng, S. (2006). A mixture model with random-effects components for clustering correlated gene-expression profiles. *Bioinformatics, 22*, 1745–1752.

Olivier, M. (2005). The invader assay for SNP genotyping. *Mutational Research, 573*, 103–110.

Palhares, A., Rodrigues-Morais, T., Van Sluys, M. A., Domingues, D., Maccheroni, W., Jordão, H., et al. (2012). A novel linkage map of sugarcane with evidence for clustering of retrotransposon-based markers. *BMC Genetics, 13*(51), 1–16.

Spellman, P., Sherlock, G., Zhang, M., Iyer, V., Anders, K., Eisen, M., et al. (1998). Comprehensive identification of cell cycle-regulated genes of the yeast *Saccharomyces cerevisiae* by microarray hybridization. *Molecular Biology of the Cell, 9*, 3273–3297.

Tamayo, P., Slonim, D., Mesirov, J., Zhu, Q., Kitareewan, S., Dmitrovsky, E., et al. (1999). Interpreting patterns of gene expression with self-organizing maps: Methods and application to hematopoietic differentiation. *Proceedings of the National Academy of Science USA, 96*, 2907–2912.

Tseng, G., & Wong, W. (2005). Tight clustering: A resampling-based approach for identifying stable and tight patterns in data. *Biometrics, 61*, 10–16.

Discrepancy and Choice of Reference Subclass in Categorical Regression Models

Defen Peng and Gilbert MacKenzie

Abstract For categorical regression models we derive the optimal design allocation of observations to subclasses and provide a statistic, based on generalized variance and its distribution for measuring the discrepancy between the optimal allocation and the observed allocations occurring in observational studies in the general linear model and extend our methods to generalized linear models. The focus is on techniques which maximize the precision of the resulting estimators. We explore the general form of optimal design matrix for general linear models with categorical regressors, and propose an algorithm to find the optimal design matrix for generalized linear models when the design matrix is of high dimension. We also find that the proposed statistic can be used to show whether secondary criteria for the choice of reference subclasses is required in parametric categorical regression models. The development and use of the techniques and tools are illustrated by means of simulation studies and the analysis of a set of lung cancer survival data.

Keywords Categorical variables • Design matrix parametrization • D-optimality • GLMs • Reference subclass choice • Regression models

1 Introduction

An ongoing question concerns the choice of reference subclass when encoding categorical variables in regression models. Other questions are focussed on the categorical encoding of continuous variables (Pocock et al. 2004; Altman and Royston 2006). The literature on the former issue is rather conflicting. For example, William (2005) claimed that the choice of reference category may be made on

D. Peng (✉)
The Centre for Biostatistics, University of Limerick, Limerick, Ireland
e-mail: defen.peng@ul.ie

G. MacKenzie and D. Peng (eds.), *Statistical Modelling in Biostatistics and Bioinformatics*, Contributions to Statistics, DOI 10.1007/978-3-319-04579-5_12, © Springer International Publishing Switzerland 2014

the basis of: (a) subject matter considerations which may suggest the choice of a particular category or, (b) the largest category should be chosen as it yields the smallest standard errors. On the other hand, Berk (2008), argued that there is no statistical justification for choosing one category over another. However, Frøslie et al. (2010), in the hyperglycaemia and adverse pregnancy outcome (HAPO) study, showed empirically that an unfortunate choice of reference category led to less precise estimators and noted that the largest reference category gave narrower confidence intervals.

The focus of this paper is on techniques which maximize the precision of the resulting estimators in a D-optimal sense. We found that, when the sample allocation is close to its ideal allocation in a D-optimal sense, the choice of a reference category can be regarded as arbitrary—there being no need to use a secondary criterion. In the case of a sample allocation being distant from its ideal allocation, the choice of a reference category affects the precision of estimators. Accordingly, the use of a secondary criterion is advantageous. For general linear models, we confirmed the finding of Frøslie et al. (2010). However, in the other cases the results are more complicated, see Peng and MacKenzie (2014).

The paper is organized as follows. In Sect. 2 we formulate the problem and derive an optimum allocation strategy. In Sect. 3 we develop an index measuring the "distance" any particular allocation is from the optimum. In Sect. 4 we extend the methodology to GLMs. In Sect. 5, we collect up the simulations results on which some of the earlier findings are based. In Sect. 6 we re-analyze population data on lung cancer survival in Northern Ireland before concluding with a short discussion.

2   Model and Formulation

2.1   General Linear Model

To make matters concrete we consider the general linear model

$$Y = X\beta + \epsilon,$$

where: Y is a continuous response variable, X is an $n \times p$ design matrix, β is a $p \times 1$ column vector of regression parameters. We will also assume that $\epsilon_i \sim N(0, \sigma^2)$ when required, for $i = 1, \cdots, n$, then $E(\epsilon) = 0$ and $E(\epsilon\epsilon') = \sigma^2 I_n$, where, I_n is a $n \times n$ identity matrix. It follows immediately that

$$\hat{\beta} = (X'X)^{-1}X'Y$$

and that

$$V(\hat{\beta}) = \sigma^2 (X'X)^{-1}$$

which implies, under the Gaussian assumption, that the observed information matrix is

$$I(\beta) = (X'X)/\sigma^2$$

when we assume σ^2 is known. It is also possible to consider other forms of the response variable Y, for example a binary response, leading to *binary regression* (Feldstein 1966).

If the design matrix X encodes a single categorical variable with p subclasses, the resulting cross-product matrix, $X'X$, may take one of several, essentially equivalent, patterned forms. Two main cases are, either,

$$X'X = \text{diag}(n_1, n_2, \cdots, n_p) \tag{1}$$

or, on letting $k = p - 1$

$$X'X = \begin{pmatrix} n & n_1 & n_2 & \cdots & n_k \\ n_1 & n_1 & 0 & \cdots & 0 \\ n_2 & 0 & n_2 & \cdots & 0 \\ \vdots & \vdots & \vdots & & \vdots \\ n_k & 0 & 0 & \cdots & n_k \end{pmatrix}. \tag{2}$$

In (1) we have included exactly $p = k + 1$ binary indicator variables and in (2) we have included an intercept term and exactly k binary indicator variables. Version (1) does not involve a reference category, and omits the intercept term, whilst version (2) involves treating one of the subclasses as a reference category. For example, if $x_{0i} = 1 \,\forall\, i$ is the intercept term, then for $i \in$ reference category : $x_{1i} = 0 \cap \cdots \cap x_{ki} = 0$. Version (2) occurs most frequently and is the subject on this note.

With these arrangements the coefficients in the linear regression model have the following interpretation

$$\beta_0 = E(Y|x_0 = 1, x_1 = 0, \cdots, x_k = 0),$$
$$\beta_j = E(Y|x_0 = 1, x_1 = 0, \cdots, x_j = 1, \ldots, x_k = 0)$$
$$- E(Y|x_0 = 1, x_1 = 0, \cdots, x_k = 0) \tag{3}$$

for $j = 1, \cdots, k$. In (3), the intercept, β_0 is the conditional expectation of Y in the reference subclass and the usual regression coefficients, the β_js, of primary scientific interest, are differences between two conditional expectations.

2.2 Optimum Allocation

Now we consider the idea of optimal allocation from the design perspective of D-optimality. Given n observations and $p = k + 1$ subclasses how should the observations be allocated to subclasses in order to minimize the generalized variance, $GV(\beta)$, of the parameter β? The generalized variance is defined as

$$GV(\beta) = \det[I^{-1}(\beta)] = \det[\sigma^2(X'X)^{-1}], \qquad (4)$$

where, e.g., $\det[A]$ stands for the determinant of the matrix A. Minimizing (4) is equivalent to maximizing $\det[I(\beta)]$ so that the D-optimal design may be found as

$$D_p(n^{*\prime}) = \underset{n_j s}{\mathrm{argmax}} \left\{ \det[(X'X)]/\sigma^2 \right\} \qquad (5)$$

subject to $(\Sigma_{j=1}^{p} n_j = n)$, where $X'X$ is given by (2) and $D_p(n^{*\prime})$ is the design comprising a vector of optimal subclass numbers $n^{*\prime} = (n_1^*, n_2^*, \cdots, n_p^*)$.

It is then easy to show that the optimal allocation is uniform. It follows that the D-optimal design matrix is

$$(X^{*\prime}X^*) = \begin{pmatrix} n & n_1^* & n_2^* & \cdots & n_k^* \\ n_1^* & n_1^* & 0 & \cdots & 0 \\ n_2^* & 0 & n_2^* & \cdots & 0 \\ \vdots & \vdots & \vdots & & \vdots \\ n_k^* & 0 & 0 & \cdots & n_k^* \end{pmatrix},$$

where $n_j^* = n/p$, $j = 1, \cdots, p$ are corresponding to the D-optimal design matrix X^*. Moreover, the minimum generalized variance is then from (4),

$$GV^*(\beta) = \sigma^2 / \prod_{j=1}^{p} n_j^*. \qquad (6)$$

It will be recalled that the D-optimal solution does not guarantee that the $se(\hat{\beta})$ is uniformly minimal, rather it is equivalent to minimizing the volume of Gaussian theory confidence regions for β (Isham 1991).

This is a useful result when we can control the allocation, but in observational studies this is not possible. Then, of course, we might choose to view this result simply as a counterfactual experiment representing an ideal allocation and ponder how distant any sample allocation is from this ideal.

3 Measures of Discrepancy

As a measure of discrepancy from $GV^*(\beta)$ we consider the general index

$$
\begin{aligned}
G_D(\beta) &= \log_e \left[GV(\beta)/GV^*(\beta) \right] \\
&= \log_e \left[\det[I^*(\beta)]/\det[I(\beta)] \right],
\end{aligned}
\tag{7}
$$

where $I^*(\beta)$ is the observed information matrix, corresponding to the D-optimal design matrix X^*. The index $G_D(\cdot)$ is a random variable with support on $[0,\infty)$ and $G_D(\cdot) = 0$ implies that the sample allocation is optimal. We retain the unknown β in the notation to accommodate the GLM cases discussed later.

In order to explore how this index varies with the sample data we shall have to vary $(n_1, n_2, \cdots, n_p)$ systematically away from $(n_1^*, n_2^*, \cdots, n_p^*)$ using positive compositions. Whilst (7) is natural in context, a potential draw-back is that the distribution of the index, over the finite set of positive compositions, is unknown, although it can always be obtained by direct enumeration (below). For a single categorical variable with $p = k + 1$ subclasses in the model, from (4) and (6),

$$
\begin{aligned}
G_D(\beta) &= \log_e \left[\sigma^2 \det(X^{*'} X^*) / \sigma^2 \det(X'X) \right] \\
&= \sum_{j=1}^{p} \log_e (n_j^*/n_j),
\end{aligned}
\tag{8}
$$

a very simple form.

However, there are other, contending indices, one of which is the generalized Chi-squared test statistic X^2. For a single categorical variable with $p = k + 1$ subclasses in the model, the X^2 is the ordinary Chi-squared *goodness-of-fit* test of $H_0 : n' = n^{*'}$, versus the alternative hypothesis of discrepancy, $H_1 : n' \neq n^{*'}$,

$$
X^2 = \sum_{j=1}^{p} [n_j - n_j^*]^2 / n_j^*
$$

from which the null distribution of discrepancy is readily available, although the adequacy of this approximation needs to be checked in the current context. When H_0 is rejected, we may choose to regard χ_ν^2, where $\nu = p - 1 = k$, as a measure of standardized squared distance that n' is from $n^{*'}$.

3.1 Compositions

First we consider some computational issues involving integers associated with this problem. For p subclasses, the set of integer numbers, $(n_1, n_2, \cdots, n_p)$, falling in

Table 1 Distributions of measures of discrepancy

Index	Null	n	p	Non-Null
$G_D(\cdot)$	$\gamma(\alpha_0, \eta_0)$			
		≤ 500	$= 2$	$\gamma(0.5, 1)$
			> 2	$\gamma(\alpha_1, \eta_1)$
		> 500	$[2-9]$	$\gamma(\alpha_1, \eta_1)$
X^2	χ_ν^2			$\chi_{\nu,\lambda}^2$

$p = k + 1$, $\nu = k$ and, (α_0, η_0) and (α_1, η_1) can be found by simulation, $\gamma(\cdot, \cdot)$ is the Gamma distribution and $\chi_{\nu,\lambda}^2$ is the non-central Chi-squared distribution

the subclasses forms a positive composition ($n_j > 0$, $\forall j$) of the total sample size n. For example, for $n = 3$ and $p = 3$ there are ten compositions; $(3, 0, 0), (0, 3, 0), \cdots, (1, 1, 1)$, nine of these involve zero cells and one, the last, the only positive composition, does not. For general n and p there are exactly $\binom{n+p-1}{n}$ compositions of which $\binom{n+p-1}{n} - \binom{n-1}{p-1}$ involve zeros and are rejected by algorithms generating positive compositions. Such algorithms are required in order to study the variation in the indices proposed above. Moreover, the set of positive compositions, when they exist, is symmetric around $n^{*\prime}$, so that in practice only half need be generated. Nijenhuis and Wilf (1978) give Fortran algorithms which we translate into R software scripts (Appendix 1) and use to generate positive compositions by rejecting all compositions involving zeros. The second script generates random positive compositions and is useful in simulation studies. As we need to consider the distribution of the indices on the Null hypothesis of optimal allocation, i.e., their *Testing Distributions*, we generate positive compositions using the multinominal function in R, which enables us to control the cell probabilities.

3.2 Indices and Their Distributions for a Single Category

The results of a comprehensive simulation study (later) showed that the Null distribution of the index, $G_D(\cdot)$, follows a Gamma(α_0, η_0) distribution, where (α_0, η_0) depend on n and p in a way described in the simulation section. In the non-Null case, the distribution of the index is generally Gamma(α_1, η_1), where the parameter α_1 and η_1 are fractional and depends on n and p in a way described in the simulation section. When $n \leq 500$ and $p = 2$ we found that $2G_D(\cdot) \sim \chi_\nu^2$, where $\nu = 1$. See Table 1 for more details and the simulation section below.

A key finding from the simulation is that the Null distribution of the ordinary Chi-squared statistic, $X^2 = \sum_{j=1}^{p}[n_j - n_j^*]^2 / n_j^*$ is well described by a χ_ν^2 distribution where, as expected, $\nu = p - 1 = k$ degrees of freedom. And the non-Null distribution is the corresponding non-central Chi-squared with parameters $(p-1, \lambda)$, where the non-centrality parameter, λ, is defined in the simulation section.

The two indices are implicitly functionally related, viz

$$G_D(\cdot) = \sum_{j=1}^{p} \log_e \left(\frac{n_j^*}{n_j}\right) = - \sum_{j=1}^{p} \log_e \left(1 + \frac{1}{2}\frac{\partial X^2}{\partial n_j}\right), \tag{9}$$

but are not easily separable. However, this equation shows that the two indices measure the same underlying discrepancy. We may also conclude that the distribution of the index $G_D(\cdot)$ is inherently more complicated than its Chi-squared competitor. The values of the α_1 and η_1 parameters, which depend on n and p, must be known in advance in order to use the index; for example, as given in this paper (later). Secondly, the extension to multiple categorical variables requires us to formulate and compute the ideal allocation, i.e., to find $n^{*'}$, for the general case.

3.3 General Expression for the Ideal Allocation

In order to pursue the comparison of the indices, we must find $(X^{*'}X^*)$ representing the ideal allocation when there is more than one categorical variable in the model. Accordingly, suppose there are m categorical variables in the model $X_1, \cdots, X_m$, such that each variable has p_ℓ subclasses, $\ell = 1, 2, \cdots, m$. Then, it can be shown that the optimal design matrix takes the general form

$$(X^{*'}X^*) = n \begin{pmatrix} 1 & v_p \\ v_p' & M \end{pmatrix}, \tag{10}$$

where $v_p = (\frac{1}{p_1} \cdot 1_{p_1}', \frac{1}{p_2} \cdot 1_{p_2}', \cdots, \frac{1}{p_m} \cdot 1_{p_m}')$, a vector with dimension $(\sum_\ell p_\ell - m)$, and 1_{p_ℓ} are $(p_\ell - 1)$ vectors with element 1, $\ell = 1, 2, \cdots, m$. M is a symmetric matrix with diagonal elements $\frac{1}{p_\ell} I_\ell$, I_ℓ is $(p_\ell - 1) \times (p_\ell - 1)$ identity matrix, $\ell = 1, 2, \cdots, m$, while the elements in the upper triangle are $\frac{1}{p_i p_j} 1_{ij}$, where 1_{ij} is $(p_i - 1) \times (p_j - 1)$ matrix with element 1, $i = 1, 2, \cdots, m - 1, j > i$.

This general pattern was derived by considering lower order cases and using multiple Lagrange multipliers to deal with the defining constraints and recognizing that, whatever the number of categorical variables included, finally, only one substitution is permitted. This finding was also confirmed for higher order cases by simulation which showed that, as the sample allocation departs from (10), the value of det[$(X'X)$] becomes smaller.

We present two simple examples of the pattern: (X_1, X_2) with $(2, 2)$ subclasses and three categorical variables (X_1, X_2, X_3) with $(2, 3, 4)$ subclasses, respectively to illustrate the construction. The ideal allocation design matrices are then

$$(X^{*'}X^*)_{(2,2)} = \begin{pmatrix} n & n_1^* & n_2^* \\ n_1^* & n_1^* & n_{12}^* \\ n_2^* & n_{12}^* & n_2^* \end{pmatrix} = \begin{pmatrix} n & \frac{n}{2} & \frac{n}{2} \\ \frac{n}{2} & \frac{n}{2} & \frac{n}{4} \\ \frac{n}{2} & \frac{n}{4} & \frac{n}{2} \end{pmatrix} = n \begin{pmatrix} 1 & \frac{1}{2} & \frac{1}{2} \\ \frac{1}{2} & \frac{1}{2} & \frac{1}{4} \\ \frac{1}{2} & \frac{1}{4} & \frac{1}{2} \end{pmatrix},$$

where n_1^* is associated with X_1^*, n_2^* is associated with X_2^* and n_{12}^* is the cross term between X_1^* and X_2^*, $\Sigma x_{1i}^* x_{2i}^* = n/(p_1 p_2) = n/4$ (Appendix 2) and similarly

$$(X^{*'}X^*)_{(2,3,4)} = n \begin{pmatrix} 1 & 1/2 & 1/3 & 1/3 & 1/4 & 1/4 & 1/4 \\ 1/2 & 1/2 & 1/6 & 1/6 & 1/8 & 1/8 & 1/8 \\ 1/3 & 1/6 & 1/3 & 0 & 1/12 & 1/12 & 1/12 \\ 1/3 & 1/6 & 0 & 1/3 & 1/12 & 1/12 & 1/12 \\ 1/4 & 1/8 & 1/12 & 1/12 & 1/4 & 0 & 0 \\ 1/4 & 1/8 & 1/12 & 1/12 & 0 & 1/4 & 0 \\ 1/4 & 1/8 & 1/12 & 1/12 & 0 & 0 & 1/4 \end{pmatrix}$$

from which we note that within each categorical variable: (a) the ideal allocation is inversely proportional to the corresponding number of subclasses and (b) the cross terms are zero. Finally, the cross terms between any two categorical variables are inversely proportional to the product of the numbers of subclasses involved. Thus, these findings allow us to generalize the index, $G_D(\beta)$ to models with multiple categorical variables.

The availability of a general expression for the ideal allocation for the index allows us to compute the value of the corresponding X^2 statistic, compare the Null distributions and compute the power functions for the two indices in the simulation section. Meanwhile, we turn now to investigate reference subclass choice.

4 Generalized Linear Models

We consider the canonical generalized linear model (Cox and Snell 1989) for independent responses Y_i with $E(Y_i) = \mu_i = g(\theta_i)$, where $\theta_i = \sum_{u=0}^k x_{ui}\beta_u$ is the linear predictor, $g(\cdot)$ is the link function, for $i = 1, \cdots, n$ independent observations and $u = 0, \cdots, k$, representing the p unknown regression parameters. The log likelihood is $\sum_i (s_i\theta_i - K(\theta_i))$, where s_i is a function of Y_i. Then the observed information matrix for β is

$$I(\beta) = (\nabla_\beta \theta^T)(\nabla_\theta \nabla_\theta K)(\nabla_\beta \theta^T)^T = (\nabla_\beta \mu^T)(\nabla_\theta \nabla_\theta K)^{-1}(\nabla_\beta \mu^T)^T. \quad (11)$$

Table 2 Canonical link functions and the form of w_i

Distribution	Density(mass) function	Link function	w_i
Normal	$f(y; \mu, \sigma) = \frac{1}{\sqrt{2\pi}\sigma} e^{\frac{-(y-\mu)^2}{2\sigma^2}}$	$x\beta = \mu = \theta$	σ^{-2}
Exponential	$f(y; \lambda) = \lambda e^{-\lambda y}$	$x\beta = \mu^{-1} = \theta$	$(x_i'\beta)^{-2}$
IG	$f(y; \mu, \lambda) = (\frac{\lambda}{2\pi y^3})^{\frac{1}{2}} e^{\frac{-\lambda(y-\mu)^2}{2\mu^2 y}}$	$x\beta = \mu^{-2} = \theta$	$\frac{\lambda}{4}(x_i'\beta)^{-3/2}$
Poisson	$f(y; \lambda) = \frac{\lambda^y}{y!} e^{-\lambda}$	$x\beta = \log(\mu) = \theta$	$\exp(x_i'\beta)$
Binomial	$f(y; n_i, p) = \binom{n_i}{y} p^y (1-p)^{n_i - y}$	$x\beta = \log(\frac{\mu}{(1-\mu)}) = \theta$	$\frac{n_i \exp(x_i'\beta)}{(1+\exp(x_i'\beta))^2}$
Geometric	$f(y; p) = (1-p)^{y-1} p$	$x\beta = \log(\frac{\mu}{(1-\mu)}) = \theta$	$\frac{1}{1+\exp(x_i'\beta)}$

Cox and Snell (1989) commented that this completes the close formal and conceptual connection between maximum likelihood estimation and generalized or weighted least squares estimation (WLS).

When the β_0 is the intercept, (11) can be expressed as the $(p \times p)$ matrix

$$I(\beta_0, \beta_c) = (X'WX) = \begin{pmatrix} \sum_i w_i & \sum_i x_{ci}' w_i \\ \sum_i x_{ci} w_i & \sum_i x_{ci} x_{ci}' w_i \end{pmatrix}, \quad (12)$$

where: $p = k + 1$ and we have partitioned $x_i' = (x_{0i} = 1, x_{ci}')$, where $x_{ci}' = (x_{1i}, \cdots, x_{ki})$ represents the k binary indicator variables and $\beta_c' = (\beta_1, \cdots, \beta_k)$ their effects. Moreover, $W = \nabla_\theta \nabla_\theta K$ is a diagonal matrix with the elements $w_i = h(x_i'\beta)$. In Table 2 we list some special cases from this family with their corresponding link functions and structural weights, w_i, derived in the next section below. These quantities play a key role in the sequel.

4.1 Covariance Matrix: One Categorical Variable

Suppose we have only one categorical covariate with exactly $p = k + 1$ categories with p parameters $(\beta_0, \beta_1, \cdots, \beta_k)$, the observed information matrix (12) becomes

$$I(\beta_0, \beta_c) = \begin{pmatrix} \sum_i w_i & \sum_{i_{[1]}} w_i & \sum_{i_{[2]}} w_i & \cdots & \sum_{i_{[k]}} w_i \\ \sum_{i_{[1]}} w_i & \sum_{i_{[1]}} w_i & 0 & \cdots & 0 \\ \sum_{i_{[2]}} w_i & 0 & \sum_{i_{[2]}} w_i & \cdots & 0 \\ \vdots & \vdots & \vdots & & \vdots \\ \sum_{i_{[k]}} w_i & 0 & 0 & \cdots & \sum_{i_{[k]}} w_i \end{pmatrix},$$

taking the general form

$$
= \begin{pmatrix}
n_r h(\beta_0) + \sum_j n_j h(\beta_0 + \beta_j) & n_1 h(\beta_0 + \beta_1) & n_2 h(\beta_0 + \beta_2) & \cdots & n_k h(\beta_0 + \beta_k) \\
n_1 h(\beta_0 + \beta_1) & n_1 h(\beta_0 + \beta_1) & 0 & \cdots & 0 \\
n_2 h(\beta_0 + \beta_2) & 0 & n_2 h(\beta_0 + \beta_2) & \cdots & 0 \\
\vdots & \vdots & \vdots & & \vdots \\
n_k h(\beta_0 + \beta_k) & 0 & 0 & \cdots & n_k h(\beta_0 + \beta_k)
\end{pmatrix}
\tag{13}
$$

and the inverse of (13) is

$$
I^{-1}(\beta_0, \beta) = \frac{1}{n_r h(\beta_0)}
\begin{pmatrix}
1 & -1 & -1 & \cdots & -1 \\
-1 & 1 + (q_1 \times \frac{n_r}{n_1}) & 1 & \cdots & 1 \\
-1 & 1 & 1 + (q_2 \times \frac{n_r}{n_2}) & \cdots & 1 \\
\vdots & \vdots & \vdots & & \vdots \\
-1 & 1 & 1 & \cdots & 1 + (q_k \times \frac{n_r}{n_k})
\end{pmatrix},
\tag{14}
$$

where $i[j]$ means subject $i \in j$th category, whence $x_{ij} = 1$ for $i \in j$th category, and $q_j = h(\beta_0)/h(\beta_0 + \beta_j)$, n_r and n_j are allocated numbers in the reference category and the other categories respectively, $j = 1, 2, \cdots, k$. This matrix is an obvious generalization of the inverse arising in the general linear model.

4.2   Optimal Allocation and $G_D(\cdot)$

Now, in the GLM family, with one categorical variable and using multiple Lagrange constraints we can show that the optimal allocation is still uniform, namely: $n_1 = n_2 = \cdots = n_{k+1} = n/(k+1)$, and does not depend on β_0 or on any of the other βs. Moreover, for GLMs involving a single categorical variable, from (7) and (13) the general index is

$$
\begin{aligned}
G_D(\beta_0, \beta_c) &= \log_e \left[GV(\beta_0, \beta_c)/GV^*(\beta_0, \beta_c) \right] \\
&= \log_e \left[\det(I^*(\beta_0, \beta_c))/\det(I(\beta_0, \beta_c)) \right] \\
&= \sum_{j=1}^{p} \log_e (n_j^*/n_j)
\end{aligned}
$$

which is identical to (8). Under this condition, the distributional properties of $G_D(\cdot)$ for all the GLMs listed in Table 2 are exactly those presented in Table 1.

4.3 Two or More Categorical Covariates

When we have more than one categorical covariate in the GLMs, the ideal allocation is no longer uniform. In this case the ideal allocations depend on the unknown parameters and the problem of their construction is therefore necessarily more complicated than that for classical linear models or for GLMs with one covariate. The construction of optimal designs in GLMs is an active area of current research. Our approach is to fix $\beta = \hat{\beta}$ and use numerical methods to obtain the optimum allocation of the n_js. Thus, similar to (5), we obtain the optimal design as

$$D_{p^*}(n^{*\prime}) = \operatorname*{argmax}_{n_j s} \left\{ \det[(X'WX)] \right\},$$

where $p^* = \sum p_\ell$, $\ell = 1, 2, \cdots, m$. Having found the optimal allocation we may proceed to compute the general index, $G_D(\cdot)$, given in (7).

For the canonical GLMs listed in Table 2 with some fixed parameters, we found that both the testing distributions and the non-Null distributions of $G_D(\cdot)$ are still well described by Gamma(α, η). See more details in the simulation section.

4.4 Indices and Choice of Reference Subclass

From the study above we know that, the distribution of the $G_D(\cdot)$ or X^2 corresponding to a particular null and alternative hypothesis can be explicitly determined by numerical methods, then they can directly be used to form decision regions (to accept/reject the null hypothesis). When we have a sample allocation, if the test results on the indices show that this sample allocation is far away from its ideal allocation significantly, then a poor choice of reference category may lead to a loss of efficiency of the regression parameter, otherwise, choice of reference category may be arbitrary, in a D-optimal sense. We present more details in the simulation section.

5 Simulation Studies

5.1 Distribution of the Index

We investigated the distribution of the index by conducting a detailed simulation study covering the following scenario space. For one categorical variable in the linear regression model, we consider the number of subclasses: $p = 2, 3, 4, 5, 6, 7, 8, 9$, and $n = 50, 100, 200, 500, 1,000$. In practice, greater values of p are unusual. When p and n are small, we use the exact distribution which

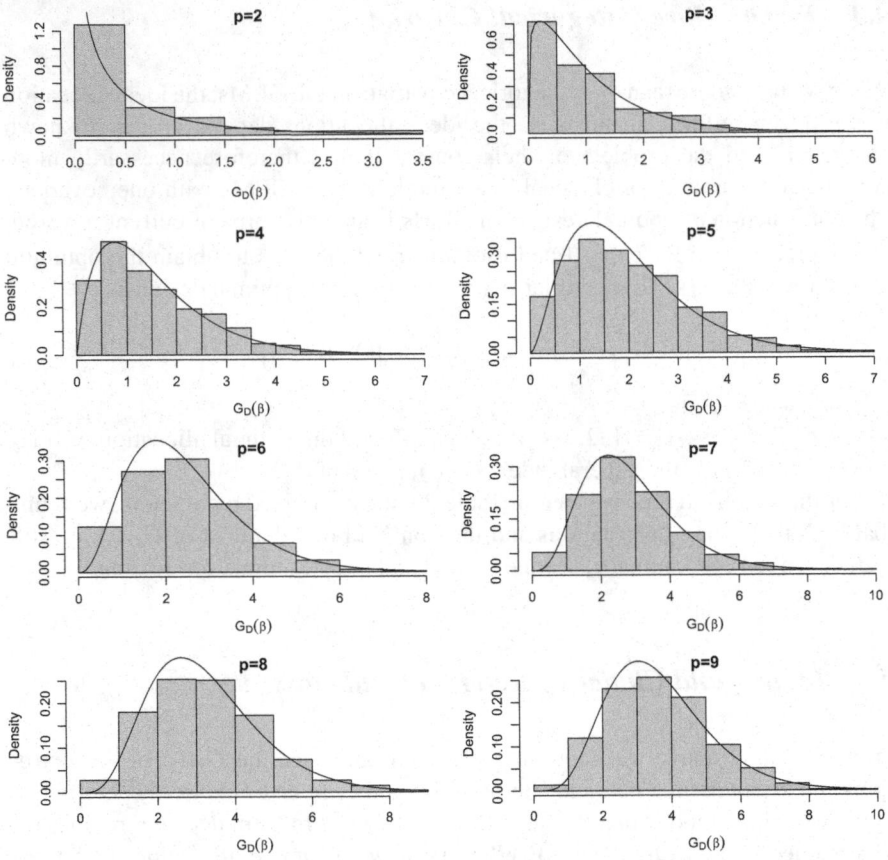

Fig. 1 Histogram of $G_D(\beta)$ index with different numbers of subclasses p for (n=100); Gamma distribution shown as *smooth curve*

is enumerable and take the number of replications, to be the exact number of positive compositions obtained (Appendix 1). For larger p and n, we use 1,000 replicates in the simulation algorithm to generate the positive compositions randomly (Appendix 1).

Figure 1 shows just eight scenarios from our simulation with a single categorical regressor in the model confirming that the histograms of the index $G_D(\cdot)$ in the non-Null case change with different p. Here $n = 100$, which we consider to be a relatively small sample size. For larger sample sizes the fit improves. The smooth curve in the histograms is the density curve of Gamma($\hat{\alpha}, \hat{\eta}$) (density $f(x) = \frac{x^{\alpha-1}}{\Gamma(\alpha)\eta^\alpha} e^{-x/\eta}$ for $x \geq 0$ and $\alpha, \eta > 0$), where $\hat{\eta} = \mathrm{Var}(G_D(\cdot))/\mathrm{mean}(G_D(\cdot))$ and $\hat{\alpha} = \mathrm{mean}(G_D(\cdot))/\hat{\eta}$ are the estimators from the Gamma distribution density with the simulated $G_D(\cdot)$. The results in Fig. 1 show that the distribution of $G_D(\cdot)$ in the non-Null case is well described by a Gamma(α_1, η_1) when $p > 2$, and χ^2_1 when

$p = 2$. The other two histograms (not shown) indicate that the distribution of $G_D(\cdot)$ in the Null case is well described by a Gamma(α_0, η_0) and the distribution of X^2 in the Null case is well described by a $\chi^2_{(p-1)}$ random variable.

5.2 Testing Goodness of Fit

We carried out some statistical hypothesis tests for each scenario: the null and alternative hypotheses were: H_0: the data follow the specified Gamma or Chi-squared distribution, and H_1: the negation of H_0. We adopted the Chi-squared *goodness-of-fit* test, Anderson–Darling test of fit and Kolmogorov–Smirnov test. For the Chi-squared *goodness-of-fit* test, we created categories such that the minimum expected cell frequency was attained. For Anderson–Darling test, we computed the p-value from the simulated data because there are no tabulated critical values available for the Gamma distribution for this test. Moreover, since the parameters are estimated from the sample data, we tested whether the cumulative distribution function follows the standard uniform distribution (Shapiro 1980).

5.3 Results: Single Categorical Variable

All three tests, the Chi-squared *goodness-of-fit* test, Anderson–Darling test and the Kolmogorov–Smirnov goodness of fit test we have conducted are in agreement on our finding shown in Sect. 5.1. It appears that the Gamma(α_1, η_1) distribution provides a reasonable fit to the proposed index $G_D(\cdot)$ in the non-Null case. And when $p = 2$, $n \leq 500$, it is distributed as χ^2_1.

To find the testing distribution (Null distribution) of $G_D(\cdot)$ and X^2, the procedures are: (a) generating the sample compositions from multi-nominal distribution by setting the cell probabilities equal to the proportions of the subclass obtained from the ideal allocation (here, uniform), (b) calculating the corresponding index $G_D(\cdot)$ and X^2 by using the formulae given above, (c) using the test methods described in Sect. 5.2 to test whether $G_D(\cdot)$ and X^2 follow some distributions. The three tests also showed that both testing distributions, i.e., the proposed index $G_D(\cdot)$ and X^2 in the Null case are well described by a Gamma(α_0, η_0) and $\chi^2_{(p-1)}$ respectively. We have summarized our findings in Table 1.

In order to estimate (α_1, η_1) and (α_0, η_0), we carried out a multiple regression analysis with ($Y = \hat{\alpha}$, or, $Y = \hat{\eta}$, $X_1 = n$, and $X_2 = p$) based on three blocks of the simulated data, 120 values for Null distribution, while 108 values by deleting $p = 2, n = 50, 100, 200, 500$ for non-Null distribution. The results are presented in Table 3.

Thus, for fixed p and n, we can find or estimate α and η in the corresponding Gamma distribution with Tables 1 and 3.

Table 3 Formulae for estimating parameters on the distributions of $G_D(\cdot)$

$\hat{Y}$	Formulae	R^2
Non-NULL:		
$\hat{\alpha}_1 =$	$0.9076p - 0.1569 \log(n) - 0.0372p \log(n)$	0.9966
$\hat{\eta}_1 =$	$-0.0237p + 0.1752 \log(n)$	0.9947
NULL:		
$\hat{\alpha}_0 =$	$0.2741p - 0.0565 \log(n) + 0.0294p \log(n)$	0.9929
$\hat{\eta}_0 =$	$\exp\left[1.1572 \log(p) - 1.0262 \log(n)\right]$	0.9978

R^2 in Table 3 is the multiple correlation coefficient. We noted that $\hat{\alpha}_0$ and $\hat{\eta}_0$ are very close to those estimates obtained in the simulation with the corresponding p and n, and using them to check the significant level 5 %, the testing results are similar to those obtained by using $\chi^2_{(p-1)}$. Further, we conducted the power of analysis by using the distributions of $G_D(\cdot)$ and $\chi^2_{(p-1)}$ respectively. On the Null hypothesis, in the Multi-nominal with p categories, $H_0 : \pi_1 = \pi_2 = \cdots = \pi_p = \pi_o$, while on H_1: at least $\pi_i \neq \pi_j$, for some $i \neq j$, $1 \leq i, j \leq p$ where $\sum_{i=1}^{p} \pi_i = 1$.

For the X^2 index we calculated the exact power at 100 different values of the effect size, $\triangle$, by using the non-central $\chi^2_{(p-1,\lambda)}$ distribution, where $\lambda = \sum_{i=1}^{p}(n\pi_i - n\pi_0)^2/n\pi_0$ (Cohen 1988) and accordingly, $\triangle = \sqrt{\lambda/n}$ (cran.r project 2009). For the analysis involving $G_D(\cdot)$, we estimated the nominal significance level ($\triangle = 0$) and power by simulation, repeating $m^*=1000$ statistical tests of the null hypothesis at each value of the effect size in H_1. Recall that under H_0, $G_D(\cdot) \sim \text{Gamma}(\alpha_0, \eta_0)$ where (α_0, η_0) are estimated by using the formulae listed in Table 3. Figure 2 shows the power functions for $G_D(\cdot)$ and X^2, against effect size. They have very similar behaviour, showing that the two indices are equivalent.

Thus, for a single categorical variable in the LM, one can use the formulae listed in Table 3 to obtain the parameters for testing the Gamma distribution and then test the discrepancy.

5.4 Results: Two or More Categorical Variables

When we have $m > 1$ categorical variables, each one has p_ℓ, $\ell = 1, 2, \cdots, m$ subclasses, to be regressed. In our simulation scenarios we considered p_ℓ, $\ell = 1, 2, \cdots, m$ running from 2 to 9, $n = (50, 100, 200, 500, 1,000)$, and replicating 1,000 times. To find the distribution of the index $G_D(\cdot)$, we used the general findings on the ideal allocation (10) in Sect. 3.3 and sampled from the Multinominal distribution with the cell probabilities which guaranteed the exact cross terms in $(X'X)$. We set the cell probabilities equal to the proportions of subclasses obtained from the sample allocation (Appendix 1) to find the non-Null distribution of $G_D(\cdot)$, and equal to the proportions of subclasses obtained from the ideal allocation to

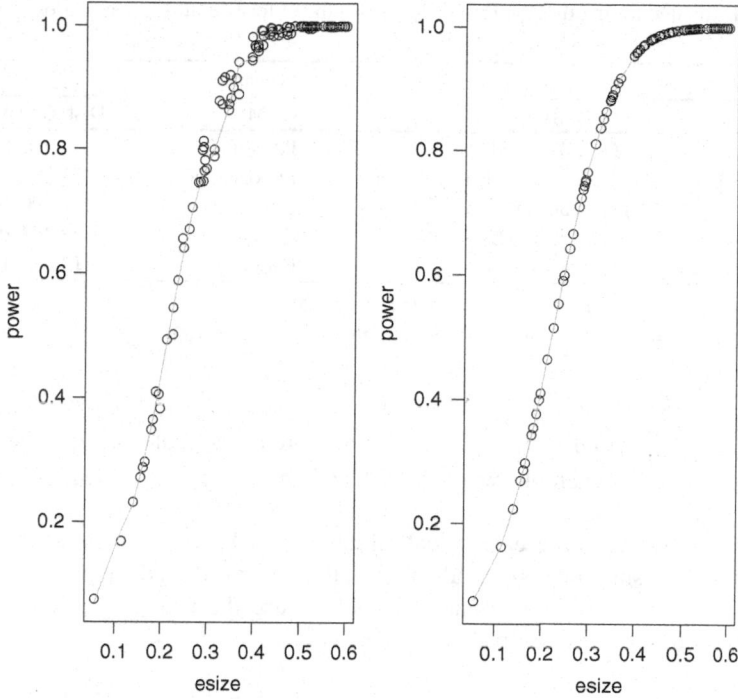

Fig. 2 Power as a function of effect size; $n = 100$, $p = 3$, esize=Δ. *Left panel*: power of $G_D(\cdot)$; *right panel*: power of X^2

find the Null distribution of $G_D(\cdot)$ respectively. The procedures are similar to those described in Sect. 5.3.

When $m = 2$, the Kolmogorov–Smirnov goodness of fit test showed that the distribution of the index $G_D(\cdot)$ in the non-Null case was well described by a Gamma(α, η) distribution except for the cases in $n = 50$, $p_1 \geq 4$, $p_2 \geq 4$. Similarly, (α, η) are the function of n, p_1, p_2 approximately, and for some special cases, $\eta = 1$. The distribution of the index $G_D(\cdot)$ in the null case was well described by a Gamma(α, η) distribution, again, (α, η) are functions of n, p_1, p_2 approximately (not shown). The simulation procedure and the corresponding findings can be extended to $m \geq 3$ categorical variables.

That $X^2 = \sum_{j=1}^{p_1+p_2} [n_j - n_j^*]^2 / n_j^* \sim \chi_\nu^2$, with $\nu = [(p_1 - 1) + (p_2 - 1)]$ in the null case with $m = 2$ is not surprising. Since $m = 2$, the n_js are the marginal frequencies from the corresponding two-dimensional contingency table. The finding holds when varying the second categorical variable in the range $[2, 9]$. We extended the procedure to $m = 3$, and found that $X^2 \sim \chi_\nu^2$, with $\nu = [(p_1 - 1) + (p_2 - 1) + (p_3 - 1)]$, when we varied the second and the third categorical variable in the range $[2, 9]$. Accordingly, suppose there are m categorical variables in model $X_1, \cdots, X_m$, such that each variable has p_ℓ subclasses, $\ell = 1, 2, \cdots, m$, then, for the generalized

Table 4 Estimated testing distribution of $G_D(\cdot) \sim \gamma(\alpha, \eta)$ for two different scenarios in various GLMs

Scenario 1[a]		Scenario 2[b]	
GLM	Dist. $G_D(\cdot)$	GLM	Dist. $G_D(\cdot)$
Poisson	$\gamma(1.7247, 0.0315)$	Poisson	$\gamma(5.3968, 0.0332)$
Exponential	$\gamma(4.5642, 0.0347)$	Exponential	$\gamma(23.892, 0.0349)$
Binomial	$\gamma(1.4750, 0.0206)$	Binomial	$\gamma(2.5490, 0.0239)$
Geometric	$\gamma(1.5251, 0.0255)$	Geometric	$\gamma(2.6363, 0.0327)$
IG(λ=1)	$\gamma(2.6408, 0.0348)$	IG(λ=1)	$\gamma(12.655, 0.0350)$

[a] Scenario 1=($\beta_0 = 0.5$, $\beta_1 = -0.3$, $\beta_2 = 0.3$, $n = 100$)
[b] Scenario 2=($\beta_0 = 0.5$, $\beta_1 = -0.3$, $\beta_2 = 0.3$, $\beta_3 = -0.5$, $n = 100$)

$X^2 = \sum_{\ell=1}^{m} \sum_{j=1}^{p_\ell} (n_{j\ell} - n_{j\ell}^*)^2 / n_{j\ell}^*$ we conjecture is distributed as χ_ν^2, where $\nu = (\sum_{\ell=1}^{m} p_\ell - m)$. For example, when $m = 4$, and $(p_1, p_2, p_3, p_4) = (2, 3, 4, 5)$, then $\nu = 10$, etc.

Thus, for two or more categorical variables in LM, one can find the testing distribution by using the general ideal allocation form (10) and similar procedures described in Sect. 5.3, or alternatively, one can use the Chi-squared distribution found above to test the discrepancy.

5.5 Results: Two or More Categorical Variables in GLMs

As mentioned earlier the determinant of the observed information matrix $(X'WX)$ depends on the unknown parameters. Accordingly, in order to find the distribution of $G_D(\cdot)$ we conducted a small simulation study, fixing the values of β in the scenario space.

Suppose we have two binary covariates X_1 and X_2 in the GLM models listed in Table 2 and let the scenario space be: $\beta_1 \in [-0.5, \ 0.5]$, $\beta_2 \in [-0.5, \ 0.5]$, $\beta_0 = 0.5$, $n = 100$, and replicating 1,000 times. We used R function "optim" to find the ideal allocation within each scenario.

Table 4 lists the results corresponding to two scenarios (complete results not shown). The main findings are that the approximate testing distribution of $G_D(\cdot)$ is well described by a Gamma(α, η) distribution. In Scenario 2 the first categorical variate has three subclasses. The approximate distribution of $G_D(\cdot)$ under non-Null is also well described by a Gamma(α, η), but the details are omitted.

We just showed that for two or more categorical variables in a GLM for lower dimensional cases of $(X'WX)$ one can use the R function "optim" to find the ideal allocation and a similar procedure to that described in Sect. 5.3 to find the testing distribution. However, for higher dimensional cases of $(X'WX)$, for example when $p > 8$, we used the following Monte Carlo algorithm.

We suppose there are m categorical variables in model $X_1, \cdots, X_m$, such that each variable has p_ℓ subclasses, $\ell = 1, 2, \cdots, m$, our algorithm to find an ideal allocation is,

1. Initialize allocation $\tilde{n} = (\tilde{n}_1, \cdots, \tilde{n}_\ell, \cdots, \tilde{n}_m)$, $\tilde{n}_\ell = (n_{\ell,1}, \cdots, n_{\ell,p_\ell})$, $\ell = 1, 2, \cdots, m$.
2. Use the proportions $\tilde{r}_{n_\ell} = (n_{\ell,1}/n, \cdots, n_{\ell,p_\ell}/n)$ as cell probabilities for the multinominal distribution, to generate sets of binary variables X_ℓ, for $\ell = 1, 2, \cdots, m$., thus building the design matrix X.
3. For the fixed (given) β, compute $\det[I(\beta)] = \det(X'WX)$.
4. Find $n_\ell^* = (n_{\ell,1}^*, \cdots, n_{\ell,p_\ell}^*)$ maximizing $\det[I(\beta)] = \det(X'WX)$.
5. Set $\tilde{n}_\ell = n_\ell^*$, and $\tilde{r}_{n_\ell} = (n_{\ell,1}^*/n, \cdots, n_{\ell,p_\ell}^*/n)$.
6. Repeat steps (2)–(5) until convergence.

The initial allocation can be sample compositions generated by using the code in Sect. 7 in Appendix 1 for each categorical variable, however, by taking the uniform allocation as the starting allocation, the search is faster. We cross-checked the results of the algorithm with the R function "optim" for lower dimensional case of $(X'WX)$, and found that the methods always agreed for GLMs fitted.

In addition, the distribution of X^2, utilizing the ideal allocation numbers as the expected values, still followed a χ_v^2 distribution as in Sect. 5.4. However, we note that in these cases the central Chi-squared distribution approach for testing discrepancy is not suitable, see the illustrative example in Sect. 5.6 below for the explanation.

5.6   Results: Illustrative Example—Drawback of X^2 in Complicated GLMs

In this example, we choose three compositions from the simulated compositions (using algorithm in Sect. 7 in Appendix 1). The example illustrates, inter alia, the use of the $G_D(\cdot)$ and X^2 and the testing results based on Poisson regression model with two binary covariates with $n = 100$ and two settings, $\beta = (0.5, -0.3, 0.3)$ and $\beta = (0.5, -0.3, 1.5)$ assumed, respectively. The results are presented in Table 5. The approximate ideal allocations and the corresponding testing distributions are obtained by using the similar procedure described in Sect. 5.5.

In the Poisson GLM setting with two binary covariates the simple link between X^2 and $G_D(\cdot)$ as (9) is lost. For example, X^2 rejects the first composition chosen, but $G_D(\cdot)$ does not. Also in the lower panel of Table 5 where the value of β_2 has been changed from 0.3 to 1.5, increasing the weight of the second binary variable, we note that the values of X^2 and $G_D(\cdot)$ no longer rank the second and third compositions similarly. For example, the index ranks the second composition closer to the ideal allocation, while X^2 ranks the third composition closer to the ideal allocation. Recall that the β information is incorporated in the determinants defining the index, while

Table 5 An example showing the $G_D(\cdot)$, and X^2 statistics, based on simulated Poisson GLM data with two binary covariates[a]

| Model-Composition(X_1; X_2; X_{12}) | $G_D(\cdot)$ | X^2 | Critical values | |
			$G_D(\cdot)$	X^2
$\beta = (0.5, -0.3, 0.3)$ -			0.1354	5.9914
Ideal-(45.544, 54.456; 54.456, 45.544; 25.984)				
(68, 32; 56, 44; 15)	0.1115	20.189		
(30, 70; 23, 77; 14)	0.9426	49.057		
(4, 96; 48, 52; 35)	1.9317	73.786		
$\beta = (0.5, -0.3, 1.5)$ -			0.2733	5.9914
Ideal-(38.479, 61.521; 64.076, 35.924; 32.364)				
(68, 32; 56, 44; 15)	0.2402	39.799		
(30, 70; 23, 77; 14)	1.5213	79.476		
(4, 96; 48, 52; 35)	2.1485	64.943		

[a] With $\beta = (0.5, -0.3, 0.3)$ and under H_0, $G_D(\cdot) \sim \text{Gamma}(1.7247, 0.0315)$ from Table 4, and with $\beta = (0.5, -0.3, 1.5)$, $G_D(\cdot) \sim \text{Gamma}(5.3663, 0.0283)$ from simulation, $X^2 \sim \chi^2(v)$, $v = (2-1) + (2-1) = 2$

X^2 uses the ideal allocation numbers generated by maximizing the determinant of the information matrix which appears in the index.

We conjecture that this lack of concordance in ranking persists for two more categorical variables. Accordingly, we prefer to rely on the index $G_D(\cdot)$ as a measure of discrepancy for the complicated GLMs.

5.7 Results: Illustrative Example—$G_D(\cdot)$ and the Choice of Reference Subclass

As an illustrative example, we choose three compositions and the corresponding values of $G_D(\cdot)$ from the simulated results when $n = 100$ and one single categorical variable with $p = 4$. The example illustrates, inter alia, the use of the index $G_D(\cdot)$ and the choice of reference subclass in the linear and Poisson regression model. The results are presented in Table 6.

From the foregoing analytical work, that the index, $G_D(\cdot)$, takes the same values on the compositions in the LM and GLM Poisson regression model, and $X^2 \sim \chi^2_3$ can be used too. With $n = 100$, $p = 4$, using the formulae listed in Table 3, we have $\hat{\alpha}_0 = 1.3778$ and $\hat{\eta}_0 = 0.0441$, i.e., the testing distribution of $G_D(\cdot)$ is Gamma(1.3778, 0.0441) approximately. Comparing with the critical values 0.1629 and 7.8147 at 5 % significant level obtained from the two testing distributions, i.e., Gamma(1.3778, 0.0441) and χ^2_3, with $n = 100$, $p = 4$, respectively, only the first allocation, which is close to ideal allocation, is not rejected.

To show the relationship between the indices and the choice of reference subclass, we used V_r, called total variance of the estimators as a measure of precision

Table 6 An example showing the $G_D(\cdot)$ statistic and the choice of reference category, based on simulated Poisson GLM data with two binary covariates

Composition	$G_D(\cdot)$ (X^2)	Switch r_{max}[a] $\rightarrow r$	Linear model V_r	GLM(Poisson) V_r
(18, 33, 26, 23)	0.0950	2→2	0.2587	0.1482
	(4.5446)	2→3	0.2832	0.1920
		2→4	0.2982	0.1582
		2→1	0.3345	0.1891
(22, 48, 5, 25)	1.0849	2→2	0.3688	0.2896
	(36.941)	2→4	0.4263	0.3112
		2→1	0.4427	0.3202
		2→3	0.9063	0.8535
(2, 3, 34, 61)	3.4465	4→4	0.9283	0.4254
	(95.396)	4→3	0.9674	0.4546
		4→2	1.8791	0.7760
		4→1	2.3791	1.1510

[a] r_{max} represents that the reference is the most numerous group

of the estimators, where $V_r = \sum_j [Var(\hat{\beta}_j)]$ and the subscript r represents the corresponding reference. In LM, we calculated V_r by setting $h(\beta_0) = 1$ and $h(\beta_j) = 1$ in form (14) where $k = 3$ and ignore σ^2. In the Poisson GLM case, we assumed $\beta_0 = 0.5$, $\beta_1 = 0.1$, $\beta_2 = -0.2$, $\beta_3 = 0.3$, and simulated response variable y from Poisson distribution with rate $\exp(X\beta)$, where X is the design matrix which is determined by the three chosen sample compositions. With y and X we fitted the Poisson GLM under different choice of reference subclass, accordingly, the estimated V_r were obtained, see Table 6. The results show that, when the allocation is close to the ideal, the V_r are very close with each other for each possible reference chosen. In this case, a choice of reference subclass can be arbitrary for both LM and Poisson GLM considered. However, as the allocation becomes further away from its ideal allocation, the corresponding total variance, V_r changes when switching from the largest subclass to the smallest subclass, and hence the penalty on the precision of the estimators increases. In these two cases, a poor choice of reference category may lead to a loss of efficiency of the regression parameter, and choosing the reference category with the largest number of observations for each categorical variable is the optimal strategy.

6 Application

A prospective epidemiological study designed to measure the annual incidence of lung cancer in Northern Ireland was carried out between October 1st, 1991, and September 30th, 1992 (Wilkinson 1995; MacKenzie 1996). During this 1-year period, 900 incident cases were diagnosed and followed up for nearly 2 years. Comprehensive clinical including information on treatment and prognosis were abstracted from the hospital and the general practitioner's records. Despite extensive enquires, the outcome could not be determined in 25 cases, and in another 20 cases the diagnosis was made at the post mortem. In total there were 855 (95 %) cases on whom survival information was complete and these cases are analyzed here.

The following nine factors were selected for study in order to determine their influence, if any, upon survival: (a) Patient Characteristics; age, sex, smoking status, (b) Disease Status/Markers; WHO performance status, cell type, metastases, sodium and albumen levels and (c) Treatment Details; surgery, radiotherapy, chemotherapy, or palliative treatment. Further details of the categorical factors studied may be found in Wilkinson (1995) and in Table 7.

We analyze survival time T, the time from diagnosis to death from lung cancer or censoring, using Cox's proportional hazards regression model (Cox 1972), in order to identify the independent effect of factors studied simultaneously. The 5 % level of statistical significance was used in performing statistical tests and in the construction of confidence intervals (CIs).

To estimate the model we first choose the natural reference category for each factor, construct the corresponding design matrix and apply a stepwise backward algorithm to the nine factors studied in order to estimate the reduced model. The natural reference subclass for a categorical is usually the least or most hazardous. Later, we switch the reference subclasses to the most numerous subclasses and re-estimate the model parameters, their standard errors and corresponding p values.

Of the nine factors studied, only seven were found to independently influence survival. In particular, survival did not depend on the gender of the patient, nor, rather surprisingly, on the age of the patient. The results for the reduced model, using the natural subclasses are shown in the left panel of Table 7. In the right hand side panel we present the effect of switching the reference to the most numerous subclass. The numbers of patients in each subclass are shown in brackets.

For these data, $(p_1, p_2, p_3, p_4, p_5, p_6, p_7) = (5, 5, 4, 3, 3, 3, 4)$, and choosing the $\hat{\beta}$ based on the model with most numerous reference subclasses, we used the Monte Carlo algorithm given in Sect. 5.5 with 10,000 replications to maximize $\det[I(\beta)]$ associated with Cox's proportional hazard model. We found that the approximate ideal allocation (cross terms omitted) to be:

$$n^* = (194, 183, 138, 207, 133; 189, 198, 155, 77, 236; 180, 219, 230, 226;$$

$$269, 260, 326; 294, 248, 313; 325, 247, 283; 233, 208, 220, 194).$$

Under H_0, using the similar procedure described in Sect. 5.5, the finding testing distribution $G_D(\cdot) \sim$ Gamma(8.3699, 0.0697) approximately, which has a critical value 0.9503 associated with a 5 % significant level. The calculated $G_D(\cdot)$ for these data corresponding to the ideal allocation is 11.2443 $>>$ 0.9503. Hence, the allocation of these data is significantly far away from the ideal allocation. In this case, the choice of reference category is not arbitrary and choosing the most numerous subclasses as references, reveals the $\hat{\beta}$ has the smallest variances (see Table 7).

Table 7 Results of PH regression analysis: backwards solution involving seven of nine factors: natural and most numerous reference subclasses

Natural reference				Largest subclass as reference			
Model (n)	$\hat{\beta}$	se($\hat{\beta}$)	p-value	Model	$\hat{\beta}$	se($\hat{\beta}$)	p-value
1. Treatment							
Pall. (441)	–	–	–	*Pall.* (441)	–	–	–
Surg. (79)	−1.209	0.249	< 0.01	Surg. (79)	−1.209	0.249	< 0.01
Chemo. (45)	−0.487	0.209	0.020	Chemo. (45)	−0.487	0.209	0.020
Radio. (256)	−0.296	0.100	0.003	Radio (256)	−0.296	0.100	0.003
C + R. (34)	−0.908	0.237	< 0.01	C + R. (34)	−0.908	0.237	< 0.01
2. WHO							
Normal (78)	–	–	–	*No Work* (286)	–	–	–
Light work (278)	0.091	0.184	0.619	Light work (278)	−0.443	0.102	< 0.01
No work (286)	0.534	0.185	0.004	Normal (78)	−0.534	0.185	0.004
Walking (191)	1.014	0.197	< 0.01	Walking (191)	0.480	0.104	< 0.01
Bed/Chair (22)	1.680	0.285	< 0.01	Bed/Chair (22)	1.146	0.232	< 0.01
3. Cell							
Squamous (247)	–	–		*Other* (379)	–	–	–
Small (121)	0.729	0.154	< 0.01	Small (121)	0.518	0.141	< 0.01
Adeno ca (108)	0.313	0.141	0.026	Adeno ca (108)	0.102	0.130	0.436
Other (379)	0.211	0.102	0.039	Squamous (247)	−0.211	0.102	0.039
4. Sod. mmol/l							
≥ 136 (505)	–	–	–	*≥ 136* (505)	–	–	–
< 136 (310)	0.327	0.085	< 0.01	< 136 (310)	0.327	0.085	< 0.01
Missing (40)	−0.093	0.219	0.672	Missing (40)	−0.093	0.219	0.672
5. Alb. g/l							
≥35 (458)	–	–	–	*≥ 35* (458)	–	–	–
< 35 (315)	0.421	0.091	< 0.01	< 35 (315)	0.421	0.091	< 0.01
Missing (82)	0.460	0.165	0.005	Missing (82)	0.460	0.165	0.005
6. Metastases							
No Met. (188)	–	–	–	*Met* (428)	–	–	–
Met (428)	0.771	0.120	< 0.01	No met (188)	−0.771	0.120	< 0.01
Missing (239)	0.351	0.132	0.008	Missing (239)	−0.421	0.096	< 0.01
7. Smoking							
Non-smoker (88)	–	–	–	*Current* (416)	–	–	–
Current (416)	0.384	0.139	0.006	Non-smoker (88)	−0.384	0.139	0.006
Ex-smoker (330)	0.252	0.142	0.076	Ex-smoker (330)	−0.132	0.085	0.119
Missing (21)	0.298	0.273	0.275	Missing (21)	−0.086	0.253	0.734

We also noted that switching the reference subclass in the WHO performance status variable affected the survival time significantly, however, a similar switch in Cell Type did not. Overall, switching the reference subclasses, increases precision and hence yields narrower confidence intervals compared with retaining natural reference subclasses. Our findings, show clearly the magnitude of the penalty in precision associated with choosing the so-called "natural" reference subclasses.

Clearly, in such an observational study one has some freedom to choose the reference subclasses and one general approach may be to select the largest subclasses, hence minimizing the variance of the estimators.

7 Discussion

In this paper we have tried to collate existing knowledge and develop some new tools from a mathematical statistical perspective with a view to clarifying decision making in this arena.

We were led first to create $G_D(\cdot)$, an index which measures the discrepancy between observed categorical distributions and the corresponding D-optimal ideal allocation. We have shown that the index and its distribution is invariant across GLMs in the case of a single categorical covariate. When we have more than one covariate in the model the properties of the index are more complicated, but we can still obtain its null distribution as a Gamma(α, η) distribution, or, alternatively, make use of the testing distribution of the X^2 statistic which follows a χ_ν^2 distribution in the Linear Model case based on the general form of the ideal allocation (10) found. However, for GLMs with two or more categorical variables, we must obtain the ideal allocation by numerical methods and $G_D(\cdot)$ is preferred.

In relation to the choice of subclass we have shown that the strategy of choosing the largest subclasses as references is optimal both in the Linear Model case and in other GLMs when a test on $G_D(\cdot)$ showed that the sample allocation is far away from its ideal allocation significantly. Otherwise, the choice of reference subclass could be arbitrary. It may be argued that we have ignored the covariance terms when defining V_r, the total variance, but, overall the results are similar when they are included.

There is a relationship between proportional hazards models and Poisson regression models. For example, McCullagh and Nelder (1989) has a chapter on converting PH models to GLM models. We have also found an observed information matrix with a similar structure to (12) when working on the interval censored data with an Exponential regression model (MacKenzie and Peng 2013). This implies that all of the findings from the GLMs hold for PH regression models. Yet another extension of GLMs are generalized additive models (GAMs) and we conjecture that the findings may also hold for some regression models in this class.

In further work we have shown that in the linear model switching to the most numerous subclasses also has the beneficial effect of reducing multi-collinearity among the columns of the design matrix as measured by the condition number of $(X'X)$.

Finally, we hope our findings will clarify some of the issues surrounding reference subclass choice and impact positively on practice in regression analysis.

Acknowledgements The work in this paper was supported by two Science Foundation Ireland (SFI, www.sfi.ie) project grants. Professor MacKenzie was supported under the Mathematics

Initiative, II, via the BIO-SI (www.ul.ie/bio-si) research programme in the Centre of Biostatistics, University of Limerick, Ireland: grant number 07/MI/012. Dr. Peng was supported via a Research Frontiers Programme award, grant number 05/RF/MAT 026 and latterly via the BIO-SI project.

Appendix 1: R Script to Generate Compositions

Generating Compositions

```
#
# Algorithm nexcom - generates compositions one at a time
#
nexcom<-function(n,k,r,t,h,Qtest)
{
if (Qtest == TRUE)
{ if(t > 1) {h <-0}
                        { h <- h+1
                          t<-r[h]
                          r[h] <- 0
     r[1] <- t-1
                          r[h+1] <- r[h+1]+1
                          Qtest <- (r[k] != n)
                          return(list(Comp=r,Ind= Qtest, Tee=t, Hee=h))}
                      }
else if (Qtest==FALSE)
                        {
                        #set up 1st pass
                        r[1]<-n
                         t<-n
         h<-0
                        if (k ==1){ Qtest <- (r[k] != n)
                                      return(list(Comp=r,Ind= Qtest, Tee=t, Hee=h))}
                        {r[2:k]<-0
       Qtest <- (r[k] != n)
                              return(list(Comp=r,Ind= Qtest, Tee=t, Hee=h))}
   }

}
#
# Example
#
#choose  n<-6 ;k<-3 -  pouring 6 balls into 3 urns
n<-6 ;k<-3
#compute myrow =number of compositions
myrow<-choose(n+k-1,n)
#initialise generation parameters
r<-rep(NA,k);Qtest<-FALSE; t<-NA; h<-NA
#
#set up matrix to hold compositions
compos<-matrix(NA,nrow=myrow,ncol=k)
#
# generate all possible compositions
#
for (i in 1:myrow)
{
test<- nexcom(n,k,r,t,h,Qtest)
```

```
r<-test$Comp
compos[i,]<-r
Qtest<-test$Ind
t<-test$Tee
h<-test$Hee
}
compos<-data.frame(compos)
#
# Create a binary indicator for positive compositions
#
z<-rep(NA, myrow)
for (i in 1:myrow)
{
tst<-all(compos[i,1:k]>0)
z[i]<-ifelse(tst, 1,0)
}
#
# Reject non-positive compositions
#
compos<-cbind(compos,z)
attach(compos)
poscompos<-subset(compos,z==1)
poscompos
npos<-dim(poscompos)[1]
npos
```

Generate Random Positive Compositions

```
#
# Algorithm simcom - generates random positive compositions one at a time
#
simcom <- function(n,p)
{
              x <- seq(1, n+p-1)
              freq <- c(rep(0, p))
              while(any(freq == 0))
       {
        rand <- sample(x, size=p-1)
        rand <- sort(rand)
        freq[1] <- rand[1]-1
        if(p>2)
       {
        for(j in 2:(p-1))
        {freq[j] <- rand[j]-rand[j-1]-1}
        freq[p] <- n+p-1-rand[p-1]
       }
        else
         {freq[p] <- n+p-1-rand[p-1]}
       }
              return(list(Iter=n,Comp=freq))
}
test<-simcom(6,3)
numsim<-test$Iter
numsim
resmat<-test$Comp
resmat
```

Appendix 2: Derivation of Optimal Allocation with Two Binary Covariates

Proof. To find the optimal allocation when we have (X_1, X_2) with $(2, 2)$ subclasses, we need to maximize $\det(X'X) = n n_1 n_2 + 2n_1 n_2 n_{12} - n_1 n_2^2 - n_1^2 n_2 - n n_{12}^2$ subject to two equivalent constraints $n_1 + n_{10} = n$ or $n_2 + n_{20} = n$, where n_{12} is the cross term of $(X'X)$, n_{10} and n_{20} are the numbers at $X_1 = 0$ and $X_2 = 0$ respectively. Using the method of Lagrange multipliers, we have

$$\Lambda(n_1, n_{10}, n_2, n_{12}, \lambda) = n_{10}n_1 n_2 + 2n_1 n_2 n_{12} - n_1 n_2^2 - n_1 n_{12}^2 - n_{10}n_{12}^2 - \lambda(n_1 + n_{10} - n).$$

Setting $\nabla_{n_1, n_{10}, n_2, n_{12}, \lambda} \Lambda(n_1, n_{10}, n_2, n_{12}, \lambda) = 0$, we have

$$n_{10}n_2 + 2n_2 n_{12} - n_2^2 - n_{12}^2 - \lambda = 0, \tag{15}$$

$$n_1 n_2 - n_{12}^2 - \lambda = 0, \tag{16}$$

$$n_{10}n_1 + 2n_1 n_{12} - 2n_1 n_2 = 0, \tag{17}$$

$$n_1 n_2 - n_1 n_{12} - n_{10}n_{12} = 0, \tag{18}$$

$$n_1 + n_{10} - n = 0. \tag{19}$$

From (15) and (16), we have

$$n_{10} - n_1 + 2n_{12} - n_2 = 0, \tag{20}$$

and from (17) and (20), we have $n_1 = n_2$. From (18) and (19) and the finding $n_1 = n_2$, after some algebra, we have $n_{12} = n_1^2/n$. Finally, from (17), (19) and the findings $n_1 = n_2$ and $n_{12} = n_1^2/n$, after some algebra, we have $n_1 = n/2$. Thus, for the optimal allocation for this case we found that $n_1^* = n_2^* = n/2$, $n_{12}^* = n/4$.

References

Altman, D. G., & Royston, P. (2006). Statistics notes - the cost of dichotomising continuous variables. *British Medical Journal, 332*, 1080.

Berk, R. (2008). *Statistical learning from regression perspective*. New York: Springer.

Cohen, J. (1988). *Statistical power analysis for the behavioral sciences* (2nd ed.). Hillsdale: Lawrence Erlbaum.

Cox, D. R. (1972). Regression models and life-tables (with discussion). *Journal of the Royal Statistical Society, 34*, 187–220.

Cox, D. R., & Snell, E. J. (1989). *The analysis of binary data* (2nd ed.). London: Chapman & Hall.

cran.r project. (2009). *R project. Retrieved 2010*, R Package "pwr". http://cran.r-project.org/web/packages/pwr/pwr.pdf.

Feldstein, M. S. (1966). A binary variable multiple regression method of analysing factors affecting peri-natal mortality and other outcomes of pregnancy. *Journal of the Royal Statistical Society, Series A, 129*, 61–73.

Frøslie, K. F., Røislien, J., Laake, P., Henriksen, T., Qvigstad, E., & Veierød, M. B. (2010). Categorisation of continuous exposure variables revisited. A response to the hyperglycaemia and adverse pregnancy outcome (hapo) study. *BMC Medical Research Methodology, 10*, 1471–2288.

Isham, V. (1991). *Statistical theory and modelling by edited by Hinkley, D. V., Reid, N. and Snell, E. J.*. London: Chapman & Hall.

MacKenzie, G. (1996). Regression models for survival data: The generalised time dependent logistic family. *Journal of the Royal Statistical Society, 45*, 21–34.

MacKenzie, G., & Peng, D. (2013). Interval-censored parametric regression survival models and the analysis of longitudinal trials. *Statistics in Medicine, 32*, 2804–2822.

McCullagh, P., & Nelder, J. A. (1989). *Generalized linear models* (2nd ed.). London: Chapman & Hall.

Nijenhuis, A., & Wilf, H. S. (1978). *Combinatorial algorithms for computers and calculators* (2nd ed.). London: Academic.

Peng, D., & MacKenzie, G. (2014, forthcoming). Choice of reference subclass in parametric regression models with categorical variables.

Pocock, S. J., Collier, T. J., Dandreo, K. J., De Stavola, B. L., Goldman, M. B., Kalish, L. A., et al. (2004). Issues in the reporting of epidemiological studies: A survey of recent practice. *British Medical Journal, 329*, 883–887.

Shapiro, S. S. (1980). How to test normality and other distributional assumptions, *Statistical Techniques, 3*, 1–78.

Wilkinson, P. (1995). *Lung cancer in northern Ireland* (MD thesis). Queen's University, Belfast.

William, G. J. (2005). *Regression III: Advanced Methods*. Lecture notes. East Lansing, MI: Department of Political Science Michigan State University. Accessed 28 Dec 2010 http://polisci.msu.edu/jacoby/icpsr/regress3.

Part IV
Applied Statistical Modelling

Statistical Methods for Detecting Selective Sweeps

David Ramsey

Abstract The emigration of humankind from Africa and the adoption of agriculture have meant that the selective pressures on humankind have changed in recent evolutionary times. A selective sweep occurs when a positive mutation spreads through a population. For example, a mutation that enables adults to digest lactase has spread through the Northern European population, although it is very rare in the African population. Since neutral alleles that are strongly linked to such a positive mutation also tend to spread through the population, these sweeps leave a signature, a valley of low genetic variation.

This article reviews the development of statistical tests for the detection of selective sweeps using genomic data, particularly in the light of recent advances in genome mapping. It also points out directions for future research.

Keywords Coalescent theory • Computational statistics • Genome mapping • Selective sweeps

1 Introduction

The genetic code of a sample of individuals gives us information about the present population. Since these codes result from the evolutionary and demographic processes within a population, they also contain information regarding these processes. Selection pressure on humankind has changed in the recent past due to the emigration from Africa and later adoption of agriculture. Previously neutral or deleterious alleles may become positive in such a new environment and thus spread through a population. A strong selective sweep occurs when a positive mutation that

D. Ramsey (✉)
Department of Computer Science and Management, Wrocaw University of Technology, Wrocaw, Poland
e-mail: david.ramsey@pwr.wroc.pl

G. MacKenzie and D. Peng (eds.), *Statistical Modelling in Biostatistics and Bioinformatics*, Contributions to Statistics, DOI 10.1007/978-3-319-04579-5_13,
© Springer International Publishing Switzerland 2014

187

was previously not observed in a population spreads. A weak selective sweep occurs when a previously neutral variant that is already present in a population becomes positively selected for. The lower the initial frequency of such a variant the more such a sweep will resemble a strong selective sweep.

When a sweep occurs, neutral variants that are tightly linked to such a positive variant will also spread through the population. Thus immediately after such a sweep, there will be a "valley" of low genetic variation around the site affected by selection. During such a sweep, the population will be split into those that have the positive mutation and those that do not. As above, those individuals with the positive mutation will tend to have very similar genetic codes around the site affected by selection. The remaining individuals will tend to have much more varied genetic codes around this site. Hence, there will be an association between the variant at the site affected by selection and the variants at surrounding sites. This phenomenon is known as linkage disequilibrium.

The layout of the article is as follows. Section 2 briefly describes the data used, nucleotide sequences, and commonly used descriptive statistics based on this data. Other forms of data can be used, but are not considered here. Section 3 considers the Wright–Fisher model, which models the evolution of a population under the assumptions of fixed population size, random mating and no selection. Section 4 considers coalescent processes. A coalescent tree is a way of modelling evolution in reverse from a sample of individuals back to a common ancestor. All the information relevant to the evolutionary processes involved in defining the genetic makeup of the sample is contained in such a coalescent tree. The standard coalescent is based on the Wright–Fisher model, but this model has been generalised to allow for selection, population structure and changes in population size. At the end of this section the effects of demographic changes and selective sweeps on the genetic makeup of a population are briefly considered. Section 5 considers classical tests for selective sweeps within a population, which were developed before the era of genome scanning. The intuition behind these tests is explained using coalescent theory. Section 6 briefly considers a classical test for differential selection in different subpopulations. Section 7 considers models that have been developed in recent years that use data from genome scans. Section 8 outlines some of the challenges and possible areas of development in the near future.

2   The Genetic Data Used

The data used consist of strings of nucleotides, which are the building blocks of the genome. There are four nucleotides: adenine, thymine, cytosine and guanine, denoted A, T, C, and G, respectively. Recently, Consortium (2003) and Project (2004) have provided extensive maps of the genome of samples of humans from different subpopulations. At a large majority of the sites observed, all the individuals have the same nucleotide. Sites at which variation is observed are called *segregating sites*. At virtually all such sites just two nucleotides (variants) are observed. The variation observed at a segregating site is termed a *single nucleotide polymorphism* (SNP). Suppose the genomes of n individuals are scanned. The following are commonly used as summary statistics:

1. The non-polarised frequency spectrum. This is made up of the frequencies of the least common (minor) variant at each of the k segregating sites, together with the position of each segregating site. The non-polarised frequency at a segregating site is between 1 and $\lfloor \frac{n}{2} \rfloor$, where $\lfloor x \rfloor$ is the integer part of x.
2. The polarised frequency spectrum. This is made up of the frequencies of the wild type variant (assumed to have been the prevalent variant in a recent ancestral population) at each of the k segregating sites, together with the position of each segregating site. The polarised frequency at a segregating site is between 1 and $n - 1$.
3. Measures of linkage disequilibrium between segregating sites.

Let p_1 and q_1 be the frequencies of chosen variants at sites 1 and 2, respectively. Let p_{11} be the frequency with which these variants are observed together. Define $D = p_{11} - p_1 q_1$. The standardised coefficient of linkage disequilibrium is $D_S = \frac{|D|}{D_{max}}$, where $D_{max} = \min\{p_1(1-q_1), (1-p_1)q_1\}$. This measure does not depend on which variants are chosen. Clearly, if the variants at these two sites are independent, then the standardised coefficient of linkage disequilibrium is equal to zero.

Two individuals are said to have the same *extended haplotype* over an interval of the genome, if they have the same sequence of nucleotides on that interval.

3   The Wright–Fisher Model

The Wright–Fisher model assumes:

1. The population is of constant size $2N$ alleles (i.e., N diploid individuals).
2. Generations do not overlap and reproduction is asexual.
3. There are no mutations, recombination or selection (i.e., alleles may be understood to be very short nucleotide sequences).
4. Each allele in generation j is the parent of a randomly chosen allele in generation $j + 1$ with probability $\frac{1}{2N}$ (i.e., reproduction in one generation is independent of what happens in other generations).

It follows from these assumptions that the number of offspring of allele i in generation j, $X_{i,j}$, has a $\text{Bin}(2N, \frac{1}{2N})$ distribution. For reasonably large N this distribution can be assumed to be $\text{Poisson}(1)$.

It should be noted that since the population size is fixed, for a given j the random variables $X_{i,j}$ are not independent. The correlation between the numbers of offspring of different alleles is negative; given that one allele has a large number of offspring, the expected number of offspring of the remaining alleles is less than 1. However, for large N these correlations will be very small.

Fig. 1 A realization of the
Wright–Fisher Process

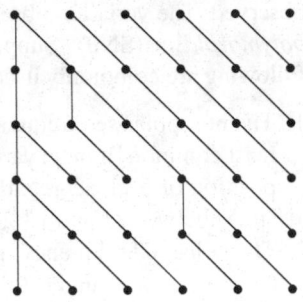

An example of a realization of the Wright–Fisher model is given in Fig. 1. Lines indicate parentage.

In this example, all the alleles in the final generation are descendants of the allele on the top left. It should be noted that Cannings (1974) generalized these models.

Suppose there are two alleles, denoted A and a (which may be understood to contain all the alleles which are not A). Define the frequency of A alleles in generation j to be P_j. According to the Wright–Fisher model, the number of A alleles in generation $j + 1$ has a binomial distribution and

$$E(P_{j+1}|P_j = p_j) = p_j; \quad Var(P_{j+1}|P_j = p_j) = \frac{p_j(1 - p_j)}{n}.$$

The variance of the frequency of the A allele is a measure of genetic drift. The *effective size of a population* is defined to be the size of a population which reproduces according to the Wright–Fisher model and exhibits the same level of genetic drift as observed in the population of interest. That is to say, for a fixed actual population size the higher the variance in the number of offspring, the lower the effective population. In practice, the effective population is estimated by assessing the time to the most recent common ancestor (MRCA) of a sample of individuals by observing mitochondrial DNA (which passes down the matrilineal line) or Y-chromosomes (which pass down the patrilineal line). In both cases no recombination occurs. The relation between the time to the MRCA and the effective population size will be considered in Sect. 4.

4   Coalescent Trees

For a more detailed account of applications of coalescent processes in statistical genetics, see Hein et al. (2004).

Fig. 2 A realisation of the
Common Ancestor Process

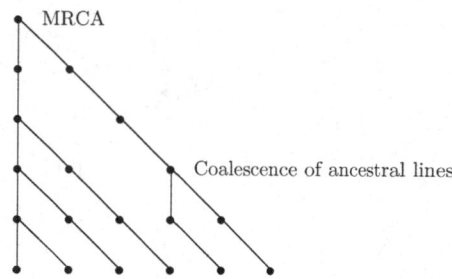

4.1 The Standard Coalescent

Consider a sample of alleles. Looking back far enough in history, these alleles have a MRCA. The birth–death process starting from this individual contains all the information regarding this sample. This process is called the common ancestor process (CAP). The realisation of this process corresponding to the realisation of the Wright–Fisher model given in Fig. 1 is illustrated in Fig. 2.

These lines contain all the information regarding the genetic composition of the present population.

The standard coalescent process models the CAP in reverse time. The present will be denoted as time 0 and time i will denote i generations ago. Suppose the evolution of a population follows the Wright–Fisher model. In reverse time these lines coalesce when two individuals have a common ancestor in the previous generation. Let G_k be the number of generations for which k distinct ancestral lines exist. We now consider the distribution of G_k when the population size is large.

First we consider G_2, the time until two ancestral lines coalesce. The probability that two randomly chosen alleles in the population have different "parents" (i.e., one individual has a different parent from the other) is $1 - \frac{1}{2N}$. Since reproduction in a given generation is independent of reproduction in other generations, it follows that the probability that two alleles have distinct ancestors i generations in the past is $(1 - \frac{1}{2N})^i$. Hence,

$$P(G_2 > i) = (1 - \frac{1}{2N})^i.$$

Now suppose the unit of time t is defined to be $2N$ generations (i.e., $t = 1$ corresponds to $2N$ generations, thus $i = 2tN$). Let T_2 be the time to coalescence of these two lines measured in these units. Then,

$$\lim_{N \to \infty} P(T_2 > t) = \lim_{N \to \infty} (1 - \frac{1}{2N})^{2tN} = e^{-t}.$$

It follows from this that T_2 has an exponential distribution with mean 1 (i.e., $2N$ generations). Hence, the coalescence of two lines occurs as a Poisson process with

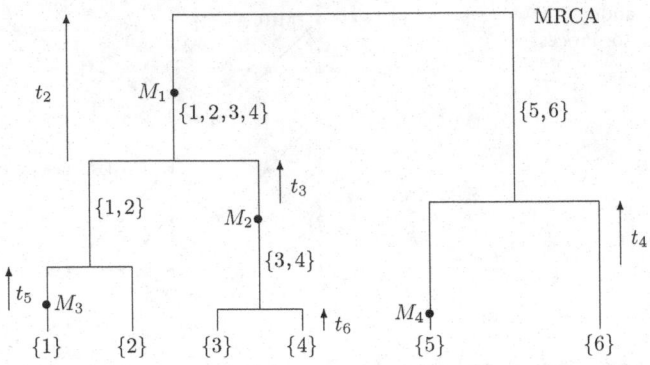

Fig. 3 A realisation of the standard coalescent

rate 1. It can be shown in a similar way that the probability of three individuals having a common ancestor in the previous generation is $O(\frac{1}{N^2})$.

Now consider T_k, this is the time (considering the reverse process) until the first coalescence of two of k ancestral lines. Each pair of lines coalesce at rate 1. Since there are $\frac{k(k-1)}{2}$ pairs of lines, it follows that $T_k \sim Exp[\frac{k(k-1)}{2}]$. It should be noted that the T_k are independent. Since the probability of three lines coalescing simultaneously is $O(\frac{1}{N^2})$, when a coalescence occurs in the limiting process, with probability one it occurs only between two lines. Hence, after such a coalescence there will be $k-1$ ancestral lines.

Figure 3 illustrates a realization of a coalescent process starting with six individuals at the present (time 0). This process can be thought of as a tree. Each vertical line represents an ancestral line. A horizontal line represents the coalescence of two lines. Each set denotes the individuals from the sample corresponding to a line.

4.2 Mutations Within the Coalescent Tree and Polarity

In the absence of mutations and recombination, the descendant alleles would be identical to the most common ancestor. Mutations can be introduced in a very simple way. The simplest model is the infinite sites model, which assumes that the number of sites in an allele is very large and the mutation rate is small. Hence, every mutation that occurs in a genetic tree occurs at a different site. This site may be chosen by generating a number at random from the uniform distribution on $[0, 1]$. Let u be the probability that a mutation occurs. It is assumed that u is of order $\frac{1}{N}$. Set $\theta = 4Nu$. In the limiting process (as $N \to \infty$ and 1 unit of time is $2N$ generations), mutations occur in the coalescent process as a Poisson process of rate $\frac{\theta}{2}$ along each ancestral line. This is illustrated in Fig. 3.

Mutation M_1 is common to individuals 1–4, mutation M_2 is common to individuals 3 and 4. Mutations M_3 and M_4 each only appear in one individual (1 and 5, respectively). Such mutations as M_3 and M_4 are called singletons and occur in the external line of a tree. Under the infinite sites model, the individuals at the end of each line only show variation at the sites of these mutations. Such sites are called *segregating sites*. The number of segregating sites is thus equal to the number of mutations in the coalescent tree.

A more advanced model for generating mutations is the finite sites model. The simplest such model assumes that mutations are equally likely to occur at each site. Improvements to this model have been made by assuming, e.g., that the mutation rate is greater in non-coding regions than in coding regions. Since a mutation can occur at a site more than once, the number of mutations is at least the number of segregating sites. However, if the mutation rate is reasonably small and the number of sites large, the infinite sites model will be a reasonable approximation.

Since it is assumed that only two variants can appear at a site, the genetic code of the descendants may be described by a binary code whose length is equal to the number of segregating sites. Two types of coding systems are used:

Non-polarised The most common variant at a segregating site is coded using 0.

Polarised The code for the most recent common ancestor is assumed to be made up of zeroes. Mutant variants are represented by ones. It should be noted that when dealing with data, it is often assumed that the ancestral code is the most common code in the most similar ancestral species or an ancestral population (i.e., nucleotide sequences for the African human population can be used to define the ancestral code for the European human population).

The non-polarised frequency at a site is the frequency of the minor variant. The polarised frequency is the frequency of the derived (mutant) variant.

Suppose the order of the sites of the mutation along the nucleotide sequence is M_1, M_2, M_3 and M_4. Then the polarised codes of the six descendants are: Individual 1—1010, Individual 2—1000, Individuals 3 and 4—1100, Individual 5—0001, Individual 6—0000.

Since mutation M_1 is the only mutation seen in the majority of individuals, the non-polarised codes are obtained by swapping 0 with 1 in position 1. The polarised frequency at site 1 is 4, while the non-polarised frequency is 2.

One simple test of the infinite sites model without recombination is based on the pattern of possible sequences under this model. Suppose mutation M_1 occurred before M_2. There are two possibilities: (a) mutation M_2 occurs on a lower branch that emanates from the branch in which M_1 occurred, (b) mutation M_2 occurs on a branch that does not emanate from the branch in which mutation M_1 occurred. In the first case, there is no individual who does not have mutation M_1, but has mutation M_2. In the second case, there is no individual who has both mutations. Hence, only three of the four possible codes for these two positions (00, 10, 01, 11) can occur. If all four possibilities occur at any pair of sites, then the infinite sites model without recombination cannot hold.

4.3 Population Size Variation over Time

The assumption of a population of fixed size may be relaxed by assuming that
the population size t units of time ago was $2N(t)$ alleles, where one unit of time
represents $2N(0)$ generations. The rate of convergence of ancestral lines at time t
relative to the rate of convergence in the standard coalescent is $N(0)/N(t)$ (since the
probability of the coalescence of lines is inversely proportional to population size).
The coalescent tree starting with n lines can be generated using the fact that the first
coalescence of any two of k lines occurs as a non-homogeneous Poisson process of
rate $\frac{k(k-1)N(0)}{2N(t)}$. In this case, the times between coalescent points are not independent.
For example, suppose a population is expanding (i.e., $N(t)$ is decreasing in t, as
we are considering the reverse process). If the time to the first coalescent point is
relatively long, then the expected time to the next coalescence is relatively short,
since going back in time the coalescence rate is increasing for fixed k.

The coalescent tree for an expanding population will tend to have relatively long
external branches and short upper branches. Hence, for expanding populations we
expect a larger number of singletons and a smaller number of mutations that occur
in a large number of individuals.

4.4 The Introduction of Recombination into the Coalescent Tree

It is more difficult to introduce recombination into a coalescent tree. Looking back in
time, when recombination occurs an allele will have two parents. One of the parents
contains the information to the left of the recombination point and the other contains
the information to the right of the recombination point. Hence, recombination is
represented by the splitting of one ancestral line into two. Suppose the probability
of recombination along an allele, r, is of order $\frac{1}{N}$. Then setting $\rho = 2rN$, each
ancestral line is subject to recombination according to a Poisson process of rate ρ.
The recombination point is chosen at random. Since the rate of coalescence is of
the order of the square of the number of lines, with probability one the number
of ancestral lines will fall to one in finite time. Using the coalescent tree, we
can trace which information was passed on. Suppose m recombinations occur in
such a coalescent tree and the order of the recombination points along the tree
is $R_1, R_2, \ldots, R_m$. Let R_0 and R_{m+1} denote the end points of the allele. Since
no recombination occurs between R_i and R_{i+1}, it follows that the ancestral lines
corresponding to this section can be described by a standard coalescent tree. Hence,
the coalescent process with recombination can be described by a set of $m + 1$
standard coalescent trees. Figure 4 gives a simple example starting with just two
individuals. The genetic information contained in A is in light grey. The genetic
information in B is denoted in dark grey. Black denotes material that is passed
down to both individuals. White denotes material that is of unknown source when

Fig. 4 The coalescent tree
with recombination

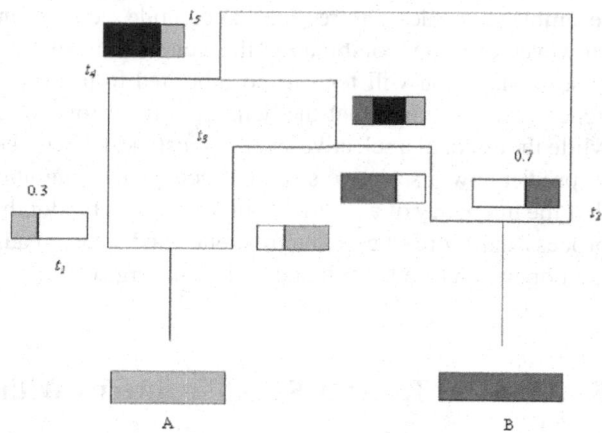

the initial tree is being generated. The source of this material becomes apparent
at coalescent points. For example, at t_3 the two central lines converge and so
must contain the same genetic information. From the graph the central section is
transferred to both A and B, hence the material is common to both.

Suppose the recombination points are at 0.3 and 0.7, in the standard coalescent
tree corresponding to the left hand section the two lines coalesce at time t_4. In the
case of the central and right hand sections, the coalescent times are t_3 and t_5,
respectively. Mutations can be added to these standard coalescent trees as before.

It should be noted that these models have been extended to account for population
structure (see Slatkin 2000) and different forms of selection (see Neuhauser and
Krone 1997). Various computer programs are available to simulate samples of
nucleotide sequences under various assumptions regarding population structure and
selection. Hudson (2002) made available a program that carries out such simulations
under various demographic scenarios when selection does not act. Spencer and
Coop (2004) extended this to models that included selection.

4.5   Selective Sweeps and the Coalescent Tree

A selective sweep occurs when a mutation that was previously not present in the
population spreads throughout the population. Variants at sites that are closely
linked to such a positive mutation will tend to also spread. This process is known
as hitchhiking. Suppose such a selective sweep has just finished. Consider the
coalescent tree for the nucleotide sequence immediately surrounding the positive
mutation. Due to a lack of recombination between neighbouring sites, the genetic
information in the present population will have been inherited from the individuals
in the population that carried the positive mutation. These individuals form a
subpopulation which grows rapidly in size. Hence, the coalescent tree will tend to

resemble the coalescent tree for a nucleotide sequence in an expanding population. However, due to recombination the genetic information at sites not linked to the positive mutation will tend to be inherited from the population as a whole. The general conclusion is that the demographic history affects the genome uniformly, while the effect of a selective sweep is just local. Coalescent theory has been applied to predict how a selective sweep affects genetic variation. It is normally assumed that the frequency of a positive mutant changes randomly according to a birth/death process, until it reaches some frequency and then spreads deterministically through the population (see Durrett and Schweinsberg 2004).

5   Classical Tests for Selective Sweeps Within a Population

In this section we will describe a classical test for a selective sweeps: Tajima's test (Tajima 1989) and mention some others. In order to do this, we first consider some statistical properties of the standard coalescent tree and two related measures of diversity, which can be used to estimate the mutation rate under the standard coalescent model.

5.1   The Height and Length of a Standard Coalescent Tree

The height of a standard coalescent tree starting from n lines, H_n, is the time required for all the lines to converge. Since T_k is the time to the first coalescence of any pair of lines from k lines and the T_k are independent, it follows that

$$E[H_n] = \sum_{k=2}^{n} E[T_k] = \sum_{k=2}^{n} \frac{2}{k(k-1)} = 2 - \frac{2}{k},$$

$$Var[H_n] = \sum_{k=2}^{n} Var[T_k] = \sum_{k=2}^{n} \frac{4}{k^2(k-1)^2}.$$

Hence, under the standard coalescent the expected time to the most common ancestor is always less than two time units ($4N$ generations). For large n, $Var[H_n] \approx \frac{4\pi^2}{3} - 12$.

Another important measure is the length of a coalescent tree, L_n. This is the sum of the lengths of the branches. It can be seen from Fig. 3 that k lines exist for time T_k. It follows that

$$E[L_n] = \sum_{k=2}^{n} k E[T_k] = \sum_{k=2}^{n} \frac{2}{k-1} = 2 \sum_{k=1}^{n-1} \frac{1}{k}.$$

$$Var[L_n] = \sum_{k=2}^{n} \frac{4}{(k-1)^2}.$$

For large n, we may use the approximations $E[L_n] \approx \ln(n) + 0.577$ and $Var[L_n] \approx \frac{2\pi^2}{3}$.

Since mutations occur along each line as a Poisson process with rate $\frac{\theta}{2}$, it follows that the expected number of mutations, $E(S)$, is given by $E(S) = \frac{\theta E[L_n]}{2}$.

It should be noted that under the infinite sites model without recombination, the number of mutations is the number of segregating sites. Under this model, we can estimate the mutation rate from a sample of n nucleotide sequences using

$$\hat{\theta}_L = \frac{2S}{E[L_n]} = \frac{S}{\sum_{k=1}^{n-1} 1/k}.$$

5.2 Nucleotide Diversity

The Hamming distance between sequence i and sequence j, $D_{i,j}$ is the number of positions at which the sequences differ. The nucleotide diversity, Π, of a set of n nucleotide sequences is defined to be the average Hamming distance between pairs of sequences, i.e.

$$\Pi = \frac{2}{n(n-1)} \sum_{i<j} D_{i,j}. \tag{1}$$

According to the standard coalescent tree, the expected Hamming distance between two nucleotide sequences is the expected number of mutations on a coalescent tree starting with two lines. Since the expected length of such a tree is one, the nucleotide diversity is an estimator of the mutation rate i.e. $\hat{\theta}_{\Pi} = \Pi$.

5.3 Tajima's Test for Selection

It should be noted that these estimators are only valid when the Wright–Fisher model holds, i.e., there is no selection and the population size does not vary in time. As argued above, after a selective sweep the number of singletons is expected to be relatively high and the number of mutations that are common to many lines relatively low compared to the standard coalescent. Each of these mutations corresponds to a segregating site, but affects the measure of nucleotide diversity in different ways. A singleton mutation will increase the Hamming distance between the individual in which it occurs and the remaining $n - 1$ individuals by one (i.e., increase the sum in Eq. (1) by $n-1$). Consider the following extreme case in which a mutation occurs when there are only two lines and both of these lines correspond to $\frac{n}{2}$ individuals. This difference will be counted in $\frac{n^2}{4}$ comparisons (and hence increase the sum in Eq. (1) by $\frac{n^2}{4}$). It can thus be seen that when a selective sweep occurs, the estimator of the mutation rate based on the number of segregating sites, $\hat{\theta}_L$, is expected to be larger than the estimator based on the nucleotide diversity, $\hat{\theta}_\Pi$.

Tajima noted that under the Wright–Fisher model for reasonably large samples there is almost no correlation between $\hat{\theta}_L$ and $\hat{\theta}_\Pi$. He introduced the standardised D statistic to test for the effect of selection, where

$$D = \frac{\hat{\theta}_\Pi - \hat{\theta}_L}{\sqrt{\hat{Var}(\hat{\theta}_\Pi - \hat{\theta}_L)}}.$$

Under the null hypothesis that the standard coalescent model holds:

$$\hat{Var}(\hat{\theta}_\Pi - \hat{\theta}_L) \approx e_1 S + e_2 S(S - 1),$$

$$e_1 = \frac{n + 1}{3a_n(n - 1)} - \frac{1}{a_n^2},$$

$$e_2 = \frac{1}{a_n^2 + b_n} \left[\frac{2(n^2 + n + 3)}{9n(n - 1)} - \frac{n + 2}{na_n} + \frac{b_n}{a_n^2} \right],$$

where $a_n = \sum_{i=1}^{n-1} \frac{1}{i}$ and $b_n = \sum_{i=1}^{n-1} \frac{1}{i^2}$.

Large negative realisations of the test statistic are assumed to be evidence that a selective sweep has occurred. Tajima observed that assuming that D has a standard normal distribution leads to a conservative test (i.e., when the standard coalescent model holds, the probability of rejecting the null hypothesis is less than the nominal significance level). He observes that a scaled beta distribution gives a better fit to the distribution of D, but the resulting test is still conservative.

However, Tajima's test does not distinguish between effects of demography and selection, since we also expect negative realisations of the test statistic D given that a population is rapidly expanding. The effect of such demographic changes should be uniform over the genome, while the effect of a selective sweep will be local. However, before the age of gene mapping it was difficult to practically make use of this idea.

The assumption that a selective sweep is complete is also important. Macpherson et al. (2008) note that partially completed sweeps may be associated with positive values of Tajima's D statistic, as at intermediate frequencies a positive mutation is likely to be linked with other alleles at intermediate frequency and thus the nucleotide diversity is likely to be relatively large. Also, varying recombination rates may produce a signal, since areas of low recombination tend to be characterised by low genetic variation.

5.4 Other Classical Tests for a Selective Sweep Within a Population

Fu and Li (1992) proposed a test based on estimating the mutation rate in two ways using the number of non-singleton and singleton mutations, ξ and $\zeta = n - \xi$, respectively. Under the Wright–Fisher model, the coefficient of correlation between these two estimators is smaller than the coefficient of correlation between $\hat{\theta}_{\Pi}$ and $\hat{\theta}_L$. They suggested that the standardised difference between these two estimators should be used to test the standard coalescent model. As before, if there has been a recent selective sweep there will be a relatively large number of singletons. Hence, we would expect large negative realisations of the test statistic. However, this is also true if the population is expanding. Also, Achaz (2008) notes that the number of singletons is very sensitive to the probability of wrongly reading a nucleotide and so such a test will not be reliable.

Fu and Li note that other estimates of the mutation rate can be used to test the standard coalescent model in the same way. Zeng et al. (2007) base tests on the joint distribution of such statistics. The joint distribution is estimated using simulations based on the Wright–Fisher model.

However, all such tests suffer from not being able to separate demographic effects from the effects of a selective sweep, although the tests of Zeng et al. (2007) are somewhat more robust to changes in population size. Möller et al. (2007) also note that such tests are sensitive to the choice of population. For example, species wide measures of D give lower average values of D than measures based on carefully defined subpopulations. Including several subpopulations in one sample tends to increase the number of SNPs, as many will be specific to just one population. Hence, the number of segregating sites will be large in relation to the nucleotide diversity.

Another problem is that different forms of selection have different effects on the pattern of variation in a population. A soft selective sweep would not have such a clear signature. This signature is also affected by whether the favoured allele is dominant, co-dominant or recessive. The appropriate signal to use depends on the development of the sweep. When a sweep is in progress the level of linkage disequilibrium will be a clearer signal than the frequency spectrum, which is more useful at the end of or after a sweep.

6 A Classical Test for Differential Selection in Subpopulations

Consider the case in which an ancestral population has split into n subpopulations each occupying some specified environment. Suppose the frequency in subpopulation i of a variant at a site is p_i. Due to genetic drift, $p_1 \neq p_2$. Mutations counteract the effect of genetic drift (if the frequency of A increases, then there will be more mutations from A to the other variant). Hence, if there is no selection, the frequency of the variants in each subpopulation will be similar. Lewontin and Krakauer (1973) introduced a test for differential selection using a measure, F_{ST}, of the difference between the subpopulations using $F_{ST} = \frac{s_p^2}{\overline{p}(1-\overline{p})}$, where s_p^2 is the variance in the frequency of A between subpopulations and $\overline{p}$ is the mean frequency of A in the population as a whole. In order to carry out such a test, it is necessary to estimate the average value of F_{ST} at sites where two variants are relatively common (by assumption most of these sites are unaffected by selection). Denote this estimate by $\overline{F}$. They noted that under the Wright–Fisher model the test statistic $T = \frac{(n-1)F_{ST}}{\overline{F}}$ has approximately a χ_{n-1}^2 distribution. Large realisations of T indicate differential selection, i.e., A is relatively more favourable in one of the environments. However, there are some problems associated with this approach:

1. The test does not work well when the (effective) sizes of the subpopulations are very different.
2. The test is sensitive to changes in the size of subpopulations.
3. If A is selected for (or against) in both environments to a similar extent, then this test is unlikely to detect selection.

7 Tests of Selection in the Era of Genome Mapping

McVean et al. (2005) outline many possibilities arising from the existence of the HapMap data. One of the obvious advantages is that there is enough data to be able to differentiate between the local effect of selection and the global effect of the demographic history of the population. New methods of detecting selecting sweeps can be broadly separated into two main classes: (1) empirical methods and (2) composite likelihood methods.

7.1 Empirical Methods

Using such an approach a score is calculated for all the sites along a chromosome. For example, the score for a site might be Tajima's D statistic calculated using data from all the sites in a specified neighbourhood. If the population is growing, then we would expect negative scores. However, if an area is affected by selection, then all the scores in a region are expected to be particularly low. Thus the intuition behind the empirical approach is to select a small proportion of the genome (say 1–5 %) as areas that seem to have been affected by a selective sweep and use then use biological methods to further investigate these regions.

Carlson et al. (2005) use a score based on the approach described above using a 100 kb window around a site. They investigated human populations of African, European and Chinese origin and selected the 1 % of genes (taken over the three groups as a whole) for which the lowest scores were observed. They concluded that recent selection seems to have played a lesser role in the African population and has acted in clearly distinct ways in the three populations. According to their criterion, they selected 7 genes thought to be subject to selection in the African population, 23 in the European population and 29 in the Chinese population. Only four genes were thought to be subject to selection in at least two populations. As in the case of Tajima's test, this method is not robust to varying recombination rates.

Voight et al. (2006) use a different procedure based on the concept of extended haplotype homozygosity (EHH) introduced by Sabeti et al. (2002). The EHH for a given interval of the genome is defined to be the probability that two randomly chosen individuals from a population have the same nucleotide sequence on that interval. This measure will fall to 0 as the length of this interval grows. Their method is designed to detect an incomplete strong sweep, hence the site affected will be an SNP. Denote by D the (derived) variant that is suspected to be favoured by selection at an SNP. The other (ancestral) variant is denoted by A. If D is in reality favoured by selection, then the individuals which have D will show less variation around that site than those who have A. Define iHH_A to be the sum of the estimates of EHH over all the intervals centered around an SNP for which EHH > 0.05 in the subpopulation which has variant A. The measure iHH_D is defined analogously based on the subpopulation that has the variant D. Their standardised score, calculated for each SNP at which the frequency of the least common variant is $>5\%$, is given by

$$iHS = \frac{\ln\left(\frac{iHH_A}{iHH_D}\right) - E_p\left[\ln\left(\frac{iHH_A}{iHH_D}\right)\right]}{SD_p\left[\ln\left(\frac{iHH_A}{iHH_D}\right)\right]},$$

where $E_p\left[\ln\left(\frac{iHH_A}{iHH_D}\right)\right]$ and $SD_p\left[\ln\left(\frac{iHH_A}{iHH_D}\right)\right]$ are the estimates of the expected value and standard deviation of $\ln\left(\frac{iHH_A}{iHH_D}\right)$ based on the empirical observations. Large negative values of this score indicate that individuals with the derived variant show less variation around that site. This is an indication that the site is affected by selection. They note that the empirical distribution is close to normal and there may be errors in determining which of the variants is the derived variant. Hence, they consider any absolute score of above 2.5 (around 1 % of the scores) as being an indication of selection. When selection occurs, it is expected that these high scores will be clustered so they also use windows of length 100 kb to illustrate the variation of scores over a whole chromosome.

They note that since the score is based on a ratio of homozygosity measures, then this method is less sensitive to local changes in the recombination rate than the method described above. This is due to the fact that low recombination rates will lead to low measures in both subpopulations, which does not greatly affect the score. They considered three human subpopulations: from East Asia, Nigeria and Europe. Unlike Carlson et al. (2005), they found that more sites in the African population were selected as candidates for sites affected by selection than in the other two populations (note this test is more sensitive to incomplete sweeps).

Akey et al. (2002) adapt the method of Lewontin and Krakauer (1973). They estimated F_{ST} for each of 25 549 SNPs based on three human populations: of African, European and East Asian origin. The average measure of F_{ST} was 0.123. Compared to simulations based on a model with migration but no selection, there was an excess of low and high F_{ST} scores, which is in agreement with the action of natural selection. Also, extreme values of the estimates of F_{ST} based on the data tended to be highly clustered.

The authors chose sites where the F_{ST} score was greater than the 97.5 % quartile of the empirical distribution to be candidates for sites affected by a selective sweep. This led to 174 candidate genes, among those were a gene associated with cystic fibrosis and a gene associated with diabetes.

Kimura et al. (2007) adapt the concept of EHH to the problem of detecting the site of a selective sweep that affects a particular subpopulation. They use sequences from two populations, where one is assumed to be the ancestral population. They define the most frequent haplotype homozygosity (MHH) to be the probability that two individuals in a subpopulation both have the most frequent haplotype over a given interval. For the ancestral population and derived population, this measure is denoted as MHH_A and MHH_D, respectively. Blocks of low variation in the derived population are defined to be intervals for which $MHH_D \geq 0.9$ that include at least two sites where variation is seen in the two populations as a whole. They define $HTMH_D$ to be the probability that two individuals in the derived population have the same haplotype as the most common haplotype in the ancestral population. From this they calculate the relative most frequent haplotype homozygosity (rMMH) for the two populations as $rMHH = \frac{HTMH_D}{MHH_A}$. A very small value of rMHH for a block indicates that the most common haplotype in the ancestral population is rare in the derived population. Hence, such a block may have been affected by selection. Similarly, the relative extended haplotype homozygosity (rEHH) is defined as $rEHH = \frac{EHH_A}{EHH_D}$, where EHH_A and EHH_D are the EHH over a chosen block in the ancestral and derived population, respectively. If selection has only occurred in the derived population, then this measure will also be small. Using results from simulations, the authors defined candidate blocks as those for which $rMHH < 0.05$ and $rEHH < 0.3$. They found that such a test compared favourably with using a test based on estimating F_{ST}. Unlike the test of Voight et al. (2006) this test is aimed at detecting complete or almost complete sweeps, since the chosen blocks must display very little variation in the derived population. It should be noted also that the test is designed to detect a sweep specific to the derived population. If there was a similar sweep at a site in both populations, the observed value of rEHH would be relatively large, since EHH_A would be large.

7.2 Advantages and Disadvantages of Empirical Methods

One of the obvious advantages of an empirical approach is simplicity. However, there are serious disadvantages. Teshima et al. (2006) reviewed the reliability of empirical methods based on simulations which considered different levels of dominance and demographic histories, as well as both hard and soft selective sweeps. One problem regarding the theory based on coalescent processes is that it is normally assumed that there is no dominance. By selecting appropriate sites from these simulations, the authors obtained data sets in which a known proportion of sites were closely linked to the site of a selective sweep. They consider scores based on nucleotide diversity π, Tajima's D and EHH (see Yamasaki et al. 2005; Carlson et al. 2005; Voight et al. 2006, respectively). Candidate sites were chosen so that the proportion of candidates was equal to the proportion of sites closely linked to a selective sweep.

They conclude that the error rate is higher for methods based on D than for tests based on π or EHH. However, the authors admit that methods based on π and EHH are more sensitive to changes in the mutation rate and they assumed in their simulations that mutation rates were constant over the whole genome. Also, the methods are sensitive to the demographic history of a population. For example, the test is more sensitive if a sweep occurred after the expansion of a population rather than before.

As argued above, the stage of development of the sweep is important in determining the efficacy of such methods. Methods based on EHH are effective if a positive variant in a strong selective sweep has increased in frequency to around 40 %. However, this method is not effective for complete/almost complete sweeps. On the other hand, methods based on π and D are effective only when a sweep is almost complete. Also, since a positive recessive mutation will, in general, take longer to invade a population than an undominated mutation, the power to detect sweeps in which a recessive variant invaded a population is relatively low as a higher level of variation is maintained.

Moreover, the nature of the sweep is very important. They simulated soft sweeps in which a previously neutral variant starts to be selected for when its frequency is 5 %. The methods based on π and D detect recently completed hard selective sweeps well. When 5 % of the sites are affected by selection, the "false discovery rate" (the proportion of chosen candidates which are not strongly linked to a site affected by a selective sweep) was 8.3 % using π and 20.3 % using Tajima's D. However, these methods were poor at detecting recently completed soft selective sweeps. The corresponding "false discovery rates" were 73.8 and 82.2 %.

Innan and Kim (2004) also observe that such tests are sensitive to the type of sweep (hard or soft). In a later paper (Innan and Kim 2008), they note that tests using samples from both ancestral and derived populations are more sensitive to soft selective sweeps than tests based on samples from just one population. A soft selective sweep has a weak signature, since local variation is not reduced by as much as under a strong selective sweep. However, if a soft selective sweep occurs in a derived population, then the frequencies of the variants in the two subpopulations will be clearly different. This fact is felt to be important especially in the case of agricultural crops, where artificial selection generally occurred from standing variation. On the other hand, when a new population breaks away from its ancestral population, a population bottleneck is a very likely scenario and this might explain such differences in the frequency spectra of the two resulting populations.

Finally, there are also some technical problems associated with empirical methods. Firstly, they cannot be used to estimate the strength of a sweep. Secondly, we are unsure of the proportion of the genome that is affected by selection. Hence, choosing the threshold above which we choose a site to be a candidate is, to a large degree, guesswork. If we choose too low a threshold, we will obtain a large number of "false positives" (candidates that are not linked to sites affected by selection). By choosing too high a threshold, we will miss many sites that are affected by a selective sweep.

7.3   Composite Likelihood Methods

Unlike empirical methods, composite likelihood methods test the hypothesis that there is no selective sweep affecting a section of the genome. The procedure used is similar to a standard likelihood ratio test in which the alternative is that a selective sweep has occurred. These tests do not, in general, consider the correlation between variant frequencies at sites and for simplicity calculate the composite likelihood. This is done by multiplying the likelihoods of the variant frequencies observed at each segregating site under the appropriate hypothesis.

Kim and Stepham (2002) present such a test, in which the null hypothesis is that the population follows the Wright–Fisher model (i.e., constant population size and no selection). The distribution of the variant frequencies under this alternative was derived by Kimura (1971). The composite likelihood of the data can be calculated simply by multiplying the individual probabilities of the observed variant frequencies. Under the alternative, it is assumed that a strong selective sweep has just finished. The distribution of the variant frequencies under the alternative, which depends on the strength of selection and the rate of recombination between a site and the location of the mutation, was given by Maynard Smith and Haigh (1974). It is possible to find maximum likelihood estimates of the location and strength of a putative selective sweep using a composite likelihood function. The test statistic is based on the ratio between the composite likelihoods obtained under the two hypotheses.

Jensen et al. (2005) note that the test of Kim and Stephan is sensitive to the demographic history of a population. This is not surprising as the null hypothesis is that the Wright–Fisher model holds. For example, the authors carried out simulations in which a population had a recent, strong bottleneck, but there was no selection. Kim and Stephan's test rejected the null hypothesis around 90 % of the time. They proposed an improved version of the original test as follows: (1) Carry out Kim and Stephan's test. If the null hypothesis of no selection is rejected, then (2) they carry out a goodness of fit test in which the null hypothesis is that a selective sweep has occurred with strength and location given by the maximum likelihood estimators calculated at stage 1. If the null hypothesis is rejected in stage 2, then they conclude that demographic factors caused the changes from the predictions made under the Wright–Fisher model. Of course there are problems associated with such an approach, such as the possibility of multiple sweeps.

Nielsen et al. (2005) use an intuitive approach to deal with the problem of assumptions regarding the demographic history of a population. Since demographic history affects genetic variation at the level of the whole genome, they assume that when there is no selection the distribution of the variant frequencies is some background distribution. Any local divergence from this background distribution may be attributed to the action of selection. Under the assumption of no selection, this distribution can be estimated from the data. Consider the case in which we have non-polarised frequencies at k SNPs for n individuals. Since the non-polarised frequency is defined to be between 1 and $i_{max} = \lfloor \frac{n}{2} \rfloor$, the background distribution can be estimated by estimating the probability of a non-polarised frequency of i, p_i, using $\hat{p}_i = \frac{k_i}{k}$, where k_i is the number of times a frequency of i is observed. The composite likelihood of the data under the null hypothesis is thus $\prod_{i=1}^{i_{max}} \hat{p}_i^{k_i}$.

The alternative is that a selective sweep has occurred. The distribution of the non-polarised frequencies under such a hypothesis can be approximated using coalescent theory. This is based on an estimate of the proportion of the population that, at the end of a selective sweep, have a neutral variant that initially appeared with the original positive mutation. This probability is given by $e^{-\alpha d}$. Here $\alpha = \frac{r \ln(2N)}{s}$, where d is the distance between a site and the positive mutation, r the recombination rate, N the population size and s is the selection coefficient (see Durrett and Schweinsberg 2004). Under this assumption, one can calculate the composite likelihood under the hypothesis that there is a selective sweep of strength s at a given locus. The maximum likelihood estimator of the strength and location of a sweep on a chromosome is found by maximising over all the loci along a chromosome. This is used to define a likelihood ratio test. It should be noted that intrinsically this test involves multiple testing (the possibility of a selective sweep at each site is considered). Hence, the authors find appropriate critical values for the test by simulating the distribution of the test statistic under the hypothesis that the Wright–Fisher model holds.

They show that the test is not sensitive to demographic history using a wide range of simulations. Also, by analysing chromosome 2 for the European population (using data from the HapMap project), they show that the test identifies a selective sweep in the neighbourhood of the lactase gene. Although the alternative hypothesis is that one selective sweep has occurred, the likelihood scores do indicate that multiple sweeps have occurred on this chromosome.

In addition, they correct for the so-called ascertainment bias (see also Nielsen et al. 2004). Often, to reduce costs a small subsample of individuals is fully sequenced (the ascertainment process). The remaining individuals in the sample are only sequenced at the sites where variation was observed in the subsample. This means that there may be more SNPs in the sample than we actually observe and high frequency variants are over-represented. This correction is a relatively simple process based on Bayes' laws.

Some work has been carried out on the use of linkage disequilibrium measures. Kim and Nielsen (2004) use information from linkage disequilibrium measures in addition to data on the frequency spectrum of SNPs used in Kim and Stepham (2002), in order to detect a recently completed sweep. However, they conclude that such an approach hardly increases the power of the test. Jensen et al. (2007) consider the same problem and show that various demographic histories, such as a population bottleneck, can lead to a similar pattern of linkage disequilibrium as a selective sweep. They conclude that linkage disequilibrium measures can be useful in detecting selective sweeps, but they note that linkage disequilibrium disappears relatively rapidly after a sweep finishes. One problem with estimating linkage disequilibrium lies in the fact that such estimation tends to be inaccurate when variants are rare (as expected around the site of a selective sweep, Jensen et al. (2007) did not use singletons in their analysis). Pfaffelhuber et al. (2008) analyse the evolution of linkage disequilibrium under a selective sweep using coalescent theory. They conclude that the pattern of linkage disequilibrium observed around the site of a complete selective sweep is similar to the pattern of linkage disequilibrium around a recombination hotspot, but a selective sweep will also reduce variation.

7.4   Advantages and Disadvantages of Composite Likelihood Methods

One of the obvious advantages of such methods is that maximum likelihood estimators can be found for the strength and location of a sweep. However, one should remember that the standard assumption of such tests is that a strong sweep has just ended. Using simulations, given this assumption Nielsen et al. (2005) showed that these estimators are accurate. On the other hand, if a sweep finished some time in the past or a weak sweep occurred, the strength of the sweep will tend to be underestimated and the variance of the estimator of the location will increase. If the sweep is not close to completion, it would be better to use methods based on linkage disequilibrium or comparing two subpopulations.

More accuracy could be obtained by using the real likelihood function (which takes into account linkage disequilibrium) rather than the composite likelihood function. Although a relatively large amount of work has been done on what frequency spectrum should be expected after a selective sweep, relatively little has been done on the form of the linkage disequilibrium. Once such work has been carried out more fully, it may be possible to use ideas from covariance modelling (see Pan and MacKenzie 2003).

Another problem is that it is assumed that there was only one selective sweep on the section of the genome considered. Nielsen et al. (2005) show that their method indicates the occurrence of many selective sweeps. Also, considering the role of genes in the region of these sites, it is reasonable to assume that many of these signals are true. The effect of multiple sweeps is unknown. It may be the case that such sweeps are sufficiently rare that their effects on the frequency spectrum can be assumed to be independent. However, if two positive mutations occur at sites which are close together, the resulting effect is difficult to predict (it will depend on the order in which the mutations occurred and the time between them). This is particularly important when we consider agricultural crops, where it is likely that artificial selection caused multiple soft sweeps occurring almost simultaneously.

8   Conclusion

Jensen et al. (2008) considered the problem of detecting selective sweeps using firstly, data from whole chromosomes and secondly, using partial maps. He concluded that low density maps lower the power of tests to detect selective sweeps. Even using an initial map as a guide to decide upon areas of the genome to sequence more fully is unreliable. Hence, the availability of genome maps is undoubtedly a huge resource for the analysis of genetic data.

It has been shown that the frequency spectrum is dependent on both selection and the demographic history of the population. It is also very important whether the selective sweep originated from a positive mutation (a strong sweep) or from standing variation (a weak sweep). In the second case, the signal will be weaker. The time at which the sweep occurred is also important, as tests based on the variant frequencies are most powerful at detecting sweeps that have just completed. If a sweep is in progress, methods based on comparing the local variation of individuals with one variant at a site with the remaining individuals (or considering the level of linkage disequilibrium) are more powerful.

However, as Hamblin and Di Rienzo (2000) show, there is evidence that the frequency spectrum of a section affected by a completed selective sweep may well not resemble the one expected. They investigated a 1.9 kb section of the genome around the Duffy blood group locus. The wild type allele is thought to be FY*B, as this is observed in apes. This allele is observed in the European population. All 24 individuals from 5 sub-Saharan subpopulations were FY*O homozygous. It has been noted that such individuals are immune to vivax malaria and there is no evidence to indicate that the FY*O allele is selected against in the European population. Hence, it has been hypothesised that a selective sweep occurred after the European population split from the African one. In the section investigated there were five SNPs in the African population and at two of these sites both variants were frequent (the frequency of the minor variant was 0.23), which is very unexpected under the theory of selective sweeps. These two sites were in complete linkage disequilibrium. It is possible that the population structure plays an important role here, as the least common variant was only observed in the populations towards the southeast.

The method of Nielsen et al. (2005) seems to be relatively robust to demographic factors. However, the test is based on the assumption that one strong selective sweep has occurred, hence there are still questions to be answered. Barnes (2006) notes that inbred lines of mice exhibit linkage disequilibrium even for sites lying on different chromosomes. This indicates that selection acts on combinations of alleles. The implicit assumption of the theory presented here assumes that the effects of selection are additive and extension of the theory to include such interactions would be overly complex.

However, there seem to be areas in which advances could be made. A couple of very recent papers indicate the problem of errors in sequencing (see Achaz 2008; Johnson and Slatkin 2006). The probability of wrongly reading a nucleotide is small, however the number of nucleotides that need to be read is very large. Since most sites are not SNPs, most of these errors result in singletons, i.e., low frequency variants are over-represented due to this phenomenon. This may lead to false signals of selective sweeps. Correcting for such a bias is not as simple as correcting for ascertainment bias, as the probability of making an error needs to be estimated very accurately and more practical work needs to be done in order to do this (even a very small error rate can have a very large effect on the frequency spectrum). It is quite possible that ascertainment will not be used in the long run and so errors in reading will become the sole source of errors in the data. The expected number of false singletons increases linearly in n, the number of individuals sequenced, but the expected number of segregating sites is proportional to $\ln(n)$. This may explain to some degree the observation that the test of Nielsen et al. (2005) seems to work best for intermediate sample sizes.

The methods described above treat each site equivalently, whereas it is known that:

1. Some sections of the genome are non-coding.
2. Triples of nucleotides code for proteins, so the position of a nucleotide is significant and many mutations (especially of the central nucleotide in a triple) do not result in a change in the protein produced, these are the so-called synonymous mutations.

Williamson et al. (2005) use such an approach to simultaneously infer the effect of demographic history and selection on patterns of variation in the human genome. Since mutations in non-coding regions can be assumed to be neutral, the sequences in such sections are used to make simple inferences regarding the demographic history of the population based on coalescent theory. This seems another possible way of estimating the background frequency spectrum. Information regarding the sequences surrounding non-synonymous mutations is then used to estimate the action of selection.

The use of linkage disequilibrium measures to detect partial selective sweeps is definitely a powerful approach and linkage disequilibrium measures do seem to give a slight improvement in the power of tests based on the frequency spectrum when a sweep has recently finished. More theoretical work on the form of linkage disequilibrium at various stages of selective sweeps would be welcome and as suggested earlier this might give us the insight to adopt methods adapted from covariate modelling. Another possible approach of making use of the spatial form of the data is to adapt the theory of Markov models (see Husmeier and McGuire 2002) or change points (see Avery and Henderson 1999) to such problems.

Finally, nearly all the ideas presented here were based on coalescent theory. Simulating data using such reverse time processes is efficient, but results in a loss of accuracy. Recently, algorithms have been formulated to simulate evolutionary processes in forward time (see Hoggart et al. 2007; Padhukasahasram et al. 2008). Development of this theory will allow us to carry out more accurate simulations and develop new theory and practice.

Acknowledgements This work was carried out in the Department of Mathematics & Statistics at the University of Limerick, Ireland, and was supported by Science Foundation Ireland, Grant No. 07/MI/012 (BIO-SI project, www3.ul.ie/bio-si).

References

Achaz, G. (2008). Testing for neutrality in samples with sequencing errors. *Genetics, 179*, 1409–1424.

Akey, J. M., Zhang, G., Zhang, K., Jin, L., & Shriver, M. D. (2002). Interrogating a high-density snp map for signatures of natural selection. *Genome Research, 12*, 1805–1814.

Avery, P. J., & Henderson, D. A. (1999). Detecting a changed segment in dna sequences. *Applied Statistics, 48*, 489–503.

Barnes, M. R. (2006). Navigating the hapmap. *Briefings in Bioinformatics, 7*, 211–224.

Cannings, C. (1974). The latent roots of certain markov chains arising in genetics: A new approach, i. haploid models. *Advances in Applied Probability, 6*, 260–290.

Carlson, C. S., Thomas, D. J., Eberle, M. A., Swanson, J. E., Livingston, R. J., Rieder, M. J., et al. (2005). Genomic regions exhibiting positive selection identified from dense genotype data. *Genome Research, 15*, 1553–1565.

Consortium, T. I. H. (2003). The international hapmap project. *Nature, 426*, 789–796.

Durrett, R., & Schweinsberg, J. (2004). Approximating selective sweeps. *Theoretical Population Biology, 66*, 129–138.

Fu, Y. X., & Li, W. H. (1992). Statistical test of neutrality of mutations. *Genetics, 133*, 693–709.

Hamblin, M. T., & Di Rienzo, A. (2000). Detection of the signature of natural selection in humans: Evidence from the duffy blood group locus. *American Journal of Human Genetics, 66*, 1669–1679.

Hein, J., Schierup, M., & Wiuf, C. (2004). *Gene genealogies, variation and evolution: A primer in coalescent theory*. Oxford, UK: Oxford University Press.

Hoggart, C. J., Chadeau-Hyam, M., Clark, T. G., Lampariello, R., Whittaker, J. C., De Iorio, M., et al. (2007). Sequence-level population simulations over large genomic regions. *Genetics, 177*, 1725–1731.

Hudson, R. R. (2002). Generating samples under a wright-fisher neutral model of genetic variation. *Bioinformatics, 18*, 337–338.

Husmeier, D., & McGuire, G. (2002). Detecting recombination with mcmc. *Bioinformatics, 18*, 345–353.

Innan, H., & Kim, Y. (2004). Pattern of polymorphism after strong artificial selection in a domestication event. *Proceedings of the National Academy of Sciences, 101*, 10667–10672.

Innan, H., & Kim, Y. (2008). Detection of local adaptation using the joint sampling of polymorphism data in the parental and derived population. *Genetics, 179*, 1713–1720.

Jensen, J. D., Kim, Y., DuMont, V. B., Aquadro, C. F., & Bustamante, C. D. (2005). Distinguishing between selective sweeps and demography using dna polymorphism data. *Genetics, 170*, 1401–1410.

Jensen, J. D., Thornton, K. R., & Aquadro, C. F. (2008). Inferring selection in partially sequenced regions. *Molecular and Biological Evolution, 25*, 438–446.

Jensen, J. D., Thornton, K. R., Bustamante, C. D., & Aquadro, C. F. (2007). On the utility of linkage disequilibrium as a statistic for identifying targets of positive selection in nonequilibrium populations. *Genetics, 176*, 2371–2379.

Johnson, P. L. F., & Slatkin, M. (2006). Inference of population genetic parameters in metagenomics: A clean look at messy data. *Genome Research, 16*, 1320–1327.

Kim, Y., & Nielsen, R. (2004). Linkage disequilibrium as a signature of selective sweeps. *Genetics, 167*, 1513–1524.

Kim, Y., & Stepham, W. (2002). Detecting a local signature of genetic hitchhiking along a recombining chromosome. *Genetics, 160*, 765–777.

Kimura, M. (1971). Theoretical foundation of population genetics at the molecular level. *Theoretical Population Biology, 2*, 174–208.

Kimura, R., Fujimoto, A., Tokunaga, K., & Ohashi, J. (2007). A practical genome scan for population-specific strong selective sweeps that have reached fixation. *PLoS One, 2*, e286.

Lewontin, R. C., & Krakauer, J. (1973). Distribution of gene frequency as a test of the theory of the selective neutrality of polymorphisms. *Genetics, 74*, 175–195.

Macpherson, J. M., González, J., Witten, D. M., Davis, J. C., Rosenberg, N. A., Hirsh, A. E., et al. (2008). Nonadaptive explanations for signatures of partial selective sweeps in drosophila. *Molecular and Biological Evolution, 25*, 1025–1042.

Maynard Smith, J., & Haigh, J. (1974). The hitchhiking effect of a favourable gene. *Genetics, 23*, 23–35.

McVean, G., Spencer, C. C. A., & Chaix, R. (2005). Perspectives on human genetic variation from hapmap project. *PLoS Genetics, 1*, e54.

Möller, D. A., Tenaillon, M. I., & Tiffin, P. (2007). Population structure and its effects on patterns of nucleotide polymorphism in teosinte. *Genetics, 176*, 1799–1809.

Neuhauser, C., & Krone, S. M. (1997). The genealogy of samples in models with selection. *Genetics, 145*, 519–534.

Nielsen, R., Hubisz, M. J., & Clark, A. G. (2004). Reconstituting the frequency spectrum of ascertained snp data. *Genetics, 168*, 2373–2382.

Nielsen, R., Williamson, S., Kim, Y., Hubisz, M. J., Clark, A. G., & Bustamante, C. (2005). Genomic scans for selective sweeps using snp data. *Genome Research, 15*, 1566–1575.

Padhukasahasram, B., Marjoram, P., Wall, J. D., Bustamante, C. D., & Nordborg, M. (2008). Exploring population genetic models with recombination using efficient forward-time simulations. *Genetics, 178*, 2417–2427.

Pan, J., & MacKenzie, G. (2003). On modelling mean-covariance structures in longitudinal studies. *Biometrika, 90*, 239–244.

Pfaffelhuber, P., Lehnert, A., & Stephan, W. (2008). Linkage disequilibrium under genetic hitchhiking in finite populations. *Genetics, 179*, 527–537.

Project, S. S. (2004). *SeattleSNPs. NHLBI Program for Genomic Applications*. Seattle, WA: SeattleSNPs. http://pga.gs.washington.edu

Sabeti, P. C., Reich, D. E., Higgins, J. M., Levine, H. Z., Richter, D. J., Schaffner, S. F., et al. (2002). Detecting recent positive selection in the human genome from haplotype structure. *Nature, 419*, 832–837.

Slatkin, M. (2000). A coalescent view of population structure. In R. S. Singh & C. B. Krimbas (Eds.), *In evolutionary genetics*. New York: Cambridge University Press.

Spencer, C. A., & Coop, G. (2004). Selsim: A program to simulate population genetic data under coalescent models. *Bioinformatics, 20*, 3673–3675.

Tajima, F. (1989). Statistical method for testing the neutral mutation hypothesis by dna polymorphism. *Genetics, 123*, 585–595.

Teshima, K. M., Coop, G., & Przeworski, M. (2006). How reliable are empirical genomic scans for selective sweeps? *Genome Research, 16*, 702–712.

Voight, B. F., Kudaravalli, S., Wen, X., & Pritchard, J. K. (2006). A map of recent positive selection in the human genome using empirical scores. *PLoS Biology, 4*, e72.

Williamson, S. H., Hernandez, R., Fledel-Alon, A., Zhu, L., Nielsen, R., & Bustamante, C. D. (2005). Simultaneous inference of selection and population growth from patterns of variation in the human genome. *Proceedings of the National Academy of Sciences, 102*, 7882–7887.

Yamasaki, M., Tenaillon, M. I., Bi, I. V., Schroeder, S. G., Sanchez-Villeda, H., Doebley, J. F., et al. (2005). A large-scale screen for artificial selection in maize identifies candidate agronomic loci for domestication and crop improvement. *Plant Cell, 17*, 2859–2872.

Zeng, K., Shi, S., & Wu, C. I. (2007). Compound tests for the detection of hitchhiking under positive selection. *Molecular and Biological Evolution, 24*, 1898–1908.

A Mixture Model and Bootstrap Analysis to Assess Reproductive Allocation in Plants

Caroline Brophy, D. Gibson, P.W. Wayne, and J. Connolly

Abstract In this paper we discuss issues that arise in predicting from complex models for the analysis of reproductive allocation (RA) in plants. Presenting models of RA requires prediction on the original scale of the data and this can present challenges if transformations are used in modelling. It is also necessary to estimate without bias the mean level of RA as this may reflect a plant's ability to contribute in the next generation. Several issues can arise in modelling RA including the occurrence of zero values and the clustering of plants in stands which can lead to the need for complex modelling. We present a two-component finite mixture model framework for the analysis of RA data with the first component a censored regression model on the logarithmic scale and the second component a logistic regression model. Both components contain random error terms to allow for potential correlation between grouped plants. We implement the framework using data from an experiment carried out to assess environmental factors on reproductive allocation. We detail the issues that arose in predicting from the model and present a bootstrap analysis to generate standard errors for the predictions from and to test for comparisons among predictions.

Keywords Bias in back-transformation • Bootstrap analysis • Censored regression • Mixture model • Reproductive allocation

C. Brophy (✉)
Department of Mathematics & Statistics, National University of Ireland Maynooth, Maynooth, Co Kildare, Ireland (Current address)

UCD School of Mathematical Sciences, Environmental & Ecological Modelling Group, University College Dublin, Belfield, Dublin 4, Ireland
e-mail: Caroline.Brophy@nuim.ie

G. MacKenzie and D. Peng (eds.), *Statistical Modelling in Biostatistics and Bioinformatics*, Contributions to Statistics, DOI 10.1007/978-3-319-04579-5__14,
© Springer International Publishing Switzerland 2014

213

1 Introduction

Several statistical issues can arise in the analysis of reproductive allocation (RA) in plants and these include the occurrence of zero values and the clustering of plants in pots. A suitable framework for the analysis of RA data that deals with these issues is presented in Brophy et al. (2007). An application of this model to data from an experiment assessing environmental factors on RA is presented in Brophy et al. (2008). In this paper we present the issues that arose when predicting from the model fitted there. The model is a two-group finite mixture model (McLachlann and Peel 2000) in which the sub-model for the first group is a censored regression model (Schmid et al. 1994) on the logarithmic scale and the sub-model for the second group is a logistic regression model (Collett 1993). When predicting from this model it is desirable to predict on the scale of the original data, i.e. on the RA scale, but this can lead to bias in predictions from back-transforming model components. It is also desirable to predict at the mean RA without bias as this may reflect a plant's ability to contribute in the next generation and biased predictions here could provide misleading model inference. We present the predictions and a bootstrap analysis to calculate standard errors for the predictions and to test for comparisons among them.

2 Methods

Log-log linear allometric regression has often been used to describe the relationship between reproductive allocation (RA, defined here to be the ratio of reproductive biomass to aboveground biomass) and aboveground biomass (Harper 1977). However, frequently many plants in experiments do not reproduce. This has previously been dealt with using censored regression (Schmid et al. 1994). Censored regression is a suitable method when the sole cause of non-reproduction is small plant size; however, this may not always be the case. We propose using a modelling approach that allows for two possible groups within the RA responses (Brophy et al. 2007). The first group contains all reproducing and some non-reproducing plants, but all plants are assumed to have the ability to reproduce. The second group contains the remaining non-reproducing plants which are assumed to be unable to reproduce under their experimental conditions. This framework was applied to data from an experiment examining reproductive allocation in plants where approximately 40 % of plants did not reproduce (Fig. 1) (Brophy et al. 2008).

The experiment was carried out as follows. Seeds of *Sinapis arvensis* were directly sown into 5.5 L, 25 cm diameter, round pots. Seeds were sown at six densities: 1, 2, 4, 8, 16 and 32 plants pot^{-1} and were grown under two CO_2 concentrations, 350 or 700 L L^{-1}. There were 6 replicate pots per CO_2 by density combination, except for combinations at the lowest density which were replicated 12 times, giving 84 pots in total. Individual plants were harvested and the aboveground biomass (DM) and the reproductive biomass (flowers and fruits) were recorded for

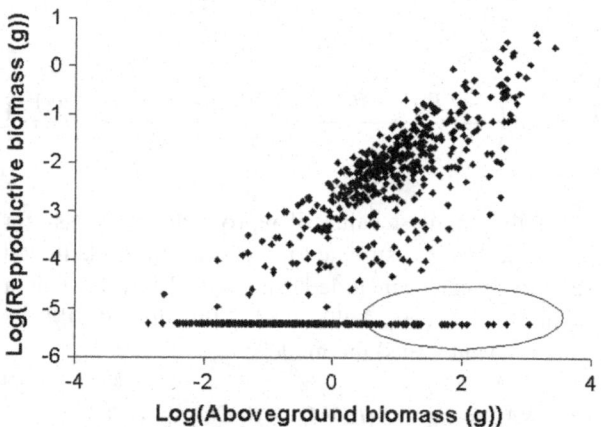

Fig. 1 Log(reproductive biomass) versus log(aboveground biomass) for individual plants of *Sinapis arvensis*. The log of non-reproducing plants is represented by −5.299 and ca. 40 % of individuals in the experiment did not reproduce. There appears to be a strong allometric relationship between log(reproductive biomass) and log(aboveground biomass); however, the *circled values* suggest a second group of values that do not follow this relationship

each of the 704 available plants. Further details are in Wayne et al. (1999). A prefix of L indicates the natural log scale, e.g. LDM = log(DM).

Figure 1 suggested two groups within the experimental data indicating that the framework of Brophy et al. (2007) would be suitable for its analysis. Using this framework we developed a mixture model (McLachlann and Peel 2000) in which the proportions of the two groups were (1-*p*) and *p* respectively. For the first group we used a variant of censored regression to model the relationship between the RA and aboveground biomass (DM) and CO_2. In the second group we modelled the proportion *p* as a logit function of DM, CO_2 and Ratio (size of an individual plant relative to the average size of plants in their pot). The model for each group included a random pot effect to allow for correlation between plants within a pot and we tested these terms using a likelihood ratio test. The likelihood function was of the form:

$$\text{Likelihood} = \prod_{RA_{ij}>0} ((1-p)f(LRA_{ij})) \prod_{RA_{ij}=0} ((1-p)F(LRA_{ij})+p), \quad (1)$$

where

$$f(LRA_{ij}) = \frac{1}{\sqrt{2\pi\sigma_1^2}} \exp\left(\frac{-(LRA_{ij}-\beta_0-\beta_1 LDM_{ij}-\beta_2 CO_2-u_j)^2}{2\sigma_1^2}\right) \quad (2)$$

and $F(LRA_{ij}) =$

$$\frac{1}{\sqrt{2\pi\sigma_1^2}} \int_{-\infty}^{\lambda-LDM_{ij}} \exp\left(\frac{-(LRA_{ij} - \beta_0 - \beta_1 LDM_{ij} - \beta_2 CO_2 - u_j)^2}{2\sigma_1^2}\right) dLRA_{ij} \quad (3)$$

and λ is the log of the smallest value of reproductive biomass for reproducing plants. Model parameters were estimated using maximum likelihood and relevant interactions were tested. p can be included in the model as a constant or as a function of experimental variables. We modelled p as a function of DM, CO_2 and Ratio giving (after testing relevant terms) the models:

$$LRA_{ij} = \beta_0 + \beta_1 LDM_{ij} + \beta_2 CO_2 + u_j + \epsilon_{ij}, \quad (4)$$

$$\log(\frac{p}{1-p}) = \alpha_0 + \alpha_1 LDM_{ij} + \alpha_2 CO_2 + \alpha_3 LRatio_{ij} + \alpha_4 LDM_{ij} * LRatio_{ij} + w_j, \quad (5)$$

where β_0, β_1 and β_2 are regression coefficients, u_j is a pot-specific random effect and ϵ_{ij} is the residual term; ϵ_{ij} and u_j are assumed to be $NID(0, \sigma_1^2)$ and $NID(0, \sigma_2^2)$ respectively. And where α_0, α_1, α_2, α_3, and α_4 are regression coefficients; w_j is a pot-specific random effect assumed to be $NID(0, \sigma_3^2)$ and its covariance with u_j is γ.

To assess the model, RA was predicted at a range of values of the covariates, CO_2, DM and Ratio. There were three steps involved in predicting from the model: predicting RA conditional on being from Group 1 using the estimated Eq. (4), predicting the probability of being in Group 2 from the estimated Eq. (5) and predicting overall RA by combining these two predictions. Several issues arose in predicting at the mean overall RA. These included the back-transformation of random and fixed components and allowing for the censored distribution of the relationship in Eq. (4). We predicted from Eq. (4) allowing for the censored nature of the relationship using first moment equations for censored distributions as described in Jawitz (2004). Using moment equations also allowed the bias caused by the back-transformation of the fixed components from the log scale McCulloch and Searle (2001) to be adjusted for. Predicting the probability of being in Group 2 was calculated by inserting the covariate values required into the estimated Eq. (5) and applying the anti-logit function. However, this predicts the probability at the median value of the random term w_j on the anti-logit scale, not it's mean. We carried out a simulation study to estimate the bias caused by this and multiplied predicted probabilities by the relevant bias adjustment.

Standard errors for predictions and relevant comparisons among predictions were calculated using a bootstrap analysis (Efron and Tibshirani 1986, 1993). Since we cannot assume independence of the individual plants due to the clustered (in pots) nature of the data, in applying the bootstrap method we sampled the data at two levels; first we sampled pots with replacement within CO_2 by density combinations and secondly we sampled plants with replacement within pots. The

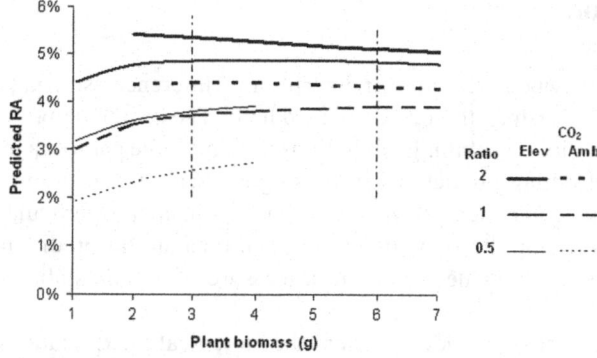

Fig. 2 Predicted RA (%) vs. plant biomass (g) for various combinations of Ratio and CO_2. The *vertical lines* aid the comparisons at 3 and 6 g discussed in Sect. 3. Adapted from Fig. 2a in Brophy et al. (2008) with kind permission of Oxford University Press. ©The Author 2008, published by Oxford University Press on behalf of the Institute of Botany, Chinese Academy of Sciences and the Botanical Society of China. All Rights Reserved

first level of sampling was done within each CO_2 by density combination to retain the structure of the original experiment design. We repeated the sampling process 1,000 times. We fitted the final model to each bootstrapped dataset and computed the prediction or comparison of interest for each fitted model. The standard error over the bootstrapped predictions estimated the standard error for the prediction from the model. Comparisons of predictions were tested for significance using BC_a confidence intervals (Efron and Tibshirani 1993).

3 Results

Predicted RA, assessed jointly from the two components of the mixture model, is presented in Brophy et al. (2008) and in Fig. 2 for a range of covariate values. The effect of CO_2 was always positive and often significant. At DM = 3 g and Ratio=1 predicted RA was 3.7 % at ambient and 4.9 % at elevated (Fig. 2) and these two values differed significantly ($p < 0.05$). We found a strong positive effect of Ratio (relative size within a pot): a plant with biomass 3 g grown at ambient CO_2 allocated 2.5 % on average to reproduction if it was half its pot average size (Ratio = 0.5) but this increased to 3.7 and 4.4 % if the plant was equal to (Ratio = 1) or double (Ratio = 2) its pot average size respectively (each of these predictions differed; $p < 0.05$). At plant biomass = 6 g and at ambient CO_2 there was a significant difference between predicted RA at Ratio = 1 and 2 ($p < 0.05$). Biological interpretations from these results are presented in Brophy et al. (2008).

4   Discussion

Many issues arise when predicting and performing inference using predictions from a complex model such as the one described here. These include predicting from a censored distribution, combining predictions from multiple parts of a mixture model and back-transforming predictions to an original scale when the model includes fixed and random components. When assessing RA data, it is particularly necessary to interpret models on the scale of the original data and to predict the mean RA without bias since RA values represent a measure of a plant's ability to continue into the next generation.

Had the biases not been adjusted here the biological interpretations would have differed significantly. In particular, the back-transformation of the fixed terms in the censored regression model from the log scale would have resulted in the RA values being underestimated by approximately 25 %. Failing to allow for the back-transformation of the random term in the logistic regression model would have also resulted in significant bias. An alternative to using the simulation study we applied here to adjust for bias in the back-transformation of the random term in the logistic regression model would be to model p using a probit analysis which has an explicit formulation for the adjustment needed in back-transforming the random term (McCulloch 1994; McCulloch and Searle 2001). While we could replace our logistic regression model with a probit model, the empirical methodology we used is a general approach for adjusting for bias in situations where explicit formulae are not available.

Acknowledgements CB is the holder of an Environmental Protection Agency (Ireland) Doctoral Scholarship, JC has received support from an Enterprise Ireland International Collaboration grant for this work, and DG received support from the United States Department of Agriculture.

References

Brophy, C., Gibson, D., Wayne, P., & Connolly J. (2007). A modelling framework for analysing the reproductive output of individual plants grown in monoculture. *Ecological Modelling, 207,* 99–108.

Brophy, C., Gibson, D. J., Wayne, P. M., & Connolly J. (2008). How reproductive allocation and flowering probability of individuals in plant populations are affected by position in stand size hierarchy, plant size and CO_2 regime. *Journal of Plant Ecology, 1,* 207–215.

Collett, D. (1993). *Modelling binary data.* London: Chapman & Hall/CRC.

Efron, B., & Tibshirani, R. (1986). Bootstrap methods for standard errors, confidence intervals and other measures of statistical accuracy. *Statistical Science, 1,* 54–77.

Efron B., & Tibshirani, R. (1993) *An introduction to the bootstrap.* New York: Chapman & Hall.

Harper, J. (1977). *Population biology of plants.* London: Academic.

Jawitz, J. (2004). Moments of truncated continuous univariate distributions. *Advances in Water Resources, 27,* 269–281.

McCulloch, C. (1994). Maximum likelihood variance components estimation for binary data. *Journal of the American Statistical Association, 89,* 330–335.

McCulloch, C., & Searle, S. (2001). Generalised, linear, and mixed models. In W. Shewhart & S. Wilks (Eds.), *In probability and statistics*. New York: Wiley.

McLachlann, P., & Peel, D. (2000). *Finite mixture models*. New York: Wiley.

Schmid, B., Polasek, W., Weiner, J., Krause, A., & Stoll, P. (1994). Modelling of discontinuous relationships in biology with censored regression. *American Naturalist, 143*, 494–507.

Wayne, P., Carnelli, A., Connolly, J., & Bazzaz, F. (1999). The density dependence of plant responses to elevated CO_2. *Journal of Ecology, 87*, 183–192.

On Model Selection Algorithms
in Multi-dimensional Contingency Tables

Susana Conde and Gilbert MacKenzie

Abstract We present a review focussed on model selection in log-linear models and contingency tables. The concepts of sparsity and high-dimensionality have become more important nowadays, for example, in the context of high-throughput genetic data. In particular, we describe recently developed automatic search algorithms for finding optimal hierarchical log-linear models (HLLMs) in sparse multi-dimensional contingency tables in R and some LASSO-type penalized likelihood model selection approaches. The methods rely, in part, on a new result which identifies and thus permits the rapid elimination of non-existent maximum likelihood estimators in high-dimensional tables.

Keywords Comorbidity • Hierarchical log-linear model • LASSO penalized likelihood • Smooth LASSO • Sparse high-dimensional contingency table • Stepwise search algorithms

1 Introduction

Our interest in model selection in contingency tables stemmed originally from an analysis of comorbidity data. A comorbidity is a disease that coexists with an index disease under study (Feinstein 1970). Typically, comorbidity data comprise several comorbidities. The scientific interest lies in the study of the dependence structure between the binary comorbidities. Such data are typically high-dimensional and sparse, which poses many challenges for the statistical analysis.

Traditionally, binary comorbidities have been measured using comorbidity indices. These are linear combinations of the comorbidities with some specified

S. Conde (✉)
Department of Mathematics, Imperial College, London, UK
e-mail: sc778@cam.ac.uk

G. MacKenzie and D. Peng (eds.), *Statistical Modelling in Biostatistics
and Bioinformatics*, Contributions to Statistics, DOI 10.1007/978-3-319-04579-5_15,
© Springer International Publishing Switzerland 2014

weights. The weights can be calculated statistically (e.g. Charlson Comorbidity Index), or decided clinically by a doctor (e.g., Davies index or others (Davies et al. 2002; Hall et al. 2004)).Thus in this modelling scheme, possible associations between comorbidities are not taken into account (Hall et al. 2004; Conde and MacKenzie 2007). When two or more diseases exist together, they can reflect a risk of mortality greater than the sum of their individual weights. Of course interaction terms could be included, but surprisingly this is rare, with no examples appearing in the literature reviewed so far (Harnett, et al., 2006, A 5 year prospective study of factors which influence selection for and survival on dialysis, unpublished; Charlson et al. 1987; Davies et al. 2002; Hall et al. 2004).

Conde and MacKenzie (2007) propose a more comprehensive statistical approach, which basically consists of constructing a multi-dimensional contingency table and using a log-linear model (Agresti 2002). Here the dependence structure is measured by interactions rather than by correlations. The latter are the natural measures for multivariate Gaussian data, but inappropriate for binary data. The log-linear modelling scheme allows a richer dependence structure between the comorbidities and can be applied to any other type of categorical variables arising in other settings. The main class of models employed is that of Hierarchical Log-Linear (HLL) models (Birch 1963; Goodman 1971; Agresti 2002). Other families of models may be useful: for example, Graphical Models (GM) (Darroch et al. 1980), which are a subset of HLL Models; Graphical Models are implemented in the Mixed Interaction Modelling (MIM) program (Edwards 2000).

In this paper we present a review of statistical approaches for analyzing such data. We focus on methods for model selection including stepwise search algorithms and penalized likelihood approaches (Conde and MacKenzie 2008; Conde 2011). First we formulate the log-linear model, describe flat tables and design matrices, and present inference in Sect. 2. Then in Sect. 3 we comment on some log-linear model classes: hierarchical, graphical, decomposable. We then describe sparseness including a new definition in Sect. 4. We review some more recent tests of goodness of fit and methods for analysing residuals in Sect. 5. Next, in Sect. 6, we describe the stepwise search algorithms and penalized likelihood model selection methods. Finally, we present some illustrations of the methods in Sect. 7 and end with a short discussion in Sect. 8.

2   Model Formulation

2.1   Contingency Table

Consider a vector of p binary random variables $(C_1, \ldots, C_p)$ where each C_r has the event space $\mathcal{X}_{C_r} = \{1, 2\}$ for $r = 1, \ldots, p$ and, for example, 1 = "absent" and 2 = "present". For the sth independent subject, $s = 1, \ldots, n$, let $(c_{1s}, \ldots, c_{ps})$ be an element of the joint event space $\mathcal{X}_C = \times_{r=1}^{p} \mathcal{X}_{C_r}$ and where $\times$ stands for

Table 1 Example of raw data

		Comorbidities			
		MI	CHF	$\cdots$	PVD
	Patient	C_1	C_2	$\cdots$	C_p
	1	1	1	$\cdots$	1
	2	2	1	$\cdots$	1
	3	1	1	$\cdots$	1
	4	1	1	$\cdots$	1
	5	2	2	$\cdots$	2
	$\vdots$	$\vdots$	$\vdots$	$\vdots$	$\vdots$
	n	2	2	$\cdots$	1

MI myocardial infarction, *CHF* congestive heart failure, *PVD* peripheral vascular disease

the Cartesian product. The cardinality of $\mathcal{X}_C$ is $q = 2^p$. Suppose $(c_{1s}, \ldots, c_{ps}) = (1, \ldots, 1)$, then the subject is not comorbid. The total number of subjects observed to be free from comorbidity is then $y_1 = \sum_{s=1}^{n} \mathbb{1}\{(c_{1s}, \ldots, c_{ps}) = (1, \ldots, 1)\}$, where $\mathbb{1}$ is the indicator function such that $\mathbb{1}\{a = b\} = 1$. The quantity y_1 is called the observed *frequency* of cell $(1, \ldots, 1)$. Similarly, y_q is the observed frequency of the last cell $(2, \ldots, 2)$.

Table 1 shows an example of a raw data set which can be transformed into a p-dimensional contingency table by counting. Table 2 presents an example of such a table formed with $p = 3$ binary variables where $\sum_{i}^{q} y_i = n$ is the total number of observations and π_i is the true, but unknown, probability of a subject belonging to cell i. The π_i, $(i = 1, \ldots, q = 2^p = 8)$ form a probability distribution and the vector of random variables $(Y_1, \ldots, Y_q)$ follows a Multinomial distribution, $\mathrm{MN}(n, \pi_1, \ldots, \pi_q)$ with probability function

$$\mathrm{pr}\left(Y_1 = y_1, \ldots, Y_q = y_q\right) = \frac{n!}{n^n \prod_{i=1}^{q} y_i!} \prod_{i=1}^{q} (\mu_i)^{y_i},$$

where $\mu_i = n\pi_i$ and $\sum \mu_i = n$.

More generally, let g_r be the number of categories of variable C_r with $g_r \geq 2$, $r = 1, \ldots, p$ so $\mathcal{X}_{C_r} := \{1, \ldots, g_r\}$. The g_r categories may be labelled $l_r^1, \ldots, l_r^{g_r}$, $r = 1, \ldots, p$. We can associate $\{l_r^1, \ldots, l_r^{g_r}\} := \{1, \ldots, g_r\}, r = 1, \ldots, p$ and consider the corresponding joint event space $\mathcal{X}_C$ containing exactly $q := \prod_{r=1}^{p} g_r$ cells. As above, we assume n independent realizations of the p variables and then, *mutatis mutandis*, we again obtain a multinomial random variable.

2.2 Bijective Mapping

In Table 2 we have written the frequencies using one index (y_i) or with multiple indices $(y_{j_1 j_2 j_3})$, where $j_r = 1, 2, r = 1, \ldots, 3$. However, in general, for p

Table 2 A three-dimensional contingency table

	$C_3(1)$		$C_3(2)$	
	$C_2(1)$	$C_2(2)$	$C_2(1)$	$C_2(2)$
$C_1(1)$	y_1 [a] $(y_{111})\,\pi_1$	$y_3\,(y_{121})\,\pi_3$	$y_5\,(y_{112})\,\pi_5$	$y_7\,(y_{122})\,\pi_7$
$C_1(2)$	$y_2\,(y_{211})\,\pi_2$	$y_4\,(y_{221})\,\pi_4$	$y_6\,(y_{212})\,\pi_6$	$y_8\,(y_{222})\,\pi_8$

[a] Design matrix notation

categorical variables each with g_r categories and $r = 1, \ldots, p$ O'Flaherty and MacKenzie (1982) showed that

$$\{1, \ldots, q\} \to \overset{p}{\underset{r=1}{\times}} \mathcal{X}_{C_r}$$

$$i \mapsto (j_1, \ldots, j_p)$$

is a bijective map. The bijective map between the two index sets is not unique (for example, leftmost, or rightmost subscript could vary fastest). When the leftmost subscript varies fastest this is known as "Standard Order" (Montgomery 2001, Chap. 6) and we adopt this convention hereafter.

Given one of the bijective mappings $i \mapsto (j_1, \cdots, j_p)$, we can define an *observed contingency table* as $y := (y_1, \ldots, y_q) \in \mathbb{R}^q$ such that $y_i = \#\{(j_1, \ldots, j_p), C_1 = j_1, \ldots, C_p = j_p\}$ representing the count of the ith element in $\mathcal{X}_C$. The quantity $\sum y_i$ is fixed. Then we can represent the contingency table as the matrix

$$
\mathcal{C}_{g_1, \ldots, g_p} :=
\begin{matrix}
C_1 & C_2 \cdots C_p & y \\
\begin{pmatrix}
1 & 1 \cdots 1 & y_1 \\
2 & 1 \cdots 1 & y_2 \\
\cdots & \cdots \quad \cdots & \cdots \\
g_1 & 1 \cdots 1 & \cdots \\
1 & 2 \cdots 1 & \cdots \\
\cdots & \cdots \cdots \cdots & \cdots \\
g_1 & g_2 \cdots g_p & y_q
\end{pmatrix}
\end{matrix}.
$$

2.3 Flat Tables

It is convenient to represent multi-dimensional contingency tables as flat tables, because the latter are more easily handled as design matrices (i.e., model matrices). See Conde (2011, p. 11) for the flat table representation of the previous example.

The flat tables produced by R contain only the *main effect* columns of the corresponding design matrix. Usually interaction effects are required and their associated columns must be generated in the design matrix. In a model with p

factors $(C_1, \ldots, C_p)$ and each with g_r levels, $r = 1, \ldots, p$, there are exactly $q = \prod_{r=1}^{p} g_r$ effects in total including the constant. A design matrix which contains the columns representing all these effects is called *saturated*. Design matrices containing interactions of any order may be generated recursively from flat tables by an algorithm (MacKenzie and O'Flaherty 1982).

2.4 Sampling Schemes

In this paper we mainly focus on the multinomial sampling scheme. Other common sampling schemes are the independent multinomial (Birch 1963) (when some sums of the y_is are fixed, for example, say some row marginal totals), or the independent Poisson (when $\sum_{i=1}^{q} y_i$ is not fixed but random; then $Y_1, \ldots, Y_q$ are independent Poisson random variables with parameters $\mu_1, \ldots, \mu_q$). A clear example of each of these schemes is in Agresti (2002, pp. 40–41).

Fisher (1922) showed that q independent Poisson random variables with parameters μ_i $(i = 1, \ldots, q)$ conditioned on $\sum Y_i = n$, have a multinomial distribution (n, π_i) where $\pi_i = \mu_i / n$. This is now a well-known result (Agresti 2002, pp. 8–9; Christensen 1997, p. 20; Bishop et al. 1975, p. 441).

2.5 Log-Linear Modelling

Let p be the number of binary comorbidities or any other variables in consideration, with p any fixed integer ≥ 2 (Conde and MacKenzie 2007). Consider the p-dimensional contingency table with exactly $q = 2^p$ cells. The possible dependencies between the p variables can be quantified using a log-linear model (Bishop 1969; Goodman 1971; MacKenzie and O'Flaherty 1982) in which the dependence is specified by the presence of interactions. In this framework, dependence is more naturally measured in terms of interactions rather than in terms of correlation.

If we define $\mu_i := E(Y_i)$, the expected value in the ith cell, we consider a log-linear regression model with k parameters (with $k \leq q$) (MacKenzie and Conde 2014; Conde and MacKenzie 2014):

$$\ln (\mu_i) = \sum_{j=1}^{k} a_{ij} \theta_j$$

(Birch 1963; Agresti 2002; Bishop et al. 1975; Christensen 1997), where

$$A = \begin{pmatrix} a_{11} & \cdots & a_{1k} \\ \vdots & \ddots & \vdots \\ a_{q1} & \cdots & a_{qk} \end{pmatrix},$$

is the $(q \times k)$ design matrix, where k is the number of linearly independent parameters and θ, is a vector of unknown parameters measuring the influence of the constant, main effects and interactions on the response, and belongs to a parameter space Θ. In general we consider models such that rank $A = k$. If the design matrix has maximal order, namely q columns, it is called *saturated*.

There are mainly two design matrix coding schemes used in this area. The Yates' coding scheme uses $(+1, -1)$ to encode the presence or absence of a comorbidity (Montgomery 2001, pp. 222–223, 242) and the binary scheme uses $(+1, 0)$. There are advantages and disadvantages to each scheme. Yates' code is D-optimal and the columns of the design matrix, A, are orthogonal which has implications for increased stability, in terms of the *condition number*, in sparse tables. On the other hand the binary coding scheme is useful for identifying inestimable effects (MacKenzie and Conde 2014).

We note that a log-linear regression model is a generalized linear model (McCullagh and Nelder 1997).

2.6 Inference

Given a sample y, the likelihood is

$$L\left(\mu_1, \ldots, \mu_q \mid y\right) = \frac{n!}{n^n \prod_{i=1}^{q} y_i!} \prod_{i=1}^{q} (\mu_i)^{y_i}$$

such that $\sum \mu_i = n$. If all the expected values are > 0 then the log-likelihood is:

$$\ell\left(\mu_1, \ldots, \mu_n \mid y\right) = \ln \left(\frac{n!}{n^n \prod_{i=1}^{q} y_i!} \prod_{i=1}^{q} (\mu_i)^{y_i} \right)$$

$$= K + \sum_{i=1}^{q} y_i \ln (\mu_i)$$

for a certain constant K and $\sum \mu_i = n$. The log-likelihood with respect to θ is

$$\ell(\theta \mid y) \propto \sum_{i=1}^{q} y_i \left(\sum_{j=1}^{k} a_{ij} \theta_j \right),$$

subject to

$$\sum_{i=1}^{q} \exp \left(\sum_{j=1}^{k} a_{ij} \theta_j \right) = n.$$

Birch (1963) showed that, if the maximum likelihood estimators $\hat{\theta}_i$ exist, they coincide for multinomial sampling, for independent Poisson (provided that $\sum_{i=1}^{q} \exp\left(\sum_{j=1}^{k} a_{ij} \hat{\theta}_j\right) = n$), and for independent multinomial sampling (provided that the parameter/s corresponding to the fixed marginal sum/s are included in the model). Then, for estimation, the independent Poisson scheme can always be used (Dobson 2002, p. 164).

The score function is

$$\frac{\partial \ell}{\partial \theta_r}(\theta) = \sum_{i=1}^{q} a_{ir} \left[y_i - \exp\left(\sum_{j=1}^{k} a_{ij}\theta_j\right)\right]$$

and the (r, s)th element of the Fisher information matrix is:

$$i_{r,s}(\theta) = E\left(-\frac{\partial^2}{\partial \theta_r \partial \theta_s} \ell(\theta)\right)$$

$$= \sum_{i=1}^{q} a_{ir} a_{is} \exp\left(\sum_{j=1}^{k} a_{ij}\theta_j\right),$$

where $1 \leq r, s \leq k$, say, where $k = \dim(\theta) \leq n$ with equality in the saturated case, i.e., $k = n$. Accordingly, the asymptotic $(k \times k)$ variance-covariance matrix is then $\Sigma(\theta) = I(\theta)^{-1}$ where $I(\theta)$ has typical element $i_{r,s}(\theta)$.

3   Model Classes

It is convenient to introduce some additional notation for the components of the parameter θ in the case of models with p binary variables. Accordingly, we denote $\theta = (\theta_1, \theta_2, \ldots, \theta_{p+1}, \theta_{p+2}, \ldots)$ by (c0, c1, ..., cp, c1c2, ...).

A *HLL model* (Birch 1963) is a log-linear model such that, if a parameter that represents an interaction is zero, the interaction is said to be null. Moreover, all the higher order interactions that include it are also null (Birch 1963; Agresti 2002). Equivalently, if an interaction is non-null, all the lower order interactions included in it (and their corresponding main effects) are non-null. For example, the model $M_1 = \{c0, c1, c2, c1c2\}$ is hierarchical. A *non-hierarchical model* is a model that is not hierarchical. The model $M_2 = \{c0, c2, c1c2\}$ is non-hierarchical because c1c2 is non-null and the main effect c1 is null.

A HLL model is characterised by its *generating set* (Krajewski and Siatkowski 1990). The generating set is the set of maximal effects, maximal in the sense of the inclusion relation, and it is unique (Edwards and Havránek 1985). For example,

Table 3 Generating sets of all the possible hierarchical models with $p = 3$

Classical set	Rest of the hierarchical models
{(*null*)}	{c1, c2}
{c1}	{c1, c3}
{c2}	{c2, c3}
{c3}	{c1, c2c3}
{c1c2}	{c2, c1c3}
{c1c3}	{c3, c1c2}
{c2c3}	{c1c2, c1c3}
{c1c2c3}	{c1c2, c2c3}
	{c1c3, c1c3}
	{c1, c2, c3}
	{c1c2, c1c3, c2c3}

model M_1 has generating set $G = \{c1c2\}$ and the model with generating set $G = \{c1, c2c3\}$ is

$$M_3 = \{c0, c1, c2, c3, c2c3\}.$$

Non-hierarchical models do not have a generating set. Furthermore, they are "scientifically uninteresting" because the significance of effects in the model *is not invariant* to the choice of design matrix (MacKenzie and Conde 2014).

Let us consider the set $\mathcal{E}_p$ of all the 2^p effects (i.e., constant, main effects and interactions) in the saturated log-linear model. For example, for $p = 3$,

$$\mathcal{E}_3 = \{c0, c1, c2, c3, c1c2, c1c3, c2c3, c1c2c3\}.$$

We define a kind of multiplication rule $*$ in $\mathcal{E}_p$ by: for all $E_1, E_2 \in \mathcal{E}_p$, $E_1 * E_2 = E_1 E_2$. where c0 is the identity element. For example, $c1 * c3 = c1c3$; $c1 * c2c3 = c1c2c3$, $c0 * c1 = c1 * c0 = c1$ from which we have that $(\mathcal{E}_p, *)$ is an Abelian group (Lang 1992).

Table 3 displays all the possible hierarchical models for three variables. In the left column, we can see the classical set, where the generating set is composed only by one element. In the right column, the rest of hierarchical models.

Lemma. *A model is decomposable if and only if it is graphical and its graph contains no chordless cycles of length exceeding three.*

The simplest nongraphical model is $\{(A, B), (A, C), (B, C)\}$ (the saturated model has the same graph of association and it is graphical). The simplest graphical model with at least one chordless cycle of length exceeding three is the model $\{AB, BC, CD, DA\}$. It follows that decomposable models are characterised by two key properties: (a) that the ML estimating equations have explicit solutions and (b) the models can be interpreted in terms of conditional independence, independence and equiprobability (Darroch et al. 1980).

The classes of models are then:

$$\{\text{Decomposable}\} \subset \{\text{Graphical}\} \subset \{\text{Hierarchical}\} \subset \{\text{Log-Linear}\}.$$

For p factors, there are exactly 2^{2^p-1} possible models, e.g., 8.988466×10^{307} possible models when $p = 10$. See Darroch et al. (1980) for the total number of hierarchical, graphical, or decomposable models for $p \leq 5$. The most appropriate model is found by searching this set.

4 Sparseness

Agresti (2002, p. 391) defined a sparse table as a table with small frequencies in some cells. For more details, see Hu (1999). Suppose a sparse table has some zeros. These can be either structural zeros, which are indeed cells for which "observations are impossible" (i.e., $\mu_j = 0$), or sampling zeros (the observed value is 0 in that sample, but $\mu_j > 0$ and then it may be non-zero in another sample).

4.1 Structural Zeros

Goodman (1968) and Mantel (1970) analyse a 2×2 contingency table with structural zeros. They define an *incomplete* table as a table with structural zeros. Mantel follows and completes the work from Goodman (1968) with respect to models of quasi-independence in 2×2 tables which are incomplete. Fienberg (1972) used quasi-log-linear models (like log-linear models but without considering the zero cells). All these authors use the method of maximum likelihood to estimate the parameters. Baker et al. (1985) note that, if the zeros are structural (in a sparse table), this does not affect the existence of the MLEs because those cells are omitted from the analysis.

4.2 Sampling Zeros

In a sparse table with sampling zeros, it may happen that the MLEs of the parameters of a log-linear model may not exist. Haberman (1970, pp. 51–52) and more recently Fienberg and Rinaldo (2006, pp. 15–17) show some examples of tables with some zeros, where the MLEs do not exist. Glonek et al. (1988) summarised the basic results about existence of MLEs in the class of HLL models. Also they determined the exact conditions which must be satisfied for the MLEs to exist (see below). Baker et al. (1985) said that the MLEs of the expected values always exist, if instead of using the equation of a log-linear model, we define the model in a more general way (constraints definition). Fienberg and Rinaldo (2006, 2012) used algebraic statistics and geometry to show the conditions of the existence of the MLEs in a (sparse) multi-dimensional contingency table with independent Poisson and product multinomial sampling schemes.

MacKenzie and Conde (2014) presents a new result concerning the nonexistence of maximum likelihood estimators. This result is based on a simple calculation that involves a binary design matrix. Hence, we can know exactly which effects have non-existent MLEs. Moreover, the result uses the properties of hierarchical models in relation to detecting non-existent MLEs.

4.3 Definition of Sparsity

If some effects cannot be estimated the saturated model cannot be fitted in the usual way, but we may consider a model which is maximal, i.e., which fits all of the available degrees of freedom. The question of how to identify the maximal model then arises. MacKenzie and Conde (2014) prove a theorem to identify the redundant columns of A and generate a design matrix for the remaining estimable effects. It turns out that the resulting maximal model is always hierarchical. This procedure is very fast for high-dimensional tables. Although it nearly always identifies the maximal model, in some pathological cases further work involving the condition number of $\Sigma(\theta)$ (Wissmann et al. 2007) is required. Backwards elimination methods can be used when a maximal model has been identified. The proposed scheme can also handle cases when the number of parameters being fitted is greater than the number of observations.

5 Goodness of Fit and Residuals

As for the goodness of fit tests of a certain model, Hu (1999) highlights that in sparse tables, the Pearson statistic (written here with the estimated expected values):

$$X^2 = \sum_{i=1}^{q} \frac{(y_i - \hat{\mu}_i)^2}{\hat{\mu}_i}$$

(Pearson 1900), or the likelihood ratio test statistic:

$$G^2 = 2 \sum_{i=1}^{q} y_i \ln \left(\frac{y_i}{\hat{\mu}_i} \right)$$

(Wilks 1935, 1938), where y_i and $\hat{\mu}_i$ are respectively the observed, and maximum likelihood estimate of the expected value in the ith cell; can be seriously flawed, and proposes, instead of the asymptotic χ^2_ν distribution for these statistics (with $\nu =$ number of free parameters), a posterior predictive check (PPC) distribution (which is asymptotically a gamma). Kim et al. (2008), for sparse tables without any structural zero, compare X^2, D^2 and L_r, where

$$D^2 = X^2 - \sum_{\substack{i=1 \\ \hat{\mu}_i>0}}^{q} \frac{y_i}{\hat{\mu}_i},$$

(Zelterman 1987); and L_r is a new goodness of fit test statistic in log-linear models with conditional independencies (Maydeu-Olivares and Joe 2005); they recommend the use of D^2 or L_r. As the contingency table becomes sparser (i.e., $2^p/n$ gets larger), the distribution of D^2 becomes more skewed.

The adjusted residuals are

$$\text{adjr}_i = \frac{\text{stdr}_i}{\left(1-\hat{h}_{ii}\right)^{1/2}},$$

where $\hat{h}_{ii}$ is the estimate of the ith diagonal element of the Hat matrix which is

$$H = W^{1/2}A(A^{\mathrm{T}}WA)^{-1}A^{\mathrm{T}}W^{1/2}$$

(Agresti 2002), where A has been defined previously and W is diagonal $(q \times q)$ with the expected values in the diagonal (for example Agresti 2002, p. 339); and

$$\text{stdr}_i = \frac{y_i - \hat{\mu}_i}{\{\hat{\text{var}}\,(Y_i)\}^{1/2}},$$

called the standardized residuals, where $\hat{\mu}_i = \exp\left(\sum_{j=1}^{k} a_{ij}\hat{\theta}_j\right)$, the estimated expected values, $i = 1, \ldots, q$.

The adjusted residuals are preferable to the standardised ones, as they have asymptotic standard normal distributions (Christensen 1997). If the random variable is a multinomial, then

$$\hat{\text{var}}\,(Y_i) = n\hat{\pi}_i\,(1 - \hat{\pi}_i)$$

$$= \hat{\mu}_i(1 - \frac{\hat{\mu}_i}{n}).$$

If the random variables are independent Poisson, then $\hat{\text{var}}\,(Y_i) = \hat{\mu}_i$; thus the standardised residuals are the square roots of the components of the Pearson statistic.

6 Model Selection Methods

We are now interested in finding a good log-linear model in terms of fit. Typically, the saturated model space containing 2^p terms must be searched to find a more parsimonious model which is "best" supported by the data. This is particularly onerous in high-dimensional problems. Thus, it can be useful to have an automatic search algorithm at our disposal.

The SPSS software package has an automatic algorithm (the HILOGLINEAR procedure) in order to find a best-fitting HLL model in a contingency table. However, the maximum number of variables that can be included in the model search, is limited to 10.

Conde and MacKenzie (2007, 2008) reimplemented the SPSS algorithm in R and constructed other similar search algorithms. The algorithms are backwards elimination, backwards elimination 2 (BE, BE2), forward selection (FS) with terminology taken from Goodman (1971); and MacKenzie–Conde Backwards Elimination (MCBE); all the algorithms can be used with any number of binary variables (but in practice available computer memory limits the performance when p becomes large).

Other approaches include penalized likelihood. For example, in regression (and using the usual least squares function), Tibshirani (1996) defined the Least Absolute Shrinkage and Selection Operator (LASSO) estimate of the parameters. The LASSO estimate finds sparse models, and does variable selection and parameter estimation simultaneously (Tibshirani 1996; Fan and Li 2001; Kou and Pan 2008). Dahinden et al. (2007) provide an extension using the LASSO penalty in a likelihood from a multinomial random variable in multi-dimensional contingency tables. Conde and MacKenzie (2012, 2014) propose other LASSO-type related penalties in this context.

6.1 Classical Stepwise Search Algorithms

These algorithms use the iterative proportional fitting algorithm (Deming and Stephan 1940) and work in a stepwise fashion eliminating (or adding) one effect at a time until they arrive at the final step. They compare two nested models at each step using the likelihood ratio criterion. See Conde (2011, Chap. 5).

Ideally one wishes to find a best-fitting model and discover the dependence structure between the categorical variables. However, in high-dimensional problems these goals may be unattainable and in practice we may be forced to consider a reduced problem involving the dependence structure of lower-order interactions such as two-way or three-way interactions.

The algorithms perform (optionally for BE2 and FS) the tests of the hypothesis that whether the m-way effects are zero, or the tests of all $\geq m$-way effects $= 0$. For

Table 4 Meaning of the tests of m-way effects are zero

m	Null hypothesis	Nested comparison	
1	H_0: All main effects	$= 0$	Compare(M_{0ways}, M_{1ways})
2	H_0: All 2-ways	$= 0$	Compare(M_{1ways}, M_{2ways})
$\vdots$	$\vdots$		$\vdots$
p	H_0: The p-way effect	$= 0$	Compare($M_{(p-1)ways}$, M_{pway})

p variables we can define: $M_{iways} :=$ the all i-ways model, where $i = 0, \ldots, p$. In Table 4 we can see the tests of m-way effects are zero, with m, the null hypotheses, and the test of comparison in the last column. In the tests of all $\geq m$-way effects $= 0$, the comparisons are always conducted with the saturated model.

Backwards Elimination starts from the saturated model, it eliminates one effect at a time, comparing the model, with the model from which the effect has been dropped. Then, eliminating one effect at a time, the effects that are eliminated always belong to the generating set of the current model in each step.

Moreover, at each step BE shows us the ≤ 10 results of the tests of comparisons of the effects that can or cannot be eliminated, both ordered decreasingly with respect to the p-values. For example, suppose that at one step, 5 effects can be eliminated, and 13 can not. BE will print, for each of the eliminable effects: the effect, the LR test statistic, degrees of freedom, and p-value of the test of the comparison, ordered from the lowest to the highest significant effect. Next, it will print at most ten effects which cannot be eliminated also ordered in the same way.

Backward Elimination 2 is akin to BE, working backwards, but starting with a model with all the *maxorder*-way interactions. This means that, for example, suppose a model with all main effects does not fit (i.e., the difference between log-likelihoods between this model and the saturated model is significantly large); and suppose a model with all the 2-way interactions does fit (this information may be available from the tests of m- or $\geq m$-way effects are zero). In this case *maxorder* $= 2$. BE2 will start its search with the model with all the 2-way interactions until we arrive at the end (i.e., until no other effect can be eliminated).

Forward Selection (FS) starts with the null model and adds one effect at a time until a model that fits the data is found. As opposed to the method in Edwards (2012), these effects can be potentially of any order and not "only" based on 2-way interactions. Another version of FS can start with the main effects model.

Conde and MacKenzie (2008) have another algorithm that calculates the tests of partial associations (Christensen 1997, pp. 217–218): here, the saturated model is always the basis for the comparisons. For each m-way effect that is present in the HLL model, these tests compare the model with all the m-way effects against a model in which the m-way effect in question is dropped out. Besides, the list is ordered increasingly with respect to the p-values, i.e., from lowest to highest.

More recently Conde and MacKenzie (2014) propose an enhanced version of the backwards elimination algorithm: MCBE, which can remove inestimable effects (that is, effects whose maximum likelihood estimator does not exist) and starts the search backwards from the remaining parameter space.

6.2 Penalised Likelihood

The idea of Penalised Likelihood (Demidenko 2004) is to attach a penalty to the usual likelihood function. Different penalties may be adopted to achieve various desirable properties: e.g., sparsity or smoothness of solutions, etc. (Hastie et al. 2001; Friedman 2008). Here we are primarily interested in encouraging sparse solutions in order to identify a more parsimonious model.

The LASSO estimate has an effect of shrinking proportionally the coefficients in the model with respect to the Ordinary Least Squares estimator. Typically, some of the coefficients go exactly to zero, depending on the regularization parameter. Thus the LASSO estimate performs variable selection and parameter estimation at the same time. Dahinden et al. (2007) use it in order to find a sparse log-linear model that fits a table where the variables involved are genetic sites (splicings of genes with presence or absence of exons).

Following the latter approach, the LASSO estimate is given by

$$\hat{\theta}_{\text{LASSO}}(t) := \arg \min_{\theta \in \Theta} \{-\ell_{\text{mult}}(\theta)\},$$

where ℓ_{mult} is the log-likelihood of a multinomial, subject to $\sum_{j=2}^{k} |\theta_j| \leq t$ for some constant t, the tuning parameter. The definition is equivalent to '

$$(\hat{\theta}_{\text{LASSO}})_\lambda := \arg \min_{\theta \in \Theta} \left\{ -\ell_{\text{mult}}(\theta) + \lambda \sum_{j=2}^{k} |\theta_j| \right\}$$

for some regularisation parameter $\lambda \geq 0$, where a large λ means that all the estimates have gone to 0; and $\lambda = 0$ means that the solution is $(\hat{\theta}_{\text{LASSO}})_0 \equiv \hat{\theta}$, the MLEs. We can name $\hat{\theta}_{\text{LASSO}}$ as the *maximum penalised likelihood estimators* (MPLEs), according to Green and Silverman (1994)'s methodology. The regularisation parameter may be estimated, e.g., by cross-validation (Dahinden et al. 2007; Conde and MacKenzie 2012) or using the Bayes Information Criterion (BIC) (Conde and MacKenzie 2012). In the literature, Yates' coding scheme is used for the design matrix, so the columns of A are orthogonal. The LASSO penalty is non-differentiable and one needs a path following algorithm such as presented in Dahinden et al. (2007). Moreover, the LASSO estimate does not automatically impose hierarchical rules and the final models selected may be non-hierarchical. Accordingly, this entire method is suspect in routine applications. Another criticism is that when the set of effects which are to be treated as null is identified, these should be eliminated from the model and the remaining effects re-estimated (non-LASSO). This step is usually forgotten and interpretation is erroneously based on the LASSO analysis.

Conde and MacKenzie (2012) consider and propose other LASSO-type related penalties such as the LASSO defined only in the interactions (in order to keep the hierarchical structure of the model), and the Smooth LASSO.

6.2.1 The Smooth LASSO

This is a new parametric, convex, analytic approximation to the LASSO. The advantage of this approximation is that for computing the solutions of the equation above, one can apply Newton–Raphson type methods thereby eliminating the need for specialized algorithms such as the method of coordinate descent (Friedman et al. 2010). Moreover, the computation of the standard errors is very easy, such as in Muggeo (2010). Conde and MacKenzie (2012) estimates λ using the method of cross-validation (Conde 2011, p. 112).

7 Applications

7.1 Classical Stepwise Algorithms

For the first application we use data comprising 48,158 subjects where the cases are patients with Chronic Obstructive Pulmonary Disease (COPD) and the age-matched controls are COPD-free. The 15 binary variables analyzed indicate the presence or absence of comorbidities. See other details of the data in Conde and MacKenzie (2007). Table 5 shows the tests that the m-way effects are zero in these data.

Next, the BE was tested using sets up to and including ten comorbidities (Conde and MacKenzie 2008) in this data set. The solutions given by BE in R were identical to those obtained by SPSS and we limited the number of variables to 10 so that we could effect direct comparison. The tables here are not sparse for small p, and they become highly sparse for larger values of p.

Figure 1 displays the (ln) timings for each program on the vertical axis, whilst the horizontal axis contain the number of comorbidities in the data set. The curves are smoothing curves, i.e., loess', formed with local quadratic polynomials (Cleveland 1979; Cleveland and Devlin 1988). From five variables upwards the times become progressively longer in R compared with SPSS; R is an interpreted language while SPSS uses compiled code in FORTRAN. Accordingly, for large values of p this combinatorial algorithm becomes infeasible and other approaches will be required. These timings refer to a standard desktop computer with 2 GHz processor and 4 GB of main memory.

Table 5 Tests of m-way effects are zero with $p = 15$ comorbidities

m	df	LR	P
1	15	689,703.2000	0.0000
2	105	5,998.8920	0.0000
3	455	480.3214	0.1198

The best-fitting model may contain some 2-way interaction terms

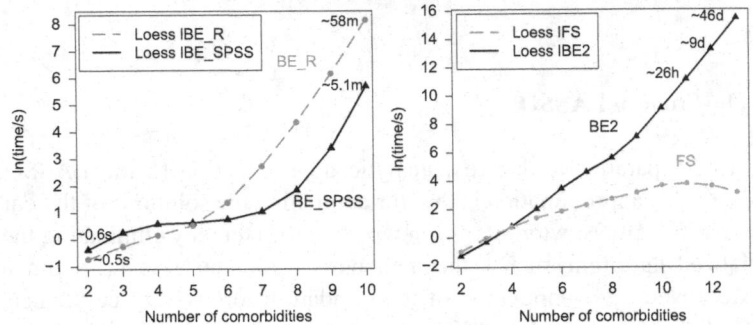

Fig. 1 Comparison of times of the algorithms

Figure 1 displays analogous ln timings for FS and BE2 (right panel), and these were obtained using a different set of (up to and including) 13 comorbidities. For $p > 4$, BE2 takes longer than BE. Note that BE2 may start with a model that contains a lot of effects in the generating set ($\binom{p}{m}$ for some $0 < m < p$), as opposed to the saturated model or the null model, which only contains one (or zero) elements respectively. For large p, FS is the fastest algorithm. However, the FS algorithm often selected models which were unsatisfactory in terms of fit, as judged by the pattern of residuals. From this perspective, the backward elimination algorithms were more satisfactory, but the final models were always more complex.

As an illustration, Figs. 2 and 3 display histograms (left panel) and Q–Q plots (right panel) of the adjusted residuals for the BE and FS solutions respectively for $p = 8$ comorbidities from the set of the left panel in Fig. 1. The final model found by BE or BE2 is {c7c8, c5c6, c2c4c5, c1c4c5, c1c3c7, c1c3c4, c1c2c4c7, c1c2c5c7, c1c2c3c5, c1c2c6c7}, with an LR= 48.9310, and 206 degrees of freedom, which is an overparameterised model. The final model found by FS is {c6, c7, c8, c1c2, c1c3, c2c4, c2c3, c4c5, c3c4}, with an LR= 276.4611, Pearson= 578.0098, and 241 degrees of freedom (i.e., a much more parsimonious model).

The graphs contain only the residuals for the cells with a non-zero frequency, and non-zero estimated value, too (for the estimated values, it was considered non-zero those >0.0001). Then the graphs contain 65 data, out of the 256. The blue curves are the graphs of the probability density functions of a standard normal rescaled such that the area under the curve coincides with that from the histogram.

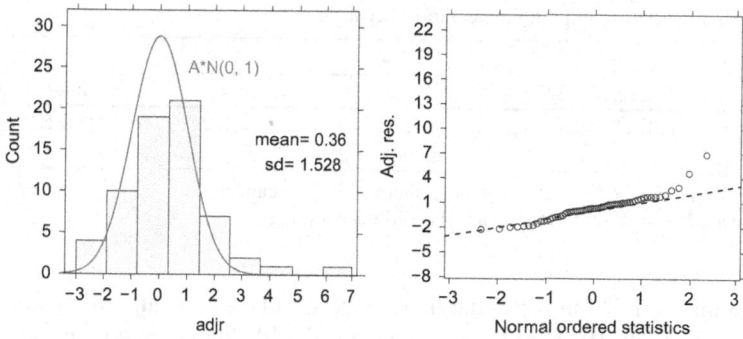

Fig. 2 Histograms and Q–Q plots of adjusted residuals for $p = 8$, set 1, BE. The quantity A is the area of the histogram

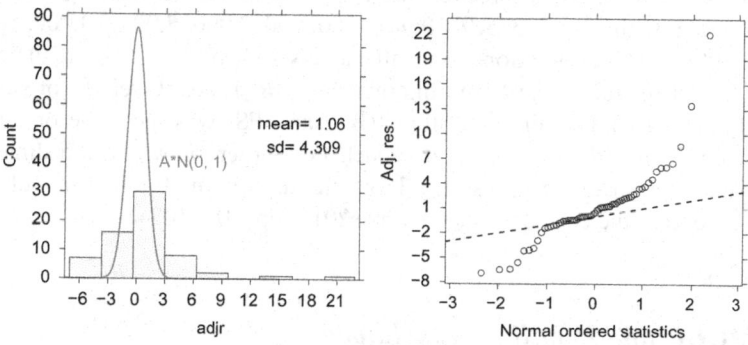

Fig. 3 Histograms and Q–Q plots of residuals for $p = 8$, set 1, FS. The quantity A is the area of the histogram. The quantity A is the area of the histogram

The distribution of adjusted residuals of Fig. 2 is a bit platykurtic compared with the normal distribution, slightly right-skewed because of the presence of an outlier corresponding to the cell in which comorbidities 2, 4, 7 and 8 were present and the rest absent, and this cell has 1 observation. There is usually some outlier (MacKenzie 2006). In the Q–Q plot the observations are approximately close to the diagonal, apart from the outlier. The Kolmogorov–Smirnov test finds a p-value of 0.04786.

Both graphs in Fig. 3 indicate clearly that the distribution of adjusted residuals is not normally distributed. The variance of the adjusted residuals in the FS solution (12.982) is more than six times greater than the corresponding variance in the BE solution (2.097). The Kolmogorov–Smirnov test has a p-value of 7.124×10^{-7}, clearly significant with the standard confidence levels.

In addition to testing with real data sets, the algorithms (BE2, FS) were tested in a comprehensive simulation study (Conde 2011, Chap. 6). A core scenario involved generating $m = 1,000$ random compositions (Nijenhuis and Wilf 1978) for $p = 2, 3, 4, 5$; $n = 100, 500$ and $m = 150$ compositions for $p = 10$; n=10,000. The

Table 6 Final models found with the comorbidity table

	MCBE, BE2, FS	LASSO		Smooth LASSO[a]
		CV	BIC	
Comorb. data	[c1, c2, c3]	[c1c2, c1c3, c2c3]	[c1c2c3]	[c1, c2, c3]

Variables mean c1: mild liver disease; c2: diabetes; c3: lung cancer
[a] We removed $\lambda^* = 0$ from the path as nlm did not converge

results of this simulation were: the final models found by the algorithms, the Wald test statistics (Wald 1943) of their parameters, the likelihood, and other quantities. For example, for $p = 2$, the algorithms always found the correct model except for the saturated case, and in the latter case the percentages of success are very high (Conde 2011, p. 98). Moreover, we also simulated tables corresponding to a specific model, with $p = 2, 3, 5, 7, 10; n = 200, 500, 2,000, 5,000, 10,000, 50,000;$ $m = 1,000$ or 100 simulations; and all models (when $p = 2$), or all models with up to and including the t-way interactions, $t = 1, 2, 3$. Overall, for small p, the final model found by the algorithms (BE2 and FS) was the same or a model in the neighbourhood of the correct model. For larger p, where the dimension of the parameter space becomes very large, the algorithms found a model in the neighbourhood of the correct model (Conde 2011, pp. 101–102).

7.2   MCBE and Penalized Likelihood

Conde and MacKenzie (2012) present an analysis of a three-dimensional contingency table from the comorbidity data and the results of a simulation study. The variables are: mild liver disease, diabetes and lung cancer. According to MacKenzie's theorem (MacKenzie and Conde 2014), the MLEs of the effects c1c2, c1c3 and c1c2c3 are non-existent. Table 6 displays the results of the final models found by MCBE and the diverse penalised likelihood approaches. Depending on the method used, the results may be very different.

The three classical algorithms and the Smooth LASSO found the main effects model, i.e., the presence of mild liver disease is not affected by diabetes and lung cancer and vice versa with all the combinations of the three comorbidities. In contrast, the LASSO method and when estimating λ by cross-validation, found a model with all 2-way interactions, i.e., there is a complicated pattern of interaction between the comorbidities. When estimating λ with the BIC, the final model is the saturated model. Moreover, the penalized likelihood approaches contain diverse effects whose MLEs do not exist in their final models.

The simulation study comprise 100 simulated random compositions with $p = 2$. Each random composition was given to MCBE, BE2, FS, LASSO using the methods of cross-validation and BIC, and the Smooth LASSO. Table 7 displays the

Table 7 Percentages of final models found; $p = 2$, in 100 simulated tables

p	n	model	% MCBE	BE2	FS	LASSO CV	LASSO BIC	Smooth LASSO[a]
2	50	null	4	8	5	0	1	23
		{c1}	11	8	13	0	3	12
		{c2}	6	5	6	3	2	9
		{c1, c2}	20	20	20	15	11	10
		sat.	55	55	52	78	79	40
		No fit[b]	4					
		Total	100	96	96	96	96	94
2	10	null	18	27	25	7	13	69
		{c1}	15	8	15	4	4	4
		{c2}	15	13	16	5	5	4
		{c1, c2}	13	13	13	14	11	0
		sat.	22	22	14	53	50	4
		No fit[b]	17					
		Total	100	83	83	83	83	81

CV: Five-fold cross-validation. BIC: BIC with a LASSO penalty. The Smooth LASSO approximation is used with $\omega = 1$ and 5-fold cross-validation
[a] We removed tables when nlm did not converge; (2, 2, respectively, in each scenario)
[b] SSM does not fit

results. By using MacKenzie's Theorem (MacKenzie and Conde 2014), to detect inestimable effects, four contingency tables in the first scenario and twenty-two tables in the second scenario had at least one inestimable effect. The acronym SSM stands for the sparse saturated model, which is the maximal model that can be fitted in a sparse contingency table after eliminating effects with non-existent MLEs detected by MacKenzie's theorem.

The classical algorithms find always hierarchical, sparser (i.e., more parsimonius) models, and those which are free of inestimable effects in the case of MCBE. On the other hand, none of the penalized likelihood approaches take into account the hierarchical rules; furthermore, these (penalized likelihood) approaches generally include effects with non-existent maximum likelihood estimators in their final models.

8 Discussion

We have presented a short review of modern methods for analysing sparse contingency tables. One of the most interesting developments concerns the elimination of non-existent MLEs by pre-processing contingency tables prior to formal statistical analysis (MacKenzie and Conde 2014). This approach is potentially very efficient and should allow the researcher to tackle higher dimensional sparse problems. Another key development is that of the Smooth LASSO which being twice differentiable simply dispenses with the need for specialised optimization algorithms such as the method of coordinate descent. An attractive feature is that it casts the analysis of LASSO problems in a classical statistical mould. A weakness with the regularization approach has been the failure of the technique to produce hierarchical solutions. Non-hierarchical solutions are not design matrix invariant and this can trap the unwary applied researcher. Another weakness of current LASSO methods is that their solutions often contain effects which may be shown not to exist in a classical analysis. This is a serious inconsistency and implies that non-existent effects should be eliminated prior to any analysis. Overall, our new approach, can in principle reconcile all of these problems by eliminating non-existent effects and fitting the Smooth LASSO optimization into a hierarchical algorithm. We expect that in time our methods will impact positively on practice.

Acknowledgements The work in this paper was conducted in the Centre of Biostatistics, Limerick, Ireland, and supported by the Science Foundation Ireland (SFI, www.sfi.ie), project grant number 07/MI/012 (BIO-SI project, www3.ul.ie/bio-si). The first author's Ph.D. scholarship was supported GlaxoSmithKline, England, UK.

References

Agresti, A. (2002). *Categorical data analysis* (2nd ed.). Hoboken, NJ: Wiley.

Baker, R. J., Clarke, M. R. B., & Lane, P. W. (1985). Zero entries in sparse contingency tables. *Computational Statistics and Data Analysis, 3*, 33–45.

Birch, M. W. (1963). Maximum likelihood in three-way contingency tables. *Journal of the Royal Statistical Society. Series B (Methodological), 25*(1), 220–233.

Bishop, Y. M., Fienberg, S. E., & Holland, P. W. (1975). *Discrete multivariate analysis: Theory and practice*. Cambridge: MIT Press, The Massachusetts Institute of Technology.

Bishop, Y. M. M. (1969). Full contingency tables, logits, and split contingency tables. *Biometrics, 25*(2), 383–399.

Charlson, M. E., Pompei, P., Ales, K. L., & MacKenzie, C. R. (1987). A new method of classifying prognostic comorbidity in longitudinal studies: Development and validation. *Journal of Chronic Diseases, 40*(5), 373–383.

Christensen, R. (1997). *Log-linear models and logistic regression* (2nd ed.). New York: Springer.

Cleveland, W. S. (1979). Robust locally weighted regression and smoothing scatterplots. *Journal of the American Statistical Association, 74*(368), 829–836.

Cleveland, W. S., & Devlin, S. J. (1988). Locally weighted regression: An approach to regression analysis by local fitting. *Journal of the American Statistical Association, 83*(403), 596–610.

Conde, S. (2011). *Interactions: Log-linear models in sparse contingency tables* (Ph.D. thesis). University of Limerick, Ireland.

Conde, S., & MacKenzie, G. (2007). Modelling high dimensional sets of binary co-morbidities. In J. del Castillo, A. Espinal, & P. Puig (Eds.), *Proceedings of the 22nd International Workshop on Statistical Modelling*, Barcelona (pp. 177–180).

Conde, S., & MacKenzie, G. (2008). Search algorithms for log-linear models in contingency tables. Comorbidity data. In P. H. Eilers (Ed.), *Proceedings of the 23rd International Workshop on Statistical Modelling*, Utrecht (pp. 184–187).

Conde, S., & MacKenzie, G. (2011). LASSO penalised likelihood in high-dimensional contingency tables. In D. Conesa, A. Forte, A. López-Quílez, & F. Muñoz (Eds.), *Proceedings of the 26th International Workshop on Statistical Modelling*, Valencia (pp. 127–132).

Conde, S., & MacKenzie, G. (2012). Model selection in sparse contingency tables: LASSO penalties *vs* classical methods. In A. Komárek & S. Nagy (Eds.), *Proceedings of the 27th International Workshop on Statistical Modelling*, Prague (pp. 81–86).

Conde, S., & MacKenzie, G. (2014). The smooth LASSO in sparse high-dimensional contingency tables (in preparation).

Dahinden, C., Parmigiani, G., Emerick, M. C., & Bühlmann, P. (2007). Penalized likelihood for sparse contingency tables with an application to full-length cDNA libraries. *BMC Bioinformatics, 8*, 476.

Darroch, J. N., Lauritzen, S. L., & Speed, T. P. (1980). Markov fields and log-linear interaction models for contingency tables. *The Annals of Statistics, 8*(3), 522–539.

Davies, S. J., Phillips, L., Naish, P. F., & Russell, G. I. (2002). Quantifying comorbidity in peritoneal dialysis patients and its relationship to other predictors of survival. *Nephrology Dialysis Transplantation, 17*(6), 1085–1092.

Demidenko, E. (2004). *Mixed models*. New York: Wiley.

Deming, W. E., & Stephan, F. F. (1940). On a least squares adjustment of a sampled frequency table when the expected marginal totals are known. *The Annals of Mathematical Statistics, 11*(4), 427–444.

Dobson, A. J. (2002). *An introduction to generalized linear models*. New York: Chapman & Hall/CRC.

Edwards, D. (2000). *Introduction to graphical modelling* (2nd ed.). New York: Springer.

Edwards, D. (2012). A note on adding and deleting edges in hierarchical log-linear models. *Computational Statistics, 27*, 799–803.

Edwards, D., & Havránek, T. (1985). A fast procedure for model search in multidimensional contingency tables. *Biometrika, 72*(2), 339–351.

Fan, J., & Li, R. (2001). Variable selection via nonconcave penalized likelihood and its oracle properties. *Journal of the American Statistical Association, 96*(456), 1348–1360.

Feinstein, A. R. (1970). The pre-therapeutic classification of co-morbidity in chronic disease. *Journal of Chronic Diseases, 23*(7), 455–468.

Fienberg, S. E. (1972). The analysis of incomplete multi-way contingency tables. *Biometrics, 28*(1), 177–202 [special Multivariate Issue].

Fienberg, S. E., & Rinaldo, A. (2006). Computing maximum likelihood estimates in log-linear models. Manuscript extracted from Rinaldo's Ph.D. thesis.

Fienberg, S. E., & Rinaldo, A. (2012). Maximum likelihood estimation in log-linear models. *The Annals of Statistics, 40*(2), 996–1023.

Fisher, R. A. (1922). On the interpretation of χ^2 from contingency tables, and the calculation of P. *Journal of the Royal Statistical Society, 85*(1), 87–94.

Friedman, J. H. (2008). Fast sparse regression and classification. In P. H. Eilers (Ed.), *Proceedings of the 23rd International Workshop on Statistical Modelling*, Utrecht (pp. 27–57).

Friedman, J. H., Hastie, T., & Tibshirani, R. (2010). Regularization paths for generalized linear models via coordinate descent. *Journal of Statistical Software, 33*(1), 1–22.

Glonek, G. F. V., Darroch, J. N., & Speed, T. P. (1988). On the existence of maximum likelihood estimators for hierarchical loglinear models. *Scandinavian Journal of Statistics, 15*, 187–193.

Goodman, L. A. (1968). The analysis of cross-classified data: Independence, quasi-independence, and interactions in contingency tables with or without missing entries. R. A. Fisher memorial lecture. *Journal of the American Statistical Association, 63*(324), 1091–1131.

Goodman, L. A. (1971). The analysis of multidimensional contingency tables: Stepwise procedures and direct estimation methods for building models for multiple classifications. *Technometrics, 13*(1), 33–61.

Green, P. J., & Silverman, B. W. (1994). *Nonparametric regression and generalized linear models: A roughness penalty approach* (Vol. 58). *Monographs on statistics and applied probability* (1st ed.). London: Chapman & Hall.

Haberman, S. J. (1970). *The general log-linear model* (Ph.D. thesis). Department of Statistics, University of Chicago, Chicago, IL.

Hall, W. H., Ramachandran, R., Narayan, S., Jani, A. B., & Vijayakumar, S. (2004). An electronic application for rapidly calculating Charlson comorbidity score. *BMC Cancer, 4*, 94.

Hastie, T., Tibshirani, R., & Friedman, J. (2001). *The elements of statistical learning*. New York: Springer.

Hu, M. Y. (1999). *Model checking for incomplete high dimensional categorical data* (Ph.D. thesis). University of California, Los Angeles.

Kim, S. H., Choi, H., & Lee, S. (2008). Estimate-based goodness-of-fit test for large sparse multinomial distributions. *Computational Statistics and Data Analysis, 53*(4), 1122–1131

Kou, C., & Pan, J. (2008). Variable selection in joint modelling of mean and covariance structures for longitudinal sata. In P. H. Eilers (Ed.), *Proceedings of the 23rd International Workshop on Statistical Modelling*, Utrecht (pp. 309–314)

Krajewski, P., & Siatkowski, I. (1990). Algorithm AS 252: Generating classes for log-linear models. *Journal of the Royal Statistical Society. Series C (Applied Statistics), 39*(1), 143–176.

Lang, S. (1992). *Algebra* (3rd ed.). Delhi: Pearson Education.

MacKenzie, G. (2006). *Screening multivariate comorbidities*. Presentation. Assess, York, http://www.staff.ul.ie/mackenzieg/Assess/assess.html.

MacKenzie, G., & Conde, S. (2014). Model selection in sparse contingency tables (in preparation).

MacKenzie, G., & O'Flaherty, M. (1982). Algorithm AS 173: Direct design matrix generation for balanced factorial experiments. *Journal of the Royal Statistical Society. Series C (Applied Statistics), 31*(1), 74–80.

Mantel, N. (1970). Incomplete contingency tables. *Biometrics, 26*(2), 291–304.

Maydeu-Olivares, A., & Joe, H. (2005). Limited- and full-information estimation and goodness-of-fit testing in 2^n contingency tables. *Journal of the American Statistical Association, 100*(471), 1009–1020.

McCullagh, P., & Nelder, J. A. (1997). *Generalized linear models*. London: Chapman & Hall.

Montgomery, D. C. (2001). *Design and analysis of experiments* (5th ed.). New York: Wiley.

Muggeo, V. M. R. (2010). LASSO regression via smooth L_1-norm approximation. In A. W. Bowman (Ed.), *Proceedings of the 25th International Workshop on Statistical Modelling*, Glasgow (pp. 391–396).

Nijenhuis, A., & Wilf, H. S. (1978). *Combinatorial algorithms*. New York: Academic.

O'Flaherty, M., & MacKenzie, G. (1982). Algorithm AS 172: Direct simulation of nested Fortran DO-LOOPS. *Journal of the Royal Statistical Society. Series C (Applied Statistics), 31*(1), 71–74.

Pearson K. (1900) On the criterion that a given system of deviations from the probable in the case of a correlated system of variables is such that it can be reasonably supposed to have arisen from random sampling. *Philosophy Magazine Series, 50*(5), 157–174.

Tibshirani, R. (1996). Regression shrinkage and selection via the lasso. *Journal of the Royal Statistical Society, 58*(1), 267–288.

Wald, A. (1943). Tests of statistical hypotheses concerning several parameters when the number of observations is large. *Transactions of the American Mathematical Society, 54*(3), 426–482.

Wilks, S. S. (1935). The likelihood test of independence in contingency tables. *The Annals of Mathematical Statistics, 6*(4), 190–196.

Wilks, S. S. (1938). The large-sample distribution of the likelihood ratio for testing composite hypotheses. *The Annals of Mathematical Statistics, 9*(1), 60–62.

Wissmann, M., Toutenburg, H., & Shalabh (2007) Role of categorical variables in multicollinearity in the linear regression model. Technical Report 008, Department of Statistics, University of Munich.

Zelterman, D. (1987). Goodness-of-fit tests for large sparse multinomial distributions. *Journal of the American Statistical Association, 82*(398), 624–629.

Obituary: Professor Ennio Isaia

In the course of preparing this book we were saddened by the unexpected news of the death of Professor Ennio Isaia of the University of Torino, following a short illness.

Ennio Isaia was a brilliant, passionate, serious statistician and a wonderful person. Ennio died in February 2010 at the age of 54. He was a prolific researcher at the Department of Statistics and Applied Mathematics "D. de Castro" in the University of Torino, the establishment where he spent most of his academic life. In his rather short life, Ennio produced many interesting research papers (over 35) in both methodological and applied statistics. He was also the author of several textbooks for the student body. His research interests were wide-ranging and encompassed:

- Robust statistics, outliers and clusters detection.
- Model selection algorithms.
- Mixture models and clustering.
- Computational statistics and high-dimensional data analysis.
- Nonparametric and semi-parametric statistical methods.
- Statistical quality and process control.

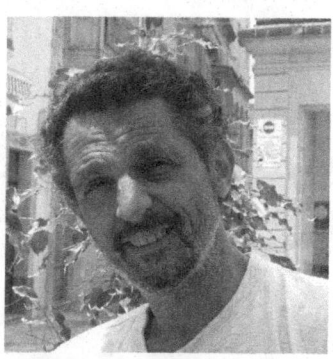

G. MacKenzie and D. Peng (eds.), *Statistical Modelling in Biostatistics and Bioinformatics*, Contributions to Statistics, DOI 10.1007/978-3-319-04579-5,
© Springer International Publishing Switzerland 2014

He had presented the results of this research at many Workshops and Conferences around the world. His last presentation was at the XIII International Conference, Applied Stochastic Models and Data Analysis (ASMDA) held at Vilnius in June 2009, entitled, *The minimum density power divergence approach in building robust regression models*.

Ennio was an active participant in International Workshops. He was also a member of the Programme Committee which helped organise the WCDM Workshop held in Torino in 2004. He was an enthusiastic supporter of the 2007 Workshop in Limerick and produced the Latex templates for that event.

Accordingly, it is with great fondness that he is remembered by his friends and colleagues.

Alessandra Durio & Gilbert MacKenzie

Autumn 2013

Printed in the United States
By Bookmasters